DECOLONIZING FEMINISMS

Piya Chatterjee, *Series Editor*

THE BORDERS OF AIDS

Race, Quarantine, and Resistance

KARMA R. CHÁVEZ

UNIVERSITY OF WASHINGTON PRESS
Seattle

The Borders of AIDS was made possible in part by grants from the Department of Mexican American and Latina/o Studies and the Office of the Vice President for Research at the University of Texas at Austin.

UNIVERSITY OF WASHINGTON PRESS
uwapress.uw.edu

LIBRARY OF CONGRESS CATALOGING-IN-PUBLICATION DATA
LC record available at https://lccn.loc.gov/2020053373
LC ebook record available at https://lccn.loc.gov/2020053374
ISBN 978-0-295-74896-2 (hardcover), ISBN 978-0-295-74897-9 (paperback),
ISBN 978-0-295-74898-6 (ebook)

Portions of chapter 4 were published in "The Necropolitical Functions of Biocitizenship: The Sixth International AIDS Conference and the U.S. Ban on HIV-Positive Immigrants," in *Biocitizenship: The Politics of Bodies, Governance, and Power*, ed. Kelly E. Happe, Jenell Johnson, and Marina Levina (New York: New York University Press, 2018), 117–32; and "Queer Migration Politics as Transnational Activism," *Scholar and Feminist Online* 14, no. 2 (2017), http://sfonline.barnard.edu/thinking-queer-activism-transnationally/queer-migration-politics-as-transnational-activism/. Portions of chapter 5 were published in "ACT UP, Haitian Migrants, and Alternative Memories of HIV/AIDS," *Quarterly Journal of Speech* 98, no. 1 (2012): 63–68.

CONTENTS

Prologue   vii

Acknowledgments   xi

Terminology   xv

Abbreviations   xvii

INTRODUCTION: The Alienizing Nation   3

PART ONE. ALIENIZING LOGIC AND STRUCTURE

1.   A Brief Rhetorical History of Quarantine   19

2.   AIDS and the Rhetoric of Quarantine   41

3.   National Common Sense and the Ban on HIV-Positive Migrants   66

PART TWO. RESISTING ALIENIZING LOGIC

4.   Boycotts and Protests of the International AIDS Conferences   103

5.   AIDS Activist Media and the "Haitian Connection"   132

CONCLUSION: Against the Alienizing Nation   157

Epilogue   167

Notes   171

Selected Bibliography   219

Index   233

PROLOGUE

It is a surreal time to be finishing a book about the AIDS pandemic and issues of quarantine, race, and resistance. As with so many books, this one has taken far too long to finish, but perhaps the universe compelled me to not finish until the middle of the COVID-19 pandemic and quarantine coupled with weeks of rebellions in defense of Black life. Unwittingly, then, I complete this project in a kairotic, opportune moment.

It would be somewhere between arrogant and silly of me to cull too many lessons from this book to help understand the moment we presently live in. The present is, after all, as Lauren Berlant reminds us, "a temporal genre whose conventions emerge from the personal and public filtering of the situations and events that are happening in an extended now whose very parameters (when did 'the present' begin?) are always there for debate."[1] We cannot pin the present down, and in extended moments when time feels more off kilter than others, more off tempo, too slow and too fast at the same time, it makes little sense to try to capture the present for anything more than a limited moment of sense-making. Nevertheless, the desire to make sense is something akin to human nature.

Many are comparing HIV/AIDS and COVID-19 by noting the similarity between AIDS originally being known as "gay cancer" or GRID—gay-related immune deficiency—and Trump's decision to refer to COVID-19 as the "Chinese virus."[2] Other comparisons abound, even as some rightfully caution about the limitations of these analogies.[3] There are some important ways that AIDS can help us understand COVID-19 that do not require analogies but instead can inform the ways we understand the deep logic of white supremacist, anti-Black, settler colonial nation-states like the United States.

AIDS reminds us that contagious or communicable disease is often used as an opportunity to further marginalize the marginalized. More to the point in the US context, Black communities suffered in wildly disproportionate ways from AIDS because it exacerbated existing violences in the forms of racism, poverty, and homophobia. The same is true with COVID-19 as Black, Indigenous, and Latino/a/x communities face more dire impacts.

The Centers for Disease Control and Prevention reports that Black and Indigenous folks are five times more likely to be hospitalized with COVID-19 than whites, and Latino/a/x people of all races are four times more likely to be hospitalized.[4] At the end of May 2020, the Black mortality rate from COVID-19 was 3.57 times that of the white mortality rate.[5] As with AIDS, disproportionate death and suffering must be contextualized within existing structural disparities so that racist explanations blaming biology and personal responsibility do not inform public health and political response. Inevitably, though, AIDS teaches us that bigoted responses will hold court in the mainstream. Politicians cannot be counted upon to address the disparate death count. Civil dialogue and respectability politics are inadequate defenses too. Agitational resistance must be the mandate of the afflicted. But until the police murder of George Floyd in Minneapolis, Minnesota, tore many away from homes and essential contact only and into the streets, the highly contagious COVID-19 seemed to make such progressive and radical resistance too dangerous to risk.[6] George Floyd's murder on Memorial Day occurred at the end of the long weekend when many US states chose to lift stay-at-home orders and "open for business"; the weeks following saw record infections, hospitalizations, and deaths in those newly opened places. Although the research appears to be mixed at the time I write this, in many cities, the protests against police have not contributed to the increase in COVID-19 cases, perhaps because protest organizers encouraged participants to wear masks and take care of one another.[7]

AIDS is also a reminder that dangerous disease is always an opportunity to foment anti-migrant and xenophobic sentiment. From the moment US mainstream media and politicians had awareness of AIDS, fingers pointed to places outside US borders and to migrant communities within them, particularly Haitians. As these pages reveal, calls to quarantine people living with HIV/AIDS resulted in criminalization of numerous, mostly Black HIV-positive people and the ban on HIV-positive migrants coming to or regularizing in the United States. Such moves are unsurprising because the United States is founded in what I call alienizing logic, and while this logic implicates not only migrant communities—those Mae Ngai calls "alien citizens" become targets too—racialized migrants are a perpetual scapegoat in US history. When Trump uses COVID-19 as a rationale to close US borders to the movement of people or demonize the Chinese, it is important to remember that he draws from a playbook that long preceded him. As people of Asian descent in the United States report an uptick in hate crimes and bias incidents in this historical moment, it is equally important to recall that disease has long been used as an opportunity to target those perceived as foreign for political ends.[8] Furthermore, reports of migrants languishing in detention centers with lack of clean water and personal protective equipment as COVID-19 runs rampant among them are eerily reminiscent of the detention camp on Guantánamo Bay that held supposedly HIV-positive Haitian migrants for nearly two years without recourse.[9]

The time period discussed in this book ends in 1993, marking the release of all the Haitian migrants from Guantánamo after a court order. At that time, 182,275 deaths had been attributed to AIDS in the United States, and prospects for a vaccine were bleak.[10] As I write, the Johns Hopkins Coronavirus Resource Center reports 163,463 COVID-19-related deaths in the United States and over 700,000 worldwide.[11] I have no idea how to make sense of either of those numbers. Perhaps the truth of the matter is that AIDS has less to teach us about COVID-19 than it has to continue to teach us about the deeply embedded, I would argue, foundational flaws inherent in these allegedly united states. Ultimately, this is a book about just that. My hope is that you learn something from it or that, at the very least, I honor the people who fought the injustices described in these pages, succumbed to them, or both.

KARMA R. CHÁVEZ
Austin, Texas
August 11, 2020

ACKNOWLEDGMENTS

When you get to a certain point in your career, it is hard to adequately acknowledge all those who have influenced your thinking, even if they have not had their hands directly on this project. Probably because of age, I'm not plagued with the same anxiety I had when I wrote the acknowledgments of my first monograph, so fearful of leaving someone out. I am sure I did then, and I am sure I will again here; after all, this book has been about a decade in the making. So, if I leave you off, please forgive me; I owe you a drink the next time we can meet in person.

Numerous awards, people, and entities directly aided in the publication of this book. The National Communication Association's 2013 Karl R. Wallace Award, the University of Wisconsin–Madison Graduate School Fall Competition, the UW Institute for Research in the Humanities Race, Ethnicity, and Indigeneity Fellowship, the UW Department of Communication Arts, the University of Texas at Austin Department of Mexican American and Latina/o Studies, the UT Center for Mexican American Studies, the UT College of Liberal Arts, the UT Office of the Vice President for Research book subvention grant, and the Bobby and Sherri Patton Endowed Professorship have financially supported this book at various stages of its development. Numerous audiences invited me to deliver earlier versions of some of the chapters, and I am grateful for the invitations, the dinners, the conversations, and all the feedback. I delivered lectures on parts of this book at the Carl von Ossietzky University, Gonzaga University, McGill University, New Mexico State University, Southwestern University, Syracuse University, University of Arkansas, University of Iowa, University of Nebraska–Lincoln, University of Nevada, Reno, University of South Carolina Upstate, the University of Texas at Austin, University of Wisconsin–Madison, University of Wisconsin–Milwaukee, Villanova University, Whitman College, and Winona State University. I also delivered versions of chapters at the National Women's Studies Association and Public Address conferences. Thank you to the staff at the GLBT Historical Society, the University of California, San Francisco Library, and the New York Public Library for assistance with the archives. Thanks to my dear friend Lisa

Flores for letting me use her password to access Colorado's databases since UT's were incredibly lacking and for opening her home for summer writing retreats, at which I wrote parts of this book (and drank far too much wine). Thanks to Sarah Schulman who assisted me very early in the project and offered strong encouragement. I also appreciate Anne-christine d'Adesky, Keith Bletzer, Kate Raphael, and James Wentzy for their willingness to talk with me about their AIDS work in the late 1980s and early 90s.

This project began in Wisconsin, and I am grateful for the support of dear friends Cindy Cheng, Kathy Villalón, and Freida Zuckerberg who helped me through an especially difficult time in my last semester there in 2016. I am thankful also to M Adams, T Banks, Cynthia Lin, Ananda Mirilli, Teresa Nguyen, Deborah Rasmussen, Kabzuag Vaj, and many others in the Madison community for giving me political home while I was there. Rob Asen, Liz Barr, Finn Enke, Nan Enstad, Maurice Gattis, Armando Ibarra, Jenell Johnson, Lori Kido Lopez, Christa Olson, Lou Roberts, Sue Robinson, Ellen Samuels, Sue Zaeske, and a number of other faculty, students, and staff helped me to thrive at UW. At Texas, I've been privileged to learn from Latino Studies colleagues CJ Alvarez, Mary Beltrán, Katy Buchanan, Cary Cordova, Richard Flores, Rachel González, Laura Gutiérrez, Marisol LeBrón, Belem López, Julie Minich, John Morán González, Deborah Parra-Medina, Lilia Rosas, Antonio Vásquez, a supportive central staff, and numerous amazing researchers. The friendship and support of UT colleagues outside of Latino Studies have also been invaluable, including that of Daniel Arbino, Nicole Burrowes, Luis Cárcamo-Huechante, Ann Cvetkovich, Shiv Ganesh, Ted Gordon, Grayson Hunt, Lisa Moore, Sharmila Rudrappa, Cherise Smith, Christen Smith, Eric Tang, Omi Tinsley, and numerous others. Sandibel Borges and Hana Masri were also important, if only temporary, UT colleagues and interlocutors throughout this process, as was Eithne Luibhéid who has supported my career in innumerable ways and supplied helpful feedback during her year in Latino Studies at UT. Thank you to Alison Kafer for all the wonderful writing dates during the pre-COVID homestretch.

Many others also deserve my thanks for various reasons. Jeff Bennett, David Cisneros, Ryan Conrad, Adela Licona, Chuck Morris, and Armond Towns offered helpful engagement with the book at different points, and Adela and Jamie Lee took good care of me when I needed it most. I am so grateful to be surrounded by a large intellectual community who make me smarter and have supported my work in different ways in the past several years: Aren Aizura, Aimee Bahng, Sirma Bilge, Jennifer Brier, Bernadette

Marie Calafell, Erica Caple James, Jara Carrington, Elora Chowdhury, Dana Cloud, Lisa Corrigan, Bryan Crable, Tara Cyphers, Jigna Desai, Patti Duncan, Dawn Durante, Joan Faber McAlister, Natalie Fixmer-Oraiz, Andie Flores, Mishuana Goeman, Mike Graupmann, Christina Hanhardt, José Herrera, Jo Hsu, Shona Jackson, Janet Jakobsen, Paul Elliott Johnson, Jiyeon Kang, J. Kēhaulani Kauanui, Deana Lewis, Maria Limón, Dana Lloyd, Jenna Loyd, Ashley Mack, Bryan McCann, John Mckiernan-González, Erica Meiners, Carlos Motta, Amber Musser, Yasmin Nair, Ersula Ore, Cate Palczewski, Erica Rand, Nance Riffe, Kat Rodriguez, Stacey Sowards, Eric Stanley, Scott W. Stern, Mary Stuckey, Jesús Valles, Anjali Vats, Kyla Wazana Tompkins, Gretchen Weber, and Naida Zukič.

My editor, Larin McLaughlin, is an incredible interlocutor who helps me think through ideas in ways that have been deeply beneficial. Her excitement about the project gave it new life. I am also grateful to series editor Piya Chatterjee for taking on the project, the anonymous reviewers for providing immensely helpful feedback that I hope they see reflected in this book, and Alja Kooistra for incredible copyediting. The entire production staff at the University of Washington Press has been tremendously supportive. Thanks to Morgan Blue for indexing and proofreading the manuscript.

I am always thankful to my family of origin for their support, love, and laughter. Along the way, eight new Chávezes have made their way into the world (with one on the way)! We've also had some health scares, but thankfully everyone is thriving in these very challenging times. I look forward to when we're all together at the farm in Nebraska again.

My best friends, Leah Mirakhor and Kimberlee Pérez, enrich my life and have enriched this project in more ways than I can express. Leah jumped in for some much-needed help with the introduction and once again saved me from myself. Thanks, dudes. HLT Quan and CA Griffith are my queer women of color family and mentors. Nothing I do is without their perpetual love. I've been kept busy over the last couple of years in Austin with my two cats, Chloe and Rico; my two dogs, Charlie and Oscar; and the nine or so feral cats that I feed every day much to the chagrin of my neighbors. They didn't help with this project, but I love them anyway.

And to Annie Hill: You found me when we were both quite low, and yet we've built this beautiful, thriving life. What a gift. You're the most brilliant and loving person I know. Thank you for everything you are.

TERMINOLOGY

The parlance concerning HIV and AIDS has more or less been worked out in the twenty-first century, but in the 1980s, this was far from the case. When first identified in gay men on the US coasts, what we now call AIDS was referred to variously, including as gay cancer, gay pneumonia, and GRID—gay-related immune deficiency. Some also initially referred to it as AID—acquired immunodeficiency. By 1982, the medical community agreed upon the term "AIDS"—acquired immune deficiency syndrome—to describe the weakened immune state, the disease that opened the body to opportunistic infections that, in the early days, would likely kill the afflicted person. When researchers and physicians began to identify a specific virus they believed caused AIDS in 1983, that virus also went by different names, including HTLV-III (human T-lymphotropic virus type III), LAV (lymphadenopathy-associated virus), and ARV (AIDS-associated retrovirus). In 1986, scientists eventually agreed upon the term "HIV"—human immunodeficiency virus—for the viral infection that under the right environmental conditions leads to AIDS.

I provide this brief summary of terminology to indicate how complicated it was even for scientists to talk about what was happening. This meant that often media and politicians were confused about the appropriate terms too. When I talk about the period prior to 1986, I either use "AIDS" or whatever term is used in a particular source. After 1986, I tend to use "HIV/AIDS" unless it makes sense to separate them or unless it is appropriate to use a term from a source. I do not use now-outdated terms like "AIDS-related complex" or ARC—a term that described a person with HIV infection and mild AIDS-like symptoms—unless used in a source. Because my interest is more cultural and political than medical, I do not get into the weeds of discussing different stages of HIV, types of opportunistic infections, or other more technical aspects of HIV/AIDS. I am sure I get things wrong, but I hope to be clear enough with my usages that my terminology does not distract from anyone's reading of the book.

Also, as a general rule, I follow Eithne Luibhéid in her use of the word "migrant" to describe all people who have crossed an international border.[1]

This means that I usually do not use "immigrant" or other legal categories like "asylum seeker" or "refugee." To use "migrant" is to deemphasize the law's categories. I also use migrant to recognize that the distinctions assigned to any one of the legal categories can be fleeting. As Luibhéid persuasively argues, there is a "shifting line" between legality and illegality, from one category to another.[2] There are occasions in this book, particularly in chapter 4 when I speak about Haitian migrants who sought refugee status in the United States, when I might use the term "refugee" to refer to them. However, that is usually only when talking in a legal context and so the distinction is relevant. Otherwise, I actively want to complicate the distinctions and the differential sympathies conjured by the different legal categories.

ABBREVIATIONS

ACLU	American Civil Liberties Union
ACT NOW	AIDS Coalition to Network, Organize and Win
ACT UP	AIDS Coalition to Unleash Power
AIDS	Acquired Immune Deficiency Syndrome
AMA	American Medical Association
amfAR	American Foundation for AIDS Research (after 2005, Foundation for AIDS Research)
ARC	AIDS-Related Complex
ARV	AIDS-Associated Retrovirus
ASFV	African Swine Fever Virus
BAM!	Black AIDS Mobilization
CBP	US Customs and Border Patrol
CDC	Centers for Disease Control (after 1992, Centers for Disease Control and Prevention)
CIRRS	Coalition for Immigrant and Refugee Rights and Services (California)
GRID	Gay-Related Immune Deficiency
HHS	Department of Health and Human Services
HIV	Human Immunodeficiency Virus
HRS	Department of Health and Rehabilitative Services (Florida)
HTLV-III	Human T-Lymphotropic Virus Type III
IAC	International AIDS Conference
IAS	International AIDS Society
INS	Immigration and Naturalization Service
IRCA	Immigration Reform and Control Act
IWG	ACT UP Immigration Working Group
LAV	Lymphadenopathy-Associated Virus
MHS	Marine Hospital Service
NGLTF	National Gay and Lesbian Task Force
PANIC	The Prevent AIDS Now Initiative Committee (later, Prevent AIDS Now In California)
PHS	US Public Health Service

THE BORDERS OF AIDS

INTRODUCTION

The Alienizing Nation

A PERSON WEARING A RONALD REAGAN MASK, BLACK SUIT, AND LONG, YELLOW rubber gloves sat casually with his ankles crossed on top of the cab of a beat-up pickup truck driving through the streets of New York. "Guards" in army green uniforms flanked the truck, donning the same gloves and what looked like N95 masks. The truck pulled a makeshift concentration camp, constructed of bars and razor wire. A watchtower protruded from the center of the camp, with yellow images of Reagan's face on all four sides, peering out like big brother. A multiracial group of "prisoners" looked out to the street from between the bars and barbed wire as other marchers walked slowly beside them carrying signs proclaiming "silence = death." This prescient performative protest at the 1987 Pride march was the brainchild of the nascent AIDS Coalition to Unleash Power (ACT UP) New York, which wanted to make a powerful statement about AIDS at the annual event.[1] Whether ACT UP members were aware is unclear, but just weeks before the Pride march, the US Senate passed a ban on HIV-positive migrants, preventing them from coming to or legalizing within the United States. Some four years later, the scene the float foreshadowed would become reality as the United States constructed a quarantine camp for intercepted HIV-positive Haitians who fled political violence after the overthrow of their president, Jean-Bertrand Aristide. Although ACT UP could not have known that they were actually predicting a future for some HIV-positive people, the ominous float made a statement about the severity of the situation for people living with AIDS, not just because opportunistic infections could be deadly but for the ways that the US government would use the disease as an opportunity to alienize already maligned people such as Haitians and homosexuals.

In a nation-state like the United States, which is founded on the creation and maintenance of a populace, a citizenry that is by definition expulsive, exterminative, and exclusionary—whether by genocide, lynching, the plantation, the reservation, the ghetto, the internment camp, the prison, the hospital, quarantine, ban, or deportation—disease becomes one of many opportunities to express this "alienizing logic." In the United States, disease has historically been an opportunity to express the state's alienizing logic when associated with particular people: Black, migrant, queer, trans, Indigenous, poor, prostitute, of color. Regardless of whether they possess US citizenship, these are alienized people; that is, they are or easily can be made alien to the nation-state. *The Borders of AIDS* is about two expressions of alienizing logic—quarantine and ban—as they manifested in the early days of the AIDS pandemic in the United States, from 1981 to 1993.

This book began, however, as a project to understand how AIDS activists engaged with the question of migration given that AIDS had always been, at least in part, about migration. I spent years thinking of the project in this way. But I eventually realized that such an approach was too limited. The more obvious question I needed to wrestle with was how did AIDS come to be associated with migration in the first place? The answer to that question became clearer as I understood how quarantine—always a concern about movement—featured in people's thinking about AIDS during the early years. Despite the fact that quarantines never made much medical or epidemiological sense to address the spread of HIV and AIDS, quarantine's centrality in the public imagination is evident in wide-ranging calls for it, extensive fears of it, and its proliferation in AIDS discourse, almost from the inception. Eventually, such rhetoric materialized in state-level quarantine laws that often emerged in response to the behaviors of supposedly recalcitrant Black sex workers. Such expressed concerns about the movement of "fugitive" Black bodies is a narrative as old as the days of fugitive slaves in the United States. The alienizing logic refined during these frenzied calls for quarantine manifested in one way with widespread passing of laws that criminalize HIV, which has disproportionately impacted Black men.[2] Although quarantine never became a law or set of laws applied to HIV-positive US citizens en masse, rhetorics of quarantine manifested in another way by animating the twenty-two-year-long US ban on HIV-positive migrants, which was only lifted in 2010. This book tells a story of how public health officials, politicians, the media, and others applied alienizing logic to people living with AIDS in the form of quarantine and ban rhetorics and how some of those most impacted fought back.

I tell this story as a rhetorical critic. To me, rhetoric is contingent discourse that usually has a public dimension (or at least an audience) and makes an argument (intentionally or not). Like other scholars who work in the archive and the field, rhetorical critics rely on a variety of sources. I draw from and analyze news reports, speeches, government documents, political propaganda, conversations, and field notes, among others. As a rhetorical critic, I attend to sources of invention, argument construction, persuasive tactics, message strategies, and the context out of which all that emerges. As such, this book contends with how people's rhetorical practices emerge from, challenge, and/or reproduce predominant cultural discourses or assumptions. As a rhetorical critic, like the creators of my sources, I tell partial and particular stories, and I make claims about the contours of the rhetorics of a particular time and place. Doing this work in this way is important because rhetoric constitutes how issues are framed, how people are imagined, and which public memories endure over time.

ALIENIZING LOGIC

To understand this story, I must first explain what I mean by "alienizing logic." A logic is a structure of thinking that thereby structures expression.[3] A logic can be expressed in innumerable ways by countless actors or entities, but who deploys a logic results in different impacts. A logic can emerge from numerous, even competing, belief systems or ideologies. What I describe as an alienizing logic refers to a structure of thinking that insists that some are necessarily members of a community and some are recognized as not belonging, even if they physically reside there.[4] The alien-outside is not a part of a simple dichotomy constituted by a firm boundary between two easily identifiable positions. This blurriness becomes clearer when looking closely at the different definitions of the noun form of "alien." Definitions are an important starting place for a scholar interested in rhetoric because the meanings of terms not only shape our understanding, but they also often form the basic grounds for claims people make and warrants they use to justify those claims. The *Oxford English Dictionary* (*OED*) provides three prominent definitions relevant to this discussion:

1a. Alien: A person who does not belong to a particular family, community, country, etc.; a foreigner, a stranger, an outsider.

2a. Alien: A person who is separated or excluded *from* a particular
community, country, custom, etc.

2b. Alien: A person who or thing which is opposed, repugnant, or
unaccustomed *to* a specified person or thing; a stranger *to*.[5]

Each relationship represented in these definitions from the *OED* help to
articulate the expansiveness of the idea of alien in the English-speaking
world and can help facilitate conceptual linkages between seemingly separate groups of people—one who does not belong to a community versus one
who is separated from or repugnant to it.

A person who does not belong: The first definition is the most familiar
one and is reflected in the many uses of "alien" to categorize people within
immigration law. It also captures the extraterrestrial made so common in
science fiction and conspiracy theory. This definition refers to a recognized
status that one possesses by virtue of their nonbelonging. It is a permanent
or quasi-permanent state of being that can only be modified by whatever
mechanism has rendered one foreign or outside, if such a mechanism exists.
At least theoretically, one can change their immigration status, but they may
not move from extraterrestrial to human or vice versa.

A person who is separated or excluded: This definition is also quite common. By force or by choice, one may become separated or excluded from a
community in which they were formerly a member. If one has chosen to
separate from a community, say by moving to another country, they
may have the option to return once again, although whether they would
be recognized as belonging upon return is an open question. The fact of
separation and exclusion changes a person whether or not they chose to
separate. If one was forcibly separated or excluded, the conditions of return
are perhaps most tenuous, as when a person returns to their community
after incarceration. The separation or exclusion, however, may not be physical; one can also emotionally or spiritually separate while remaining in the
same physical location. This definition also refers to a status, but it is a status that lacks the clarity implied by the previous definition. An exclusion
or separation can exist for any duration of time depending on the conditions that catalyzed it. Moreover, one may not be alien based on the first
definition even if they are physically separated from their community of
belonging.

A person who or thing which is opposed, repugnant, or unaccustomed: This
definition is probably the least common in usage as it implies a someone
or some entity that experiences someone else as repugnant, oppositional,

or otherwise disquieting. This definition most fully evidences the blurry boundaries between the inside and outside, as one might belong to a community yet another community member finds them unacceptable or wishes them outside of it. Perhaps a young person comes out to their family as queer or trans, and the majority of the family continues to love them, but a parent or grandparent, now knowing that the young person is queer, cannot accept them. In the eyes of that parent or grandparent, the young person opposes all that the family stands for, and the young person's real or perceived sexual practices or gender expression disgust the parent or grandparent. To that family member, the young person is alien. Because this definition suggests that a member of a community views the alienized person not just as foreign or strange but as contrary, offensive, objectionable, and perhaps even incompatible with the community, when one is rendered alien in this way, it suggests immediate danger. What lengths would someone take to remove that which is potentially inside but contrary to the entire community?

In real life, these definitions are perpetually blended together even if one understanding dominates in particular contexts. In each case, to be rendered alien involves a relationship between two or more entities and involves a recognition by one or more of those entities of a person as an alien. Taken together they provide a framework to begin to understand how alienizing logic works. We can gain a fuller understanding by turning attention to some of the scholarly conversations that have theorized the alien, particularly in relation to the citizen.

THE ALIEN AND THE CITIZEN

The term "alien" has a long history of legal and metaphorical usage in immigration law.[6] "Alien" is also politically charged and, historically, the subject of significant debate, often around using the term "illegal alien."[7] In social theory, scholars use the categories of the alien and the stranger to theorize the production of otherness. For example, Zygmunt Bauman explains that society produces strangers "who conceal borderlines deemed crucial to its orderly and/or meaningful life and are thus charged with causing the discomfort experienced as the most painful and least bearable."[8] Thus, modern states have either worked to assimilate or exclude strangers they produce, or when that does not work, states attempt to expel or destroy them.[9] In this way, the stranger is both foundational to building state order and that which must be culturally or physically annihilated.[10] Sara Ahmed explains that the production of the stranger is not always abstract, unknown, or outside, often occurring through an embodied encounter with an other who is recognized as such.[11] Katarzyna Marciniak builds upon such theorizing to explain the production of the alien as a particular kind of stranger. Aliens emerge from what she terms "alienhood," or "a highly racialized rhetorical and disciplinary apparatus that classifies immigrants, refugees, and border crossers in relation to the U.S. territory."[12] Marciniak's work investigates what she describes as the "palimpsestic signification" of the alien in US American culture as both foreigner and extraterrestrial, which has significant implications for how people deemed alien get recognized and are able to exist in society.

Marciniak points to the political-legal framework that conceptualizes the juxtaposition between the alien and the citizen. At its most basic, citizenship refers to a legal status that indicates whether one belongs to a particular political body, and in contemporary times, that body is the nation-state. Yet citizenship has always been a fraught idea with exclusion as central to its definition as inclusion.[13] Furthermore, debates exist over what citizenship is, who a citizen is, and where citizenship is practiced.[14] Linda Bosniak argues that political theory about citizenship has often fallen into two camps: those who explore the contours of the political community within borders and those who study the formation of the citizenry at national borders. In terms of the latter, scholars consider the way national borders are legally and physically fortified against international migration, which leads to the production of numerous types of aliens with varying legal statuses and relationships to the state.[15] Within the political community, alienage simultaneously defines the boundaries of citizenship and complicates those boundaries, as one defined as alien might practice what looks like citizenship without the legal status, what some have called cultural or social citizenship.[16] Furthermore, as Aihwa Ong so aptly put it, citizenship is "variegated," and how much the state values someone determines the kind of "rights, discipline, caring, and security" they enjoy.[17] Citizenship has always been differentially granted in the United States, particularly in how it has historically and consistently denied citizenship to Black and Indigenous people. Women, queer, and trans folks across racial lines, as well as Asian and Latino/a/x descended people, have historically been relegated to what has often been called "second-class citizenship," generally not a recognized legal category but a status that does not include all of the rights a citizen should have. Being relegated to this status may limit access to rights such as voting or involve unequal or disparate treatment by various political actors.[18]

The disadvantages between those the state recognizes as aliens (migrants) and the second-class citizen vary in important material ways—only the former can be legally deported, which means that tensions can arise over rights struggles for the different groups.[19] But the shared disadvantage in relation to legal citizenship status also illuminates important resonances, as revealed in what Mae Ngai calls "alien citizenship." Ngai uses the term to describe the historic status of Asians and Mexicans, whose racial and ethnic statuses have remained linked, and therefore even those with legal citizenship "remained alien in the eyes of the nation."[20] Although Ngai uses alien citizenship in very particular ways, for my purposes it is helpful to consider the idea more expansively. The alienized citizen is not foreign but does not belong to the citizenry outside of a formal status; may be excluded or separated from that citizenry by borders, bars, or other boundaries; and in some cases is actively opposed and repugnant to the citizenry, making the citizen not only alienated but also vulnerable to structural and interpersonal violence. When considering all of these discussions of the alien, it becomes clear that thinking of the alien in only the legal register as a foreign migrant is part of a divide and conquer strategy that denies a fuller meaning of alienage. The state and other official entities apply alienizing logic to citizens and migrants alike. The logic may manifest differently— genocide, lynching, the plantation, the reservation, the ghetto, the internment camp, the prison, the hospital, quarantine, ban, or deportation. Fundamentally, those with inalienable rights have the power to alienize; those without them do not.

ALIENIZING LOGIC AND DISEASE

Brett Stockdill writes of HIV/AIDS that it, like many other diseases, "has always been a problem that has severely affected those at the intersections of multiple oppressions: homophobia, racism, sexism and classism in particular."[21] His claim is important because while illness can technically afflict anyone, extreme health disparities exist between the structurally privileged and those who reside in the intersections of the structures of oppression. Disease can manifest because of structural oppression, and disease can become an opportunity to exacerbate structural oppressions through alienizing logic.[22] Fundamentally, using disease or fear of disease as an opportunity to enact alienizing logic has always been racialized and usually racist.[23] Susan L. Smith notes, for example, that in the antebellum United States, many white southerners "believed that if black people became sick it was because of an inherently weaker constitution" at the same time that some physicians maintained that "African Americans were more resistant than white people to certain diseases, such as yellow fever and malaria."[24] Either way you cut it, Black people's relationship to disease was one of the many factors white people used to alienize them, and such logic continues to the present day; many continue to believe that supposed Black inferiority explains health disparities.[25]

Other groups also suffered. For example, Nayan Shah writes, nineteenth-century public health officials saw the project of preserving the "public health" as "undercut by the reputed vile and disease-breeding qualities of Chinese settlement in the city. In the name of safeguarding the health of the entire population, public health strategies of surveillance, documentation, and quarantine generated new conceptions of Chinese behavior at odds with the standards of proper social conduct."[26] Here the concern is not about the health of the Chinese but how their allegedly unhealthy (cultural) habits might leak out, impacting the good health of the "general" population. Not all Chinese were migrants, but some were, and public health officials often put racialized migrants at the center of concerns about disease. Howard Markel and Alexandra Minna Stern note a consistent pattern in US American history of stigmatizing migrants "as the etiology of a wide variety of physical and societal ills."[27] Such a pattern can be seen starkly in historic practices at US ports of entry where migrants would be undressed and scrutinized for signs of malady and moral weakness or they and their belongings deloused to prevent their diseases from penetrating the United States.[28] From the arrival of the first ships carrying stolen Africans to the relatively present day, migrants have been quarantined to ensure their fitness to the nation. Examples are virtually endless and continue well into the twenty-first century. I elaborate on these histories in chapter 1.

Regardless of the bodies they inhabit or are thought to inhabit, illnesses have a large discursive life intermingling with the physical course they run.[29] As Susan Sontag has argued, the "reputation" of an illness adds "to the suffering of those who have it."[30] Near the end of Paula Treichler's extensive book, *How to Have Theory in an Epidemic*, she notes that AIDS "takes place in language and discourse, where *AIDS*, the word, is constructed, where it becomes a story, where it is rendered intelligible, and where it is acted upon."[31] Treichler's framing of AIDS in this way is a reminder for those whose perspectives on AIDS contend with the element of human struggle and day-to-day experience of the disease. This framing is also significant because both scholars and laypeople have tended to tell the story of HIV/AIDS in the United States primarily in relation to gay men. A majority of written US accounts of the pandemic feature most prominently the stories of gay men, often in relationship to the systems and institutions they had, and have, to navigate.[32] The most memorialized and discussed AIDS activism from the early days of the pandemic emerged from ACT UP, a group typically remembered for its use of queer political strategies on behalf of white, middle-class, urban, gay, male US citizens. US histories from a biomedical perspective, with doctors and public health officials at the center or as author, also largely emphasize the gay male community over others that were also afflicted.[33] Even as such an emphasis overlooks the breadth of communities afflicted by HIV/AIDS, it is nonetheless understandable because as the Centers for Disease Control and Prevention (CDC) reports, more than half of HIV/AIDS cases in the United States have been in men who have sex with men. The connections between AIDS, AIDS activism, a particular style of "in-your-face" queer politics, gay and lesbian identities, and heterosexism/homophobia will always remain predominant in US American imaginations of HIV/AIDS. Moreover, gay men and other queer and trans communities have long been subject to alienizing logic: through detention and deportation, incarceration and institutionalization, and estrangement and isolation from communities.[34]

This book does not minimize those connections or realities, but it emerges from a concern shared with Michele Tracy Berger, who emphasizes the obstacles faced by those living with HIV/AIDS who confront multiple axes of oppression, or "intersectional stigma." The concerns of those experiencing intersectional stigma differ from those living with HIV/AIDS who hold relative privilege based on race, class, or gender.[35] My concern extends further: How do immigration and citizenship status matter as additional sites of power and oppression that impact people's experiences with HIV/AIDS and the ways HIV/AIDS becomes an opportunity to enact alienizing logic?[36]

When I say immigration status matters to our understanding of AIDS, I refer to the fact that since the beginning of the AIDS crisis, US-based migrant communities from Haiti and Africa, as well as other parts of the Caribbean, Asia, and Latin America, were not only devastated by AIDS, but media and politicians widely stigmatized some of these groups as the supposed origins of AIDS and as high-risk groups for contracting and spreading the disease. Furthermore, laws and provisions banning migrants with

HIV and AIDS not only prevented people's movement but also forced many migrants with HIV/AIDS who were already in the United States deeply underground to avoid detection, possible detention, and deportation.

When I say that citizenship status matters, I suggest that lacking legal citizenship obviously makes a difference in how people have historically been able to live with HIV/AIDS. I also mean something much bigger, which I signaled above. We know the stories of how HIV/AIDS impacted mostly white, middle-class, US citizen gay men. As stated above, AIDS, like many diseases before it, also had dire effects on other US citizens already far removed from their supposed inalienable rights: Black, Indigenous, Asian, and Latino/a/x communities; prostitutes; drug users; the incarcerated; and the poor. Without political power by virtue of race and class privilege, these communities were not only the subject of stigmatizing rhetoric and treat- ment, but they suffered from the active neglect of their government, their communities, and the medical establishment. If not left for dead, these alien citizens were actively maligned and blamed in the US public sphere. These citizen groups and migrants alike were subject to alienizing logic in a host of forms, including the subjects of this book: quarantine and ban.

This book intervenes in the ways that historical, media, and rhetorical accounts of HIV/AIDS often racialize people living with AIDS as white, gen- der them as male, and assume their US citizenship. This monograph joins the small body of scholarly literature regarding the public memory of HIV/ AIDS in the United States that does not center the experiences of white, gay, US citizen men but focuses instead on how AIDS created an opportunity for politicians, public health officials, and mainstream media to use immi- gration status, race, and citizenship to enact alienizing logic.

METHODOLOGY

To tell this story, I center the time beginning when US media and medical publications recognized AIDS in 1981 until just after the codification of the US ban on HIV-positive migrants in 1993 while over two hundred suppos- edly HIV-positive Haitian migrants languished in an HIV detention camp on Guantánamo Bay, Cuba. This time frame shifts the usual temporality for the "early years" of AIDS in the United States, often marked as ending in 1996 as medications became available that made the disease manageable for those who could afford them. In this way, I join the authors in Jih-Fei Cheng, Alexandra Juhasz, and Nishant Shahani's edited volume, *AIDS and the Distribution of Crises*, who also complicate the way US American scholars have prioritized the start and supposed end of the "crisis" period of HIV/AIDS in the Global North.[37] Although I shift the temporality only slightly, doing so offers yet another rupture in what gets taken for granted when the most privileged people living with AIDS are centered in the stories we tell.[38]

To research this book, in addition to using digital databases for news reports and congressional records, I relied largely on AIDS activist archives. Importantly, with the exception of those consulted here, information from and about migrants, the subject of the majority of this book, is largely absent from existing archives related to HIV/AIDS. References to migrants and their experiences in the HIV/AIDS pandemic, especially as it produced conditions for detainment and detention, are found largely in ephemera—a flyer announcing an Immigration and Naturalization Service rally, a line on an agenda, or a recalled memory of a living organizer. I am sure, too, there are many memories living in people whose experiences were not documented, who no longer connect with the communities with which they organized back then out of necessity or trauma or reasons unknown, or who I did not know to ask. AIDS scholar Ted Kerr writes of an instructive incident at an AIDS symposium in Toronto:

> A black woman in her late 20s suggested that if we are going to try to represent the history of AIDS, we are going to have to do more than just visit the archives, because "no one was talking picture [sic] of the women who looked like me." She went on to share that through her work as an organizer, she had heard countless stories about the early days of AIDS in Canada from black people and other people of color, but she is sure that none of them will ever be widely known, in part because people are still dealing with their trauma around the epidemic, and in part because no one is asking them to talk.[39]

My work largely relies on archival sources, so this woman's criticisms implicate this project. But investigating archival source material with a critical lens that refuses to center the most obvious voices within that material is an important way to intervene in "how the legacy of antiblack violence shapes the project of archival recovery."[40] Furthermore, I follow Darius Boot and other Black queer and feminist scholars in the ways I represent people and center what Katherine McKittrick and Tiffany Lethabo King call "Black livingness."[41] Although this is not a book only about Blackness, the treatment of Black folks and their resistance features centrally through-out the book. Therefore, it is imperative to notice Black livingness by "reading intertextually," to ensure that new relationships, voices, and understandings can come to the surface that betray "the archive of vio-lence."[42] What that means for me in this book is that I provide accounts of Black life and resistance even when what I have to work with from the limited archive are traces and ephemera.

MAP OF THE BOOK

The Borders of AIDS unfolds through five chapters divided into two sections, with each chapter addressing an important aspect of how HIV/AIDS created an opportunity to animate alienizing logic. In the first part, "Alien-izing Logic and Structure," I emphasize how people with power to frame issues and make decisions utilize disease as an opportunity to enact alien-izing logic. This focus helps to see the development and perniciousness of this logic and how it manifests historically and in relation to HIV/AIDS. The sources I primarily draw upon are both official, including materials from the *Congressional Record*, public health conferences, statements from immigration and political officials, and mainstream, including reports and stories from major newspapers and magazines. I layer the accounts in the first part with the voices of activists and people living with HIV/AIDS. Chapter 1 maps the development of quarantine laws in the United States in relation to racialized US citizens, migrants, and supposed sexual deviants. Chapter 2 explains how the historical precedents discussed in the first chap-ter manifest in the perfect storm that is HIV/AIDS in the United States. Despite its inappropriateness as a response to HIV/AIDS, public health officials, politicians, and therefore the public widely considered quarantine a reasonable response to addressing the growing AIDS pandemic. The cre-ation and reissuing of quarantine laws largely happened on the backs of a handful of Black sex workers who became the subjects of media frenzy. Chapter 3 explores the way the alienizing logic of quarantine morphs into "national common sense" in US immigration law, as some of those most adamantly in support of nationwide quarantine in the United States became the key architects of the ban on HIV-positive immigration in 1987.

In the second part, "Resisting Alienizing Logic," I shift attention to how mostly queer AIDS activists responded to and resisted alienizing logic as it applied to migrant communities who may or may not have also been queer. As suggested above, many books have addressed queer AIDS activism, marking AIDS as the catalyst to what has become contemporary queer politics. Most of those books focus on US citizens battling on behalf of US citizens. For me, as a scholar of queer and migration politics and coalition and as someone who knows how central the questions around migration were to thinking on HIV/AIDS, telling a story that puts queer politics and migration politics into productive conversation is of vital importance in order to understand another crucial dimension to the history of HIV/AIDS in the United States. Given the power of alienizing logic in constituting the expressions of quarantine and ban, complicating the important historical archive and scholarly record of queer AIDS activism with an examination of how queer AIDS activists battled on behalf of an alienized group of which many were not a part—migrants—offers important insights into the texture of struggles against AIDS and the possibilities for innovative coalitional moments. I derived source material largely from queer and AIDS archives, including collections from ACT UP chapters, some individual ACT UP members, the National Lawyers Guild, and the International AIDS Society held at the GLBT Historical Society; the University of California, San Francisco library; the New York Public Library; and the Archives of Sexuality and Gender online database.

Chapter 4 in the book's second part explores boycotts and protests of the International AIDS Conferences in 1990 and 1992, which were both scheduled to take place in the United States. Because US immigration law excluded people living with HIV/AIDS, as well as others such as sex workers and those with criminal drug convictions, from traveling to the United States and therefore attending the conference, public health officials and nongovernmental organizations boycotted the San Francisco conference in 1990, catalyzing an organized cadre of international AIDS activists to heavily protest it. Activists further agitated against the conference scheduled for Boston in 1992, getting it moved to Amsterdam and beginning a twenty-two-year boycott of the United States by the International AIDS Conference. Chapter 5 considers Haitians' distinct relationship to HIV/AIDS through the lens of AIDS activist media. In this chapter, I argue that AIDS activist media makers provided some of the most accurate and informative reporting on the so-called Haitian connection in the early days. I also show how queer and AIDS activist media makers later became among the most prominent to document fights against the US government's extreme application of alienizing logic when it used Guantánamo Bay to detain hundreds of allegedly HIV-positive Haitian migrants.

Although the events in this book are from the past, they remain a live part of our present. As Cheng, Juhasz, and Shahani write, "With AIDS we find ourselves in the midst of long-term and still ongoing global crises."[43] Furthermore, as the moment in which I write indicates, COVID-19 has become yet another opportunity to enact alienizing logic. While, unlike HIV, we have hope that a vaccine will ensure this crisis is not protracted in the same way, the eerily similar ideological denials, fears, and governmental neglect constitute the present. The alienizing nation endures, but then and now, those at the nation's literal and figurative borders resist it. AIDS thus continues to have many lessons to teach us about our present and our presence within it.

PART ONE

ALIENIZING LOGIC
AND STRUCTURE

CHAPTER 1

A BRIEF RHETORICAL HISTORY OF QUARANTINE

THREE HUNDRED PEOPLE JOINED NOBEL LAUREATE TONI MORRISON to dedicate "a bench by the road" on Sullivan's Island, South Carolina, in the summer of 2008. The bench idea came from a 1989 interview in which Morrison lamented the dearth of suitable commemorations for the history of enslaved Africans in the United States. "There's no 300-foot tower, there's no small bench by the road," Morrison said.[1] Sullivan's Island has been referred to by some as the Ellis Island for captured Africans brought to the United States to be enslaved; some historians believe that throughout much of the 1700s, as many as 40 percent of all Africans brought across the Atlantic were medically inspected and quarantined at Sullivan's Island's pesthouses.[2] For those who survived the Middle Passage, a minimum of ten days in a 30′ × 10′ brick structure awaited them on the island.[3] The people of Charleston built the pesthouses because they worried about the possibility of introducing African diseases or the diseases that emerged from the horrific conditions of the ships. Once determined healthy enough to go to the auction block, Africans were transported to nearby Charleston to be sold. Sullivan's Island was one of the first quarantine stations in the colonies, and despite its macabre status as the gateway for the arrival of so many forced African migrants, this history is relatively unknown. Commemorated only by Morrison's bench and a small historical plaque erected a decade earlier, it is hard to find very much at all that tells this story of what is now an affluent beach town.

Sullivan's Island is a stark reminder that medical and public health practices in what would become the United States have always been deeply racialized practices and at their worst have been explicitly racist, sexist, homophobic, xenophobic, transphobic, and/or ableist. From medical experimentation on Black and Indigenous people, often without anesthesia, to involuntary sterilizations of Indigenous, Latina, and Black women, to dehumanizing treatments and medical neglect of marginalized communities, triumphs in medicine and public health often emerge on the backs of Black, Indigenous, and people of color as well as those deemed mentally unfit and migrants.[4] The development and implementation of quarantine practices share these same troubling tendencies.

In this chapter, I provide a rhetorical history of quarantine in the United States, beginning in the late eighteenth century.[5] I take cue from Richard McKay in my *longue durée* approach, which "treads lightly" over large periods of history, a move that some historians will be wary of as it "risks severing the incidents from the original interpretive frameworks that imbued them with meaning."[6] Yet, as McKay notes, "other observers have been less concerned about original context when reappropriating and recirculating older ideas."[7] For my purposes, I am interested in how ideas about quarantine traveled rhetorically from the early days of the US republic to the late twentieth century in texts that shaped the public sphere—news reports, political speech, and public health discourse. My objective is not to provide a comprehensive history of quarantine in the United States but instead to note the ways that arguments about quarantine emerge at specific moments in time and to begin to trace the constellation of ideas, beliefs, and people that consistently accompany quarantine rhetoric. Through this rhetorical history, I unpack how quarantine, as an alienizing logic, emerges primarily from concerns about mobility and migration, showing that the applications of quarantine frequently rely on rhetorical appeals premised in anxieties about foreign invasion, international migration, and migrant communities that may bring infectious disease into the larger community. In the early part of the twentieth century, the alienizing logic animates calls to quarantine alien citizen groups as quarantine begins to be applied to venereal disease, particularly to prostitutes, in what is rolled out as the infamous American Plan.[8] Even as calls to quarantine and broader anxieties about public health and contagious disease fade during the mid-twentieth century with the advancement of treatments, what I map here sets the stage for the reemergence of quarantine rhetorics in the early years of the AIDS pandemic in the United States.

QUARANTINE: A CENTURIES-OLD CONCEPT

Societies have practiced isolation and quarantine in order to protect the public health throughout time, including depictions found in the Hebrew Bible.[9] Historians generally mark formalized and systematic rules for practices of quarantine as emerging in the fourteenth century in Italy,[10] but international historian Mark Harrison locates it in "regulations devised in the Republic of Ragussa (Dubrovnik) in 1397."[11] Although the colloquial usage of isolation and quarantine are synonymous, the public health definitions differ: isolation refers to the segregation of the *ill* or infected, whereas quarantine refers to the containment of *well* people, animals, or goods that may have been exposed to a communicable infection. This distinction is partly reflected in the *Oxford English Dictionary* (*OED*) definitions of quarantine as "isolation imposed on newly arrived travellers in order to prevent the spread of disease; a period of time spent in such isolation. Later also: such isolation applied to a person or animal known to be suffering from an infectious disease or to the contacts of a such a person or animal, or to newly imported animals, plants, or inanimate objects."[12] The definitions signal the distinction, particularly as applied to newly arrived travelers, and collapse the difference in later usages, connecting it to those already ill, a point to which I return.

I want briefly to consider the dictionary definitions of quarantine because they articulate the basic dimensions of the concept—travel, temporality, economics, and politics—that continue to come up in this chapter and chapter 2. First, public health practitioners historically used quarantine at ports to prevent illness and infestation brought from distant locations. By most accounts, the word "quarantine" extends from *quarantenaria*, first used in Venice and referring to the forty-day isolation imposed on vessels arriving with travelers, animals, and goods.[13] Second, and as implied by the forty-day isolation period, the temporality of quarantine is significant as quarantines are inherently temporary; once a threat of infection is no longer live, the quarantine ends. Third, although throughout time human travelers have always been subject to quarantine, public health and maritime historians note that in the medieval era, quarantine was primarily concerned with "goods and merchandise."[14] Although this dimension of the definition appears to be only about economic concerns, controversies around quarantining goods led many to view quarantine as an evil and a political tool. As Harrison explains, "Quarantine was not maintained simply as a defence against disease. By the late sixteenth century the internal problems of countries afflicted with plague were severely aggravated by the embargoes imposed by other states. The merest hint of plague in a foreign port could be enough to trigger such bans and in some cases rumours were deliberately put about to damage the commerce of rivals."[15] Quarantine as both economic and political becomes salient for discussion in later chapters.

Only in the modern period, particularly from the nineteenth century onward, did quarantine become "more tightly tied to human movement and its regulation in the great age of intercontinental migration."[16] What emerges is a phenomenon that Alan M. Kraut refers to as "medical nativism,"[17] which describes "how the stigmatizing of immigrant groups is justified by their association with communicable disease; it implies the almost superstitious belief that national borders can afford protection against communicable disease."[18] Businesses and politicians alike often considered quarantine an expensive nuisance when applied to commerce, but as it became central to modern nation-building through immigration restriction, it gained widespread acceptance as an important and legitimate mechanism of population management. The connection with human movement has become so strong that in some circles, quarantine is used metaphorically or metonymically to refer to "border detention."[19] Each dimension of quarantine's definition implies a concern over movement. The definition reflects a literal need to contain in order to prevent the spread of disease. When coupled with histories of public health and the institution of quarantine, these definitions signal a metaphorical anxiety over the containment of national borders to protect the national body.[20] Put differently, they reflect an alienizing logic.

The collapsing of isolation and quarantine as reflected in the later *OED* definitions, while potentially problematic for public health officials, is of less concern for the analysis here. Although public health officials use isolation to describe what to do with the ill and quarantine for the well, as shown, only quarantine gets deployed to mean both in common usage, including among public health officials who know the difference. A rhetorical study of this kind is less concerned with what Thomas Goodnight called the "technical sphere" and more concerned with the public one.[21] After all, the average person is not meant to have the same technical vocabulary as a public health expert, and there are probably many terms that differ in their common and technical usages. It is also likely that the term "isolation" never caught on in the same way as quarantine due to its expansiveness: it certainly has its public health meaning but can also refer to any manner of segregation, separation, or even solitude. Furthermore, this enfolding of isolation into quarantine points to the rhetorical significance quarantine possesses that isolation does not. Quarantine raises specters of plagues, leper colonies, yellow warning flags nailed to the doors of the infected, and deadly epidemics. Quarantine is emotionally charged, capable of conjuring fear and panic. Upon every usage, quarantine arrives in public discourse with centuries of symbolic baggage, none of it good. In other words, when someone speaks of quarantine, a well-worn rhetorical path precedes them, which means the work of persuasion or shifting public discourse has already begun upon utterance. It is not merely a technical term but also a public term that despite its vast usages across time and place, is sedimented as an alienizing logic in its relation to negativity, foreignness, and preventing movement.

QUARANTINE AND FOREIGN THREATS

Quarantine has an expansive history within the United States. Rhetorics of quarantine as connected to movement and migration emerge at key moments in history within US public discourse. Dealing with epidemic disease was always a matter of concern, specifically at ports of entry and in densely populated areas, what many public health officials regarded as the external and internal classes of concern.[22] Prior to twentieth-century developments in the understanding of how disease spreads, numerous outbreaks of disease occurred, often with disastrous results. Some regions and cities enacted quarantine laws and regulations in colonial times and others in the early days of the republic. For example, after an outbreak of yellow fever in 1699, Philadelphia passed a quarantine law in 1700.[23] Charleston, South Carolina, enacted its first quarantine law in 1698 and began to build the quarantine station on Sullivan's Island in 1707.[24] The state of Virginia enacted quarantine regulations for arriving vessels as early as 1722, revising those regulations throughout the eighteenth century.[25] New York approved its first quarantine law in 1758.[26] The Maryland legislature approved a law in 1793 to appoint a health officer at the Baltimore port in order to assess all foreign and "suspected" vessels and issue a quarantine if necessary.[27]

The Maryland law undoubtedly was in response to one of the most devastating instances of disease outbreak in Philadelphia, then the US capital, in 1793. During the summer and fall of that year, roughly one-tenth of the population perished as a result of yellow fever.[28] The outbreak allegedly began as French fleeing the rebellion in Saint-Domingue (Haiti) arrived in the city. But, at the time, there was much speculation about its origins. In a letter to Thomas Jefferson, who lived in Philadelphia at the time when he was secretary of state, Jefferson's eventual secretary Henry Remsen offered his assessment: "Some think it was engendered in Philadelphia, but others, more justly perhaps, suppose it to have been imported; and this latter idea is confirmed by the circumstance of the arrival there of a vessel from Barbadoes [*sic*], while the disorder was unknown, the Captain of which and three of the crew died on the passage, and the greater part of the rest soon after they had gone into lodgings in water street. It is also now ascertained, that some months ago a very mortal fever prevailed in some of the English islands."[29] As Remsen notes, the fever likely did not originate in Philadelphia; it was likely a foreign epidemic.

Although we now know that yellow fever is spread by mosquitoes and not by air, at the time, two competing theories existed: that it was contagious by air or physical contact or that it spread due to environmental factors.[30] Persuaded at least in part by the first theory, the mayor ordered "that arriving passengers and goods be kept isolated for two to three weeks."[31] Lessons from Philadelphia were numerous, including becoming the basis for implementing quarantine stations at ports and sowing the seeds for a sanitation movement. In 1795, Philadelphia created its own board of health in order to enact sanitation and quarantine rules. The ensuing problems with enforcement across state lines set the stage for federal quarantine policies to be implemented.[32]

Throughout the eighteenth century, quarantine continued to be managed by state and local officials, even as members of the new US Congress debated whether to nationalize quarantine in the 1795–96 session. Debates about quarantine largely centered on the tensions between a state's or town's police power to regulate the entrance of goods and people who might have communicable disease and the impacts of those regulations on commerce. This debate around commerce emerged in early congressional discussions of whether to nationalize quarantine laws given that the US Constitution grants Congress the right to regulate commerce.[33] In 1796, Representative Samuel Smith of Maryland proposed "that the President of the United States be authorized to direct such quarantine to be performed on all vessels from foreign countries arriving at the ports of the United States as he shall judge necessary."[34] Others lamented that given the lag in communication time to report an outbreak, state and local officials were far better suited to manage disease at ports of entry. Eventually, the new Congress decided to keep the power of quarantine at state and local levels, with appropriate federal support.

Still, as health officials insisted on the importance of quarantine for the sake of the public health, and such orders were generally regarded prudent when issued to protect the healthy in cities and towns, quarantine continued to receive the ire of those who maintained that such regulation killed commerce at ports. Reports about quarantines regularly showed up in newspapers in port cities, and the kinds of reports varied from mundane lists of vessels detained and the numbers of ill or deceased on board to quarantine violations. Often those violations came from disgruntled ship crews. For example, in 1868, the *New York Times* reported on schooner *William Allen* of Sagua La Grande in Cuba, which a quarantine officer found to have yellow fever on board. The mate refused to go into quarantine and instead sent the body of the deceased captain floating to the shore and took to sea once again.[35] The vessel was later stopped in Philadelphia. The ire was not helped by quarantine officials who were the subject of corruption accusations, including a significant investigation in New York, as vessel crews complained of drunken officers who took elaborate bribes in order to more quickly move ships from quarantine.[36]

The efficacy of quarantine was hotly debated, prompting health officials in major port cities to assemble an American Congress for Sanitary Reform, later renamed as the Quarantine and Sanitary Convention and then the National Quarantine and Sanitary Convention, which first met in Philadelphia in 1857 and was convened by that city's board of health director, Wilson Jewell.[37] This convention was one of the precursors to the American Public Health Association and only met four times, ending at the start of the Civil War.[38] The name reflected the tension between a need for quarantine at ports for external threats and sanitation for internal ones. At the third convention, a debate emerged from a question posed in the Report on Quarantine created by the previous convention's quarantine committee and presented to the convention: "Have quarantines secured the object for which they were originally intended? If not, the reasons for failure."[39] Participants considered many sides of the question with yellow fever serving as the primary case under consideration, along with some discussion of typhus fever, cholera, and smallpox. Yellow fever raised the alarm for many participants, even causing some to abandon quarantines altogether because it was becoming clear the virus was not spread communicably. In fact, during this debate, one physician urged the convention to recognize this fact via resolution, which it did, decades before the mosquito theory was first scientifically introduced in Cuba and proven in the United States.[40]

During this debate, there was little specific focus on migrants, who other than ship crew were the ones arriving on some of the vessels in question. Because they would be staying, many quarantine regulations applied only to them so that the sick could be managed and treated.[41] As the convention went on, participants considered a next key question before them: "What reforms are required to make quarantines more efficient and less burthensome?"[42] The committee report laid out the initial answer to the question:

> While no impediment should be placed to the entrance of those sick with Typhoid and Yellow Fever into such of the public hospitals as are willing to receive them, effectual measures should be insisted upon being adopted to prevent, as far as possible, poor, squalid immigrants, of improvident and uncleanly habits, whether sick or well, from crowding together in small, unwholesome dwellings, and in unhealthy, over-populated localities. From a neglect of this precaution, it is evident that the provisions of the best devised and most rigorously executed code of quarantine regulations, as a means of preventing the introduction of disease from without, will be effectually counteracted.[43]

This is the only other mention of migrants in the over seven hundred pages of the proceedings and so cannot be said to characterize any particular viewpoint or strong position on migrants, disease, and quarantine. Yet that does not mean that quarantine did not operate by alienizing logic at this time. Throughout the proceedings, the most targeted group in need of sanitary attention was the poor. This quotation begins to connect the linkages between migrants and disease within quarantine discourse, commenting on their status as poor and their hygiene as "uncleanly." And, of course, during this time period, many of the poor who would move into crowded, "unwholesome dwellings" would be migrants. Thus, even as migrants were not of primary concern and members worked to keep a clear distinction between quarantine and sanitation, this comment foreshadows how quarantine (and sanitary powers) came to be applied through alienizing logic—whether to migrants or alien citizens.

Innumerable applications of quarantine and epidemic outbreaks occurred in the nineteenth century, and a complex set of twists and turns led to the creation of the first national quarantine law and the department known in the twenty-first century as the US Public Health Service (PHS). Some key moments in the nineteenth century are worth unpacking in order to evidence the ways that the practice of quarantine emerges from an alienizing logic, even when not applied at ports and borders. In 1878, the US Congress passed a national quarantine law for the first time, which was meant to put powers to create regulations for quarantining vessels into the hands of the Marine Hospital Service (MHS).[44] So as not to interfere with state and municipal quarantine systems, the new law authorized local officers as national authorities.[45] Congress gave the MHS no appropriations for its new task, which proved deadly within just a few months as a yellow fever outbreak originating in Cuba arrived in the southern United States, infecting more than 120,000 people and killing 20,000.[46] Fears about yellow fever and other urban and migrant diseases finally prompted Congress in 1879 to create the short-lived National Board of Health tasked with gathering all relevant information on issues impacting public health, advising government departments, and creating a plan for a nationwide organization to present to Congress.[47] Additionally, Congress gave the board quarantine power both in the interior and at ports of entry. For a variety of reasons, the board "was an impossible administrative machine," and funding for it was not renewed in 1883, returning quarantine powers to the MHS.[48] By the turn of the century, the MHS became the Public Health and Marine Hospital Service, and in 1912, it was shortened to the Public Health Service, which to this day manages, promotes, and protects public health nationwide.

Epidemic outbreaks continued on the East Coast, as did migration, particularly of so-called new immigrants from places like southern and eastern Europe. Fears of Asian migration, particularly Chinese laborers, also animated discussions of quarantine on the West Coast.[49] Concerns about the health conditions of Mexicans and others who might try to subvert US laws by crossing the southern border prompted the development of quarantine stations in the Texas-Mexico borderlands.[50] In 1875, Congress passed the Page Act, which denied the entrance of Chinese women on the fear that they were prostitutes.[51] In 1882, Congress passed two pieces of relevant legislation: the Immigration Act, which excluded any person "liable to become a public charge," and the Chinese Exclusion Act, which virtually halted migration of Chinese laborers for nearly six decades, although Chinese still arrived in relatively small numbers at the US port in San Francisco. Concerns about the health of Chinese migrants from all classes concerned the San Francisco Board of Health, which in 1880 ordered that all arriving Chinese passengers be held until they could be vaccinated for smallpox. Given that San Francisco was the port of entry for so many Asian migrants, the local board demanded of the national board, "The special character of this immigration, chiefly Chinese coolies, having no regard to sanitary laws, and bringing with them diseases of a most contagious character, render it absolutely necessary that this port should possess a quarantine station commensurate with the important position it occupies in guarding against the introduction of such diseases as small-pox and Asiatic cholera into the United States."[52] Such public health professional views about Chinese culture and cleanliness pervaded the sentiment of the time and animated the more virulent xenophobic beliefs and laws that led to rampant anti-Chinese oppression.

The Chinese were perhaps the most vilified group, but a broader anti-migrant sentiment began to characterize much Gilded Age rhetoric, including as it related to quarantine laws and regulations. Technically under federal purview according to Section I of the US Constitution, immigration controls until the mid-nineteenth century were often exercised at state levels. Several cases challenged state jurisdiction, and in 1884, the Supreme Court upheld federal regulation of immigration. From then on, immigration laws were almost entirely understood as federal matters.[53] President Benjamin Harrison, a one-term president elected in 1888, would have incredible powers to bridge the issues of immigration and quarantine. An immigration restrictionist, Harrison expressed his views in his acceptance speech for the Republican nomination in September 1888:

> While our doors will continue open to proper immigration, we do not need to issue special invitations to the inhabitants of other countries to come to our shores or to share our citizenship. Indeed, the necessity of some inspection and limitation is obvious. We should resolutely refuse to permit foreign governments to send their paupers and criminals to our ports. We are also clearly under a duty to defend our civilization by excluding alien races whose ultimate assimilation with our people is neither possible nor desirable. The family has been the nucleus of our best immigration, and the home the most assimilating force in our civilization.[54]

Harrison reflected a widespread belief at the time that the era of mass immigration needed to end as the demographics and character of the young United States changed. Harrison's juxtaposition of "proper" immigration connected to family and assimilation with that of "paupers and criminals" referred centrally to Chinese, but he had concern about other groups, too, who did not necessarily fit into that dichotomy.

In March, Harrison signed the 1891 Immigration Act, which centralized immigration controls under the office of the president and focused on groups other than the Chinese, thus expanding restrictions on immigration. The act enhanced processes of enforcement and inspection and expanded the list of those excludable and deportable. The federal government decided that all immigrants would undergo a health inspection by MHS officials before departure in their countries of origin and upon arrival to the United States.[55] Congress added this inspection because with the new law, the United States now excluded "persons suffering from a loathsome or a dangerous contagious disease."[56] Although on average only 1 percent of those attempting to enter were excluded for health-based reasons from 1890 to 1924, increasingly health was the reason why people were excluded over and against other reasons such as moral ones. Health accounted for 2 percent of exclusions in 1898 and 69 percent by 1916.[57]

Soon it became clear who those non-Chinese targets would be. In his 1891 third annual address to Congress, Harrison noted that Jews were not "beggars," but the large number fleeing Russia, rejected by most other countries due to anti-Semitism, and arriving in the United States was "neither good for them nor for us."[58] The next year, 1892, marked some profound convergences between anxieties about immigration and demands for quarantine.[59] The concerns about migrants of all kinds, but especially the allegedly unassimilable to the cultures of those descending from West Europe, were many. As outbreaks of diseases happened throughout the United States and in points of origin for would-be migrants, public health concerns continued to animate anxieties about unrestricted immigration.[60] In January 1892, Ellis Island opened as an immigration inspection station and quarantine center, and a significant number of European migrants would be processed there for the next several decades.

In May 1892, Harrison signed the Geary Act into law, which extended the Chinese Exclusion Act into the foreseeable future. Later that year, reports emerged about a cholera outbreak in Russia, followed by reports that Jews fled for the United States en masse. Media around the country sounded the alarm about the pending arrival of cholera-ridden Russian Jewish migrants, most coming through Hamburg, Germany. One report cited short dispatches from cities abroad, beginning with Hamburg, recording the number of deaths and new infections in each city.[61] Media often utilized elaborate war metaphors to describe the threat: "In view of the rapid western march of the dread Asiatic cholera," began one story.[62] One headline read, "Cholera's Onward March: Incapacity and Filth in Russia Help Its

Progress."[63] Stories pervaded the news, fueling nativist and anti-migrant sentiment. A *New York Times* editorial titled "Dangerous Immigration" insisted, "Bearing in mind the quality of a majority of the immigrants who have been coming to America from Eastern Europe by way of Hamburg, the infectious diseases they have brought heretofore, and the wide prevalence today of Asiatic cholera in the region from which many of them come, we may say that this country would be much better off if the stream could be stopped for the next twelve months or for a longer time."[64] The *Times* called for a quarantine of the entire country's borders.

As the end of August neared and the ships carrying the potentially sick migrants were about to dock, anxieties reached a fevered pitch. The *New York Times* and other major publications anxiously and increasingly angrily reported about the threat of migrants and cholera. A front-page story in the *New York Times*, which summarized cholera dispatches from around the world, wrote, "With the danger from cholera out of the question, it is plain that the United States would be better off if ignorant Russian Jews and Hungarians were denied a refuge here. What can be expected in the line of citizenship from men and women who cannot even read or write the language of their native country?"[65] Because epidemics and contagious disease had so regularly been attached to the poor, the claim expresses alienizing logic, resonating with existing beliefs about migrants and disease. Moreover, the *Times* conjured not only the possibility of denying these people refuge but also the impossibility of their ability to achieve at the level expected of a US American citizen. The author(s) also expressed a distrust in officials' ability to prevent an outbreak in the United States. The piece went on: "With the cholera killing people by the wholesale in the ports whence these creatures assemble to take passage to the United States, there is good ground for the present demand for absolute prohibition. These people are offensive enough at best; under the present circumstances they are a positive menace to the health of the country. Even should they pass the quarantine officials, their mode of life when they settle down makes them always a source of danger. Cholera, it must be remembered, originates in the homes of this human riffraff."[66] The *Times* initial concern is logical enough—if everyone is dying, then why take the risk? However, the virulent anti-migrant rhetoric takes hold as the piece continues, culminating in the charge that migrants are riffraff—not just disreputable, but human trash. Although in this time period, public health officials parse out the differences between disease spread by germs and contagion and that which is spread by improper sanitation, the *Times* collapses the distinction on the backs of the migrants: they are both—dangerous for the environments they create and dangerous for the contagions they carry. Put simply, migrants are inherently dangerous.

In a more measured editorial on September 1, 1892, *Times* staff called on President Harrison to convene Congress in special session to halt immigration altogether until the threat of cholera passed. The editorial asked, "Is it worth while [*sic*] to measure the inconvenience and distress of immigrant families against the awful consequences of a visitation of cholera? Is it worth while to consider the loss of a few thousands in foreign trade in the face of a peril that threatens to destroy pretty much all domestic trade?" Although the *Times* does not draw upon the same nativist and xenophobic discourses as its report from just a couple of days earlier, to the regular reader or the reader only familiar with the national mood, such claims do not need to be stated. Moreover, while the piece acknowledged the economic drawbacks, it becomes clear that quarantine is foremost a matter of immigration, and it is the would-be migrants, not goods and crews, that need to be the primary focus in rendering a decision not about quarantining migrants but about quarantining the country. The piece concluded, "It is our judgment that no less rigorous measure will suffice to keep out the cholera this year and next year."[67]

Amid this fervor, the pressure finally compelled President Harrison to issue a circular on September 1. Harrison did not close the US borders to immigration. Co-written by Surgeon General Walter Wyman and Treasury Secretary Charles Foster, the proclamation declared:

> It having been officially announced that cholera is epidemic in Germany, Russia, France, and at certain points in Great Britain as well as in Asia, and it having been made to appear that immigrants in large numbers are coming into this country from the infected districts aforesaid, and that they and their personal effects are liable to introduce cholera into the United States and that vessels occupying them are thereby a direct menace to the public health, and it having been further shown that under the laws of the several states quarantine detentions may be imposed upon those vessels a sufficient length of time to insure against the introduction of contagious diseases, it is hereby ordered that no vessel from any foreign port carrying immigrants shall be admitted to enter at any port of the United States until such vessel shall have undergone a quarantine detention of twenty days.[68]

Steamship operators held various opinions about the effects of this proclamation on stopping cholera. Some thought it would have no real effect at all. All lamented the loss of revenue from holding goods that happened to be on ships with migrants and from no longer being able to transport steerage passengers—the class where most disease was assumed to strike.[69] They also agreed to comply with the quarantine.

By September 29, the New York City Health Department cautiously declared the city free from cholera, although it would take some time to say for sure.[70] In the end, only 120 people in New York died during this scare, a low number considering the intensity of the rhetorical crisis. However, the effects on Jewish migrants were long-lasting, and Harrison's proclamation became the basis for the 1893 National Quarantine Act, which gave interstate quarantine powers to the federal government's office of the Treasury.[71] The placement of powers in the Treasury signals the overwhelming influence of business interests in both creating and implementing a response to contain contagious disease.[72] Although intending to once again codify a national-level response that would not negatively impact commerce, the new law continued to emphasize the need to manage migrants arriving at US ports and land borders.

Interior quarantine laws and practices continued to be refined during the turn of the century, and unsurprisingly because of alienizing logic, migrants, US citizens of color, and the poor bore the brunt. In 1894, Louisiana State Home for Lepers, now known as the Gillis W. Long Hansen's Disease Center, and colloquially just called "Carville," opened in Carville, Louisiana. The Carville hospital remained open until 1999, and its residents were legally quarantined there until the 1960s, although it continued to accept patients into the 1980s. Undoubtedly, as Susan Sontag reminds, leprosy, now known as Hansen's disease and named for the Norwegian scientist who discovered the microorganism that caused it, has been one of the most meaning-laden diseases in world history, carrying an array of moralistic stigmas.[73] Although its US origins are not known, Marcia Gaudet contends it likely came from European explorers first and by enslaved West Africans later.[74]

Fears about leprosy were long wrapped up with anti-migrant sentiment and nativism, meaning once again disease was an opportunity to enact alienizing logic. In a report on an "anti-coolie" meeting in San Francisco in 1861, one of many led by white labor organizers, most notably Denis Kearney,[75] a guest named Alfred Buetell claimed that both cholera and leprosy came from China, using this as a rationale for "peaceably if we can; forcibly if we must" not only preventing further Chinese immigration but eliminating those in the United States.[76] A commentary in 1873 in the *Idaho Signal* warned that the Chinese introduced leprosy to Hawaii and that this should be a lesson for how to treat Chinese migrants recently arrived into San Francisco. The author cautioned, "We know not how many afflicted ones may have arrived in our midst last Thursday, but we do know of two Chinese lepers who have resided in the Chinese portion of the town for many months past. Their fingers and toes are rotting off them by piece-meal."[77] Such visceral language likely incited fear among readers. This fear was exacerbated by this author's claims that leprosy was of "syphilitic origin" and transferred through sexual intercourse. Even reports that were not overtly inflammatory connected leprosy with Chinese migrants. One from the *New York Sun* that considered whether leprosy was contagious began with the question of Chinese immigration: "If it have a contagious character, Chinese immigration to the United States might be attended with a physical danger even more grave than its alleged moral or political evils."[78] Even as the article claimed that it appears the disease was non-contagious in China, the framing fed fears about Chinese immigration and the deep origins of the disease in that country. The general agreement among the scientific community by the 1880s that leprosy was not contagious did little to quell fears about the disease or about immigration.[79] The disease retained a strong connection to immigration, including at Carville. Julia Rivera Elwood notes that in the 1950s, roughly 40 percent of the residents of Carville were foreign born, with the majority being Mexicans.[80] Gaudet writes that many housed there in the 1980s were migrants without health insurance.[81]

Migrants continued to be the focus of border and interior quarantine practices as the twentieth century began. In mid-1899, reports came in that a vessel heading for San Francisco was quarantined in Honolulu because bubonic plague had been found on board, killing at least two Chinese.[82] By late that year, national papers reported on an outbreak of the bubonic plague in China's Manchuria region, killing hundreds per week.[83] And by early January 1900, there were reports of plague in Honolulu, which led public health officials to cordon off and guard the Japanese and Chinese parts of town in a "shotgun quarantine."[84] As the plague spread throughout the Hawaiian Islands, officials in San Francisco worried about its movement there. In early March, more than fifty policemen guarded Chinatown after police and a doctor decided a man's death there was from the plague and called for an immediate quarantine.[85] The dead man's body was cremated, and the entire quarter was roped off. Food and mail were passed across the ropes.[86] Within days and despite the protests of the Chinese consul, doctors confirmed the man had died of the plague and called for volunteers to help disinfect Chinatown.[87] In May, at least six deaths from the plague were reported, and sanitation and quarantine efforts began anew.[88] Shortly thereafter, federal officials took over and mandated that all Chinese be inoculated. Chinese resisted, with some believing the vaccination was actually designed by whites to annihilate Chinese.[89]

Meanwhile, the state of Texas issued a quarantine on travel from the entire state of California. While California public health officials and police lodged intense quarantine and sanitation efforts against Chinese, Secretary of the Board of Health W. P. Matthews issued a statement on May 22: "At this time there is no case of bubonic plague in California. In view of the facts our board consider your quarantine against us unwarranted and unjust, and, therefore, ask you to remove it or so modify it as to apply only to Chinese."[90] Even as Matthews appealed to other states based on the lack of the disease anywhere in California, he supported a quarantine on Chinese, despite no plague among Chinese either. Although a court sided with Chinese that the quarantine was illegal, much damage was already done.[91] As Nayan Shah details, the struggle over containing the plague and confronting Chinese demands for rights along with their efforts to police one another against the white establishment continued for many months.

Even as modern medicine was increasingly better at managing disease, the rise in eugenicist thinking, particularly as applied to concerns about the vibrancy of American stock and the status of US American labor, continued to animate alienizing logic in the form of quarantine rhetoric. Terence V. Powderly, the US commissioner general of immigration and previously longtime head of the Knights of Labor, explained in 1902 that while religious or political concerns were often the reasons why people opposed new migrants in a previous era, health should be of utmost concern now.[92] Powderly and the Knights of Labor were notoriously opposed to migrants, particularly Chinese migrants (as suggested above in the example of Kearney), with Powderly often couching his anti-migrant sentiment in health metaphors.[93] In 1888, he wrote, "Immigration is to the United States what certain kinds of food are to the human system. When its tide flows in regularly; is made up of enlightened, well disposed people; when too many are not landed at once on our shores, it cannot but prove beneficial and healthy."[94] Although he ostensibly cared in earnest about the health of the US American national body, his concerns also stemmed from the type of migrant arriving in the United States after 1860. He put it plainly, "The population which came previous to 1860 was civilized, that which comes to-day [sic] is, in great proportion, semi-barbarous."[95] Powderly noted that these migrants are filthy in their hygiene, and they not only take American jobs because they accept low wages, but they also never learn English, and the only money they put in the economy is for alcohol.

As commissioner general, Powderly's claims about the importance of health-based migrant exclusions took a more measured tone than his earlier writing. Powderly explained:

> If we remain indifferent simply because these diseases [favus and trachoma] do not prove fatal to life, we evade our duty; for the health of the nation is imperilled [sic] while one man is diseased. The old cry, "America is the asylum of the oppressed of the world," is too threadbare to withstand the assaults of disease. There is a danger that the oppressed may through the burdens they fasten on others, become oppressors. At any rate, there exists no reason why the United States should become the hospital of the nations of earth, even though it does afford an asylum for those who come here to escape oppression.[96]

Powderly inserts himself into contemporary debates of the time about the role that the United States, ostensibly a nation of migrants, should play given the range of places from which new migrants arrive. His prescient commentary signals what would, in two decades, become very restrictive immigration policies based on quotas that privileged northern and western Europeans, essentially barred all from Asian countries, and policed the US-Mexico divide. But here he premises his claims within a kind of common sense about health, shifting the burden of protection from the US American citizen to the would-be migrant.

Ten years after Powderly's writing, eugenicist thinking was in full force among those in the PHS and including those tasked with migrant inspection and quarantine.[97] In an assessment of 1911 statistics on immigration inspection at Ellis Island, Alfred C. Reed, an assistant surgeon for the PHS, touted the predominant medical perspective of the day: "It may be said that the best class is drawn from northern and western Europe, and the poorest from the Mediterranean countries and western Asia."[98] A year later, Reed argued that physically and mentally unhealthy migrants had immediate effects in terms of with whom they came in contact and long-term effects in terms of the fitness of their descendants to belong to the general public.[99] In further explaining the effects, Reed distinguished venereal disease from other dangerous and loathsome diseases, noting both the difficulty of detecting it but the utmost importance of doing so. Although he spent more time in this essay detailing the problems with other diseases, his start with venereal disease as distinct from others foreshadowed the concern with sexually transmitted disease that would, from then on, be central to quarantine, including migration exclusions.[100] Influenced by the renowned eugenicist H. H. Goddard, Reed also expressed concern about mental health, and in fact, mental health standards that Goddard developed became central to the medical inspection process at Ellis Island. Such eugenic reasoning had much to do with the quotas and restrictions passed in the 1917, 1921, and 1924 immigration acts. These points of view absolutely shaped racial groupings in the early twentieth century. For example, as Natalia Molina writes about public health practice in Los Angeles, "Rather than addressing the structural inequality that produced the unhealthy environments that hosted virulent diseases, public health departments consistently identified the root problem as racialized people who were in need of reform. By shaping racial categories and infusing them with meaning, health officials helped define racialized people's place in society."[101] Such racialized meaning-making had implications far beyond health.

Events on the US-Mexico border in 1916 to 1917 offer another illustrative example of the powerful link between disease, quarantine, and racialized migration. In March 1916, the PHS in Laredo, Texas, began marking the arms of Mexican laborers entering the United States with "admitted" in permanent ink upon passing a medical exam.[102] The tattoo provoked outrage among Mexicans but signaled the expansive, twenty-year-long quarantine program that would face Mexican laborers just a year later over fears of a typhus outbreak. Although Mexican migration had gone relatively unregulated for decades, with increased Mexican settlement in the United States, border quarantines became more common. Racialized rhetoric bolstered the justification of such quarantines. National commentator Frederic J. Haskin wrote in July 1916, "The occasional forays of Pancho Villa across the Rio Grande are not the most dangerous Mexican border raids, nor the hardest against which to defend the country. The worst menace is contained in the continuous stream of Mexican refugees who pour across the international bridge, laden with germs of smallpox and typhus."[103] Haskin drew on extensive discourses that framed Mexicans as dirty and full of germs. Eventually, health officials supported by police organizations held

Mexican laborers in quarantine facilities where officials stripped them of their clothing and baggage, which were fumigated while they too were deloused with kerosene, gasoline, and/or vinegar and inspected for lice and other signs of disease. Mexican women organized rebellions against their treatment, throwing bottles and stones at soldiers.[104] Their actions did not change the quarantine protocol, and delousing Mexicans happened well into the mid-twentieth century, including with those admitted through the Bracero program.[105]

After World War II, overt eugenicist thinking fell out of fashion in the medical establishment. As technology and diagnostics improved throughout the twentieth century, health concerns continued to preoccupy immigration officials though the landscape changed. Angel and Ellis Islands both closed by 1954 as the primary mode of travel changed from sea to air. This meant that while antibiotics and vaccines could now treat or prevent several diseases, due to the quicker travel times, illness did not have time to manifest during the course of migration. Several countries built clinics and hospitals and improved nutrition and sanitation standards, which also lessened the likelihood that migrants might arrive with communicable diseases.[106]

Yet, as Howard Markel and Alexandra Minna Stern explain, during the debates that led to the 1952 McCarran-Walter Act, the language of disease as a basis to exclude "undesirable immigrants" persisted even as it applied more broadly to physical or mental health, criminal or immoral behavior, poverty, addiction, and/or communism.[107] For example, Senator Pat McCarran (D-Nevada), a man with known racist views and the namesake of the 1952 law, offered a health-based rationale for his far-reaching legislation. The 1952 act codified numerous exclusions, including several based on health, and created an exclusion based on having a "dangerous contagious disease." McCarran rationalized his controversial legislation: "Today, Mr. President, as never before, a sound immigration and naturalization system is essential to the preservation of our way of life, because that system is the conduit through which a stream of humanity flows into the fabric of our society. If that stream is healthy, the impact on our society is salutary; but if that stream is polluted, our institutions and our way of life become infected."[108] As Markel and Stern contend, even though immigration policy in this era is generally concerned with Communist and other ideological exclusions, McCarran's rhetoric makes plain that matters of health, even if now more metaphorical and not overtly tied to concerns over "better breeding," remained central. Although migrants arriving at US borders were generally more healthy in the mid- to late twentieth century than they had ever been, and visitors or US American travelers were just as likely to spread disease into the US national body as were migrants, the link between "alien" and disease never waned in the imaginary or in immigration policy.

For our purposes, it is simply important to show that quarantine's constant connection with migrant communities and immigration discourses throughout the course of early US American history into the twentieth century reflect most starkly how quarantine is a manifestation of US alienizing logic. Furthermore, these discourses help to inform how and why quarantine emerges again in relation to HIV/AIDS in the 1980s.

QUARANTINE AND SEX WORK

A last point that is important to consider in this rhetorical history is a key shift in the target and meaning of quarantine. Certainly, diseases like the bubonic plague and leprosy held moralistic stigmas, and at least in the case of leprosy, there were suggestions that it had connections with sex. However, in the United States before World War I and when Pancho Villa and his troops crossed into United States territory at New Mexico in 1916, the problem of venereal disease and its impact on US soldier readiness became of paramount concern. Philippa Levine explains that during this time period in Britain, "VD was not seen only as affecting individuals, but as something that would weaken the 'race.' Health thus became a moral and a national problem."[109] Sexual problems were always at their core racial problems too. The same was true in the United States. As World War I approached, fears about whether soldiers would be "fighting fit" proliferated. In 1916, officials decided to develop "moral zones" around military camps that would limit access to alcohol and prostitutes. These efforts to mitigate soldiers' bad behavior had limited success and so "quarantine, detention, and internment became the new themes of the attack on prostitution."[110] Such concerns make sense in the context of the Progressive era concern over sexual health and the family, in which syphilis, and syphilitic prostitutes in particular, were seen to be an utmost threat.[111]

In July 1918, the federal government passed the Chamberlain-Kahn Act, also known as the Public Health and Research Act, which gave the federal government the power to quarantine women suspected of having venereal disease.[112] Wendy Parmet notes that right away, "health officials began to use quarantine powers against prostitutes on the presumption that they had venereal disease. This use of quarantine marked a departure from its prior use. Until then, quarantine had been used primarily against infectious diseases to which the entire community felt vulnerable." Parmet further explains that this treatment of prostitutes attached "a great stigma" to being quarantined, also making it "a complement to police work, a way of holding prostitutes longer than many criminal sentences would allow."[113] This so-called American Plan "became one of the largest and longest-lasting mass quarantines in American history," extending in some cases into the 1970s.[114] Unsurprisingly, as Scott W. Stern maintains, "nonwhite, working-class, and immigrant women were disproportionately harmed by the Plan at every stage, from arrest and examination to incarceration, sterilization, and punishment."[115] The creation and implementation of the American Plan suggests how deeply imbricated racialized gender and sexuality are with projects of war and imperialism.[116]

Although the program never fully came to fruition, President Wilson allocated $250,000 for prostitute "detention homes," and Congress provided $1 million. Such concerns though were widespread and long-lasting. For instance, in October 1918, the Texas Social Hygiene Association issued a statement that provided "an authoritative interpretation of the State quarantine law."[117] The statement went on: "Prostitution is hereby declared to be a prolific source of syphilis, gonorrhea, and chancroid, and the repression of prostitution is declared to be a public health measure. All local and state health officers are, therefore, directed to co-operate with proper officers whose duty it is to enforce laws directed against prostitution, and otherwise use every proper means for the repression of prostitution." One direct implication of this call, like the federal law, was to quarantine anyone who had or was suspected of having a venereal disease and for the sake of the public health needed to be isolated. The statement concluded that "infection with venereal disease is not in itself a felony. The crime lies in illicit relations on the one hand, or knowingly contributing disease to others on the other." The statement made it clear that this policy was not intended to make a moral claim but only a health one. Yet the connections between prostitution and immorality ensured that the American Plan always had a moral thrust and spread across dozens of states for decades.[118] Only with the advent of penicillin in the 1940s did the plan, and mass quarantine of prostitutes and other promiscuous women, subside considerably.[119]

CONCLUSION

When what is presently called the Centers for Disease Control and Prevention (CDC) took over quarantine responsibilities in the 1960s, even as quarantine stations existed at every port, threats that once preoccupied public health officials, politicians, and the media no longer seemed all that threatening. And by the 1970s, the number of quarantine stations dropped to the single digits. Even though state and federal governments still had quarantine powers on the books, these were largely seen as relics of the past.

My intention in this chapter has been to map the rhetoric of quarantine in the United States, emphasizing how it has historically been enacted as an alienizing logic and who its targets have been. Even though infectious disease was a different concern by the 1980s, questions about mobility, borders, and sexual promiscuity become salient again with the advent of the AIDS crisis, for as Peter Baldwin writes, "Path dependence has structured public health. . . . Decisions taken in the early nineteenth century to control cholera and syphilis continue to influence the response to AIDS."[120]

CHAPTER 2

AIDS AND THE RHETORIC OF QUARANTINE

PROGRESSIVE ORGANIZATIONS AND MEDIA SOUNDED AN ALARM in March 2013 over Kansas House Bill 2183, originally proposed to protect first responders who might be at risk for contracting HIV at work. As *Think Progress* put it, "But the Kansas Department of Health and Environment rewrote the language in the bill, broadly deregulating when isolation can take place and opening up the possibility that HIV positive people could be quarantined."[1] Quickly, the Kansas Department of Health and Environment issued a press release assuring the public that this was a misreading and that "contrary to recent media coverage, no version of Kansas Substitute House Bill 2183 would have ever allowed for isolation of persons infected with or quarantine of persons exposed to human immunodeficiency virus (HIV)." The state epidemiologist Charles Hunt said, "The law requires isolation and quarantine be based on what is reasonable and medically necessary, and neither of those thresholds are met with respect to HIV."[2] Despite Hunt's clear and confident assurance that HIV could never meet the thresholds required to quarantine an individual or a group of people, it should come as no surprise that AIDS advocates and other progressives demanded attention for this bill. This trauma runs deep. Thirty years earlier, politicians, public health officials, physicians, and legal scholars had no such clarity about whether people with AIDS or those at risk for contracting it should be placed into quarantine.

By December 1982, the Centers for Disease Control (CDC) had a strong sense that AIDS was "an infectious agent transmitted sexually or through exposure to blood or blood products" and not casual contact,[3] and it had confirmed by early 1983 that people had only become infected with AIDS by "intimate contact and blood transfusions."[4] Thus, from very early on, public health and medical professionals had the information before them that unlike air- or saliva-borne infections like tuberculosis, AIDS was not casually communicable. Nevertheless, the question of quarantine was prominent in debates about how to prevent the spread of AIDS throughout much of the 1980s. The loudest of these voices came from the far right, including figures such as Jerry Falwell of the Moral Majority, Orange County Republican congressman William Dannemeyer, and right-wing fringe figure Lyndon LaRouche. Yet serious considerations of quarantine filled the pages of dozens of law reviews and found their way to the editorial pages of major publications, the surveys of prominent pollsters, and the drafting tables of state public health officials and legislators. Some even suggested that the CDC quietly laid plans in preparation for a mass quarantine of people with AIDS.[5] How is it that an obviously ill-fitted approach garnered so much careful consideration? What was the nature of the rhetoric used in advocating for and resisting quarantine, and what resulted from its proliferation?

This chapter examines how alienizing logic manifested in the rhetoric of quarantine by exploring how calls for and fears of quarantining people with AIDS proliferated in US public discourse during the early years of the pandemic. I begin by situating the rhetoric of quarantine during the first years of HIV/AIDS in the United States by examining its presence in media, political, legal, religious, and gay rights discourses during the time. I explore how gay men's seemingly irrational fear about being treated like "lepers" became a proposal and fundraising mechanism for members of the religious right, a seriously debated policy among public health officials, and an issue on the ballot in the state of California. This chapter also details how even though no widespread quarantine of people living with HIV or AIDS ever came to be in the United States, a few high-profile and sensationalized cases of Black sex workers animated the creation or renewal of quarantine laws and set the stage for laws that criminalize HIV. Moreover, quarantine ultimately became national common sense in US immigration policy on HIV/AIDS, the subject of the subsequent chapter.

AIDS AS A FOREIGN, SEXUALIZED DISEASE

If, in human contexts, quarantines are employed to prevent the movement of people with infectious disease or who might be at risk of carrying an infectious agent, and the primary targets of quarantine practices in the

United States have been migrants and those engaged in supposedly deviant sexual practices, then AIDS created a perfect storm. First, AIDS in the United States was always imagined as foremost a foreign disease, spread by foreigners who engaged improperly with animals or who practiced improper sex. One only needs to think of gay Canadian flight attendant Gaëtan Dugas, the villain in Randy Shilts's *And the Band Played On*, popularly named "Patient Zero" for allegedly bringing AIDS to the United States.[6] In popular memory, the sexually promiscuous Dugas not only slept with hundreds—if not thousands—of men in every city he landed over the course of his life, but Shilts portrayed Dugas as actively spreading his disease once he knew he was ill. Only in 2016 did historical and scientific studies intervene in this record, noting that epidemiologists never named Dugas as "Patient Zero." Rather, a man later identified as Dugas was found to be near the center of a cluster of people in a sexual network who had AIDS. This man was named "Patient O," where "O" stood for "outside of California" because the man (Dugas) resided outside the state. Furthermore, genome analysis revealed that Dugas was not the origin of AIDS in the United States.[7]

Other origin myths also began outside of the United States, usually in Haiti or Central Africa. One myth questioned whether the African swine fever outbreak in Haiti during the late 1970s had somehow jumped to the human population, possibly by handling blood or eating infected meat, became AIDS, and then spread to the United States.[8] This theory perhaps explained why Haitians were uniquely vulnerable to AIDS and were one of the original groups the CDC designated as high risk. This belief about Haitian susceptibility to AIDS led to, as we see in later chapters, horrifically violent treatment of Haitians in Haiti and in the United States, including those fleeing political violence in Haiti to claim asylum in the United States. The most persistent origin story about AIDS begins in Central Africa and has been repeated in various forms.[9] The first of these emerged from Harvard scientist Max Essex, who in 1985 isolated in green monkeys of Central Africa a virus very similar to what would soon be called HIV. Essex and others theorized that also possibly by handling blood or eating infected meat, the virus jumped to the human population, eventually spreading around the globe.[10] Numerous versions of the African monkey theory have emerged over the decades with some African scientists, journalists, and politicians denouncing these theories as problematic and reflective of anti-Black racism that undoubtedly led to the mistreatment of Africans in places like the United States.[11] Thus, the supposed foreign origins of AIDS in the

United States positioned it as similar to so many of the quarantinable diseases from the past, with migrants serving as the sources and targets of stigma and blame.

AIDS was a deadly, incurable venereal disease, and in its earliest days, it was unclear how it spread. Even after experts had a clear sense that a virus was linked to AIDS and that virus was only transmitted through very limited means, the average US American was unclear about how the virus spread, with many believing it could be passed on through casual contact, kissing, or mosquito bites. Thus, if in the twentieth century it was not unusual to quarantine those who spread curable venereal diseases, it makes sense that proposals to quarantine people with AIDS would seem absolutely rational to many.

Because quarantines are a manifestation of alienizing logic, past quarantines in the United States most adversely affected communities imagined outside of the proper white citizenry, including sex workers and migrants. Although others might have been afflicted, and on occasion the reach extended further, the most well-known and documented quarantines in US history targeted these already dehumanized groups that lacked political, racial, and economic power. In the early years of AIDS, other than hemophiliacs who were always imagined as AIDS's innocent victims, the high-risk groups included precisely such stigmatized and dehumanized people: gay men, intravenous drug users, and Haitians.

Thus, even though HIV is not the kind of infection that could be prevented or controlled with mass quarantine, as a stigmatizing venereal disease affecting societal outlaws and supposedly originating elsewhere that increasingly presented a threat to the "general population," it is not surprising that some public health officials and politicians at least considered the possibility of quarantine. But before any politician or public health official mentioned quarantine as a response to growing concerns around AIDS, members of the gay community had already expressed their fears. In an August 1982 article titled "Return of the Pink Triangle?" in the gay northern California newspaper *Mom . . . Guess What?* the author noted that while experts were not completely clear on how AIDS was spread, the CDC was considering "the imposition of a quarantine on gay blood donors."[12] The author's use of "quarantine" in this sentence is not exactly right by conventional definitions, but in the sense that he feared gay men would be uniquely isolated from participating in a quintessential expression of good citizenship, the usage is not entirely improper.[13] Although federal health officials were quoted saying there were too many unknown factors to take such drastic measures, gay activists were concerned with the civil liberties and civil rights implications.

By mid-1983, the federal government first asked gay men and then required them to refrain from donating blood. Some in the gay community used the metaphor of the leper colony to describe this treatment.[14] Leper colonies have long been invoked as an analogy for all forms of medical quarantine and often function as an argument through analogy when a marginalized group decries its treatment by the majority. In addition to being an argumentative touchstone, the leper colony also functions as a lesson about the ethical risks of placing people in quarantine. As modern medicine eventually showed, Hansen's disease was not contagious through casual contact and most of those confined to leper colonies like Carville were migrants, poor, of color, or otherwise at the margins of a society that alienized them. Although health professionals in 1983 were still learning about how AIDS was transmitted, the hysteria that surrounded the disease, and the people identified as most likely to be afflicted, prompted panicked calls for quarantine that the gay community feared.

In July 1983, evangelical pastor, head of the Moral Majority, and influential friend of the Ronald Reagan administration Jerry Falwell issued a call for quarantine of all people with AIDS. According to news reports, Falwell "said federal agents may quarantine cattle in Texas to prevent an epidemic of brucellosis, but AIDS, 'the No. 2 cause of death among hemophiliacs, has not received the same radical and immediate treatment from governmental agencies or the Congress.'"[15] Falwell's argument by analogy is completely coherent within an established logic of quarantine that has targeted animals and those otherwise dehumanized: if cattle with a rare bacterial infection that can spread to humans but hardly ever kills them are quarantined, why would the government not act swiftly to isolate those with an incurable infection killing innocent hemophiliacs?[16] Daniel Villanueva, president of the conservative Christian American Family Association took the call for quarantine further. Villanueva circulated a petition to tens, if not hundreds, of thousands of people with the following demand: "Since AIDS is transmitted primarily by perverse homosexuals, your name on my national petition to QUARANTINE ALL HOMOSEXUAL ESTABLISH-MENTS is crucial to your family's health and security."[17] No doubt this petition echoes the rhetoric of fundraising letters and pamphlets sent out by far right evangelical leaders throughout the 1980s and was designed to be sensational. Still, this rhetoric reflected concerns that many US Americans held about their families' health and security in the era of AIDS.

Quarantine's entrance into AIDS discourse in the early 1980s was quite narrow: the already vilified gay community anticipated the way it would be treated and virulently anti-gay evangelical Christian leaders predictably called for extreme measures against gays and others living with AIDS.

Evangelical leaders had considerable influence in the 1980s, and they capitalized on widespread fears of the new disease. Unsurprisingly, calls for quarantine quickly became mainstream. As mentioned above, several dozen legal scholars debated the merits of quarantine for people with AIDS based on constitutional, ethical, and other factors from 1984 to the early 1990s. Between 1985 and 1987, more than a dozen publications and survey companies from the *Los Angeles Times* to Gallup polled ordinary US Americans about their beliefs surrounding AIDS and consistently asked the question about whether people with AIDS should be quarantined. Usually one-quarter to one-third of those surveyed wanted quarantine, but at some point, more than one-half thought quarantine was an appropriate response.[18] Between 1983 and 1989, institutions including jails and prisons, schools, and the US military initiated quarantine measures to isolate people with AIDS.[19] Although experts almost uniformly agreed it would not work outside of such institutions (and several questioned the value of quarantine within those institutions), quarantining people with AIDS was a mainstream idea. In the next two sections, I explore the rhetoric of quarantine in two sites: (1) among state and local public health officials who wanted to use the quarantine power in extreme circumstances for recalcitrant individuals, and (2) within political discourse, particularly in the state of California, where some politicians wanted broad punitive actions against those with AIDS, including possible widespread quarantine.

PUBLIC HEALTH DISCOURSE

The Reagan administration was generally split on how to deal with the growing AIDS crisis, reflecting deeper ideological divides among the administration's avowed conservatives. In fact, as Jennifer Brier contends, the AIDS crisis produced those fractures as officials battled over the best way to confront the pandemic.[20] Epidemics always create political dilemmas including "how to reconcile the individual's claim to autonomy and liberty with the community's concern with safety. How does the polity treat the patient who is both citizen and disease carrier? How are individual rights and the public good pursued simultaneously?"[21] Members of Reagan's cabinet like far-right Secretary of Education William Bennett believed in measures that largely ignored the rights of individuals with AIDS, advocating mandatory testing and reporting as primary ways of preventing the disease.

Surgeon General C. Everett Koop, a conservative and a Catholic, worked to strike a balance, firmly arguing that education was the best defense—and offense. This divide and Reagan's own indifference to AIDS led to a quiet administration for the first several years, particularly on Reagan's part. Nevertheless, Koop issued a national report on AIDS in 1986, which detailed a fairly progressive approach to AIDS (especially in the context of the Reagan administration). It provided matter-of-fact advice and included a clear statement about AIDS and quarantine at the very end of the report, suggesting the relevance of quarantine to discourse on AIDS. Koop wrote, "Quarantine has no role in the management of AIDS because AIDS is not spread by casual contact. The only time some form of quarantine might be indicated is in a situation where an individual carrying the AIDS virus knowingly and willingly continues to expose others through sexual contact or sharing drug equipment. Such circumstances should be managed on a case-by-case basis by local authorities."[22] That he included it in his report indicates the far-reaching nature of quarantine discourse and that Koop felt he had to address it. Because of his role as the nation's physician, he lent significant credence to positions against quarantine. In general, Koop's viewpoint reflected that of most public health officials who considered quarantine. A large-scale study of the National Academy of Sciences noted that while politicians and pundits discussed quarantine proposals, the most efficacious approach was "the least-restrictive measures commensurate with the goal of controlling the spread of infection."[23] Thus, most agreed quarantine powers should only be exercised in the most extreme circumstances: to isolate individuals with AIDS who refused to alter their risky behavior.

But because of alienizing logic, it is not surprising that the primary targets of public health officials' quarantine efforts were prostitutes or those assumed to be. Sex workers became the targets even though "hookers"[24] were never added as a fifth H to the CDC's high-risk "4-H club" (homosexuals, heroin users, hemophiliacs, and Haitians). The reasons sex workers were not identified as a high-risk group are numerous. For one, as sex workers' rights groups insist, they take sexual health more seriously than the average person.[25] For another, many sex workers were assumed to be intravenous drug users, and the CDC schema did not account well for falling into multiple categories. The same is true for gay sex workers who were likely categorized only as gay men. And for a third reason, as Paula Treichler and Gena Corea have shown, women in general were not considered in a lot of early research and epidemiological work on AIDS,[26] and thus women sex workers were surely going to be disregarded, a problem that remains in research.[27]

Even as sex workers get disregarded and erased throughout history, US public health officials have been preoccupied with them as a source of venereal disease even when there was no proof of any disease at all.[28] Given this history, it should be no surprise that the AIDS pandemic created conditions to renew such connections, and sex workers, especially Black sex workers, became a primary preoccupation for public health and medical officials. Black sex workers also became test cases for either applying existing quarantine laws and policies or creating new ones, and their stories became media sensations. Scott W. Stern explains that while such responses are not "a direct continuation" of the American Plan, which quarantined so many women assumed to be sex workers in the early and mid-twentieth century, "the response to AIDS is an obvious intellectual, legislative, and judicial successor" to it.[29] As successors, state responses to allegedly noncompliant Black sex workers living with AIDS abided by what René Esparza calls "a carceral rationality."[30] Carceral rationality operates through alienizing logic, by which contagion must be contained and expelled. Black sex workers, already viewed by the state as contaminated outlaws, become the sites of a legacy of anti-Black racialized and sexualized fears when they are determined to have AIDS. The Black sex worker with AIDS who refuses state control becomes an ultimate alien to the state, a fugitive.

MEDIA SPECTACLE AND THE INCORRIGIBLE BLACK SEX WORKER

In Douglas Crimp's essay "Portraits of People with AIDS," he discusses a protest of a 1988 museum exhibit featuring portraits of people living with AIDS. The portraits, Crimp explains, are predictable. People with AIDS (PWA) "are ravaged, disfigured, and debilitated by the syndrome; they are generally alone, desperate, but resigned to their 'inevitable' deaths."[31] The protestors, mostly from the AIDS Coalition to Unleash Power (ACT UP), engaged visitors in conversation about the problems with the exhibit's representations and handed them a flier with a statement laying out their view and ending with the following: "The PWA is a human being whose health has deteriorated not simply due to the virus, but due to government inaction, the inaccessibility of affordable health care, and institutionalized neglect in the forms of heterosexism, racism, and sexism. We demand the visibility of PWAs who are vibrant, angry, loving, sexy, beautiful, acting up and fighting back. STOP LOOKING AT US; START LISTENING TO US."[32] Clearly Crimp and the activists' critique is not merely about the exhibit but of a genre of representations that glorify suffering and supply single dimensional depictions of individuals living with AIDS. Their call for defiant images works only when coupled with the demand not only to look but to listen to those who are most impacted. The call to listen, particularly to people who refuse the decontextualized victim narrative and who insist upon a structural analysis of the causes of AIDS, is crucial not only to affirm the humanity of people living with AIDS but also to join *their* fight.

Crimp's call is even more important, in my view, when depicting Black people living with AIDS, given their disproportionate rates of HIV infection and death from AIDS and histories of racist representation—generally and in relation to disease. As Evelynn Hammonds writes, "In this culture, how we think about disease determines who lives and who dies. The history of black people in this country is riddled with episodes displaying how concepts of sickness, disease, health, behavior and sexuality, and race have been entwined in the definition of normalcy and deviance. The power to define disease and normality makes AIDS a political issue."[33] Questions about the ways in which AIDS is political and politicized in relation to Blackness are as live now as they were when Hammonds wrote in the 1980s.

Representation and definition remain at the center of such questions, which is, at least in part, why Darius Bost's work "poses a challenge to black/ queer studies that center social death as their sole interpretive framework."[34] The archive with which I am working in this section lends itself to participation in the tendency to center social death and Black fungibility. Tiffany Lethabo King writes, "To be rendered Black and fungible under conquest is to be rendered porous, undulating, fluttering, sensuous, and in a space and state at-the-edge and outside of normative configurations of sex, gender, sexuality, space, and time to stabilize and fix the human category."[35] In this way, Black fungibility is inherent to the project of constructing the Human—the supposedly universal category of white liberal imagination. Yet King goes on: "Black fungibility resists conventional understandings and deployments of fungibility as solely a space of Black death, accumulation, dereliction, and limits." It "also represents a space of alterity and possibility, or what Snorton calls 'fungible fugitivity.'"[36] Reckoning with the agentic possibilities of the fugitivity of fungibility should not obscure what Stephen H. Marshall calls the "racialization of bare life"[37] or even the persistence of what Saidiya Hartman has named as the "opacity of black pain."[38] These works call to "notice 'Black livingness'"[39] even amid and perhaps because of pernicious state and media violence targeting Black life.

In early 1984, Yale New Haven Hospital reported treating four female prostitutes and three of their male clients who manifested signs of AIDS. Although hospital staff warned the women to stop soliciting, two disappeared and one kept working.[40] Upon another arrest, local media identified one of the women as Carlotta Locklear, a twenty-nine-year-old Black woman and a drug user with a fifteen-month-old child who was under the care of the hospital. As Stern notes, the coverage terrified Locklear, who told a local newspaper, "I can't even walk to a car because I'm afraid they'll blow my head off."[41] Local AIDS activists also expressed concern about the coverage, with one worrying it "gives men a reason to resort to violence against prostitutes."[42]

In exchange for eliminating her bail, Locklear agreed to a judge-ordered drug treatment program.[43] Within days, she left the program and was reportedly seen back on the street, provoking a police and media frenzy as they searched for the "escapee" and "runaway."[44] CBS's *60 Minutes* even aired a segment on Locklear. Six days later, Locklear turned herself back in to her public defender, and she was held on $25,000 bond.[45] Prosecutors charged her with narcotics possession and disorderly conduct and reportedly sought harsher punishment for her because she "put an awful lot of people at risk."[46] In May of that year, Judge Anthony DeMayo determined that Locklear was not a public health risk as she promised no longer to sell sex.[47] He gave her probation and mandated treatment. She reportedly tried to volunteer with the AIDS Project in New Haven but was rejected.[48]

Despite the judge's determination that Locklear was not a public threat and her own investment in supporting local AIDS work, the fugitive threat that some politicians imagined Locklear to pose served as a rationale to pursue quarantine on a broader scale. Connecticut already had a quarantine law on the books for communicable diseases like tuberculosis, but state representative Richard D. Tulisano, a Democrat and civil libertarian, considered proposing quarantine legislation that would apply to people living with AIDS.[49] Tulisano was quoted as asking, "If she just has AIDS and isn't bothering anybody, what can you do? On the other hand, if she's knowingly infecting other people, what should you do?"[50] Tulisano painted an either/

or dichotomy of the options available to a sex worker who knows she lives with AIDS. Either she can isolate herself from all risky behavior and therefore quit supporting herself, or she can knowingly infect others. His comments reflected the limitations in understanding possessed by politicians and public health officials—not just about AIDS but about the material realities and safer-sex practices of sex workers.

In San Francisco, police sent a prostitute suspected of having AIDS to a clinic for screening, but staff at the overburdened clinic asked her to return at a later date because they did not have time to screen her. The woman summed up the dilemma from her point of view, telling the *San Francisco Chronicle*, "I don't like the idea of maybe giving this to someone else, but I don't have any other way to survive other than to work the street."[51] Alyson O'Daniel writes in her study on Black women surviving HIV/AIDS that "as strategies for survival, drug use and sex work may operate to mitigate some conditions of poverty even while paradoxically increasing the parties' vulnerability to HIV infection."[52] Locklear's drug use compounded her situation as she potentially engaged in risky behavior not just for work but for an addiction or to cope. Even as her drug use was a concern, what clearly drew law enforcement and public officials to Locklear was her selling sex, which is why Judge DeMayo framed his granting of her probation on the condition she stop soliciting. Initially sending her to a drug treatment program functioned to keep her from endangering people on the streets. When she fled, it could be assumed she would use drugs again. It could also be assumed she would try to work. Media and police alike capitalized on that possibility as they hurriedly searched for Locklear and reported on her "escape." It is unclear why after the media and police frenzy, DeMayo gave Locklear only probation. Locklear died in early 1985, just a few months after both houses of the Connecticut state legislature passed a quarantine bill that enabled public health officials to confine certain people living with AIDS.[53]

Across the country, fears over women sex workers, especially Black women with AIDS, catalyzed questions about quarantine: whether old quarantine laws and statutes should be applied to individual cases, whether sweeping new legislation should be developed to address the possibility of reckless sex workers, and what the ethics of quarantine measures should be. They also raised questions about the police power of public health officials and the use of criminal arrest and jail to keep people off the streets. Few, if any, public health officials or politicians quoted in the media paid any mind to the fact that for sex workers, AIDS was not just a health matter but a labor issue. Few, if any, directed any attention to the women's race, even as race obviously featured centrally in the way public health and elected officials treated these women.

In 1988, the American Civil Liberties Union (ACLU) fought the first legal challenge to an AIDS-related quarantine in *Doe v. Sercy*. In March of that year, the South Carolina Department of Health and Environmental Control quarantined the Black woman known only as Jane Doe because she was allegedly HIV positive, was an intravenous drug user with unspecified mental health challenges, and had only Social Security and prostitution for income.[54] Under South Carolina law, health officials had near absolute power to quarantine this woman, and they did so for as many as ninety days without giving her a hearing, access to legal counsel, or any other due process.[55] Reportedly, an ACT UP chapter traveled to the area to draw attention to the case after local activist DiAna DiAna sought its assistance.[56] Even with ACT UP's presence, presumably because this woman was contained, this case did not draw media attention.[57] I can find no record of what happened to Jane Doe.

By 1991, when police in Alton, Illinois, arrested twenty-one-year-old Felicia Ann Horton for allegedly offering to perform oral sex on an undercover police officer for money even though she knew she was HIV positive, *Doe v. Sercy* was the only case at least one observer could find.[58] The local prosecutor filed both a civil quarantine action and a felony charge for attempted criminal transmission of the AIDS virus, a charge that did not require proof of transmission.[59] Horton was one of the first people charged in the state of Illinois with a felony related to HIV transmission.

Horton had a hard life, as the numerous media interviews with her friends, family, and neighbors made clear. Childhood friend Anissa Womack commented that Horton was a very shy child and subject to teasing: "She just never stood up for herself; so they picked on her."[60] Horton's mother reported that she ran away at twelve and lived in foster care or the streets ever since: "She was just wild."[61] In describing how her community seemed to regard her, reporter Terry Hughes Column noted, "All of it is a bit detached, as if the subject were a wild animal that showed up around the neighborhood all the time."[62] The two uses of "wild" here are telling—one as out of control and the other as disconnected from civilization. I'm reminded of a third use of "wild" in Hartman's explanation of her methodological approach in her book *Wayward Lives, Beautiful Experiments*: "The wild idea that animates this book is that young black women were radical thinkers who tirelessly imagined other ways to live and never failed to consider how the world might be otherwise."[63] Perhaps this captures Horton's character.

After her arrest, Horton agreed to enter a treatment center at an undisclosed location in northern Illinois. On May 22, she walked away only to reappear in a Chicago ER to give premature birth after five months of evading authorities. She reportedly left the treatment center "because she didn't like it and wasn't comfortable there." While in hiding, she stayed "with another woman in Chicago, and had become such good friends with the woman that she named her baby after her. Horton said she had been receiving welfare payments under her real name through the Illinois Department of Public Aid."[64] Put differently, she seemed to make a life in plain sight outside of the law's lens.

Although in the end authorities did not pursue her for quarantine or the felony charges, so much damage was done. Her identity had been released, prompting concerns that her treatment by media and the legal system were racially motivated.[65] Horton told a reporter that the disclosure had ruined her life. "'Everybody knew about me,' she said at the time. 'I had to walk around the street with people talking about me. They humiliated me. They destroyed my life.'"[66] After more run-ins with the law over the course of the next twenty years, Horton tried to fashion another way for herself, writing in her last journal entry in May 2011, "I wish to get myself together to better my life. I am getting older now and I should give myself a chance at life."[67] She died two months later, jumping from a moving vehicle, perhaps her last fugitive act.

Black women's lives are frequently subject to surveillance, scrutiny, and confinement, and the lives discussed here show how public health and law bridged on their backs. In these early years of the AIDS pandemic, as queer/AIDS activists in groups like ACT UP insisted that "silence = death," "women of color living with HIV grappled with the reality that making noise could be just as deadly," as Celeste Watkins-Hayes notes.[68] The particular kind of attention paid to Black women sex workers' words and actions, including those of Locklear, Doe, and Horton, illustrate this point profoundly.[69]

At the same time that Black women sex workers received fevered responses in places as disparate as Connecticut, South Carolina, and Illinois, the slipperiness between men who were sex workers and promiscuous gay men in public prompted rash quarantine proposals in political speeches, state legislatures, municipal health offices, and public health departments, especially in the US South. Paul Cameron, a white man and discredited social psychologist from Lincoln, Nebraska, who ran the Institute for the Scientific Study of Sexuality, was the most notorious advocate for such proposals and had surprisingly wide political influence. Cameron weighed in against a referendum in Houston, Texas, for an employment non-discrimination ordinance that protected homosexuals. In his testimony before the Houston City Council against the ordinance, he advocated for quarantine for "urban gays," most of whom he claimed "now carry the AIDS germ."[70] His stated intention was to alert Houston's citizens of the threat homosexuals posed to the public because of AIDS, in addition to their overall risky lifestyle. Stopping AIDS, in his view, involved "quarantining gays, closing all gay bars and baths, criminalizing homosexual acts that involve exchange of bodily products, and closing the borders to homosexual travel."[71] Cameron, a notoriously anti-gay social scientist, considered by some as the grandfather of homophobic junk science, took the quarantine logic to the absolute extreme.[72] His presence in Houston drew a lot of media attention, and reportedly council members took him seriously enough to ask him questions about the implementation of his proposal. The Houston city health director, James Haughton, a Panamanian immigrant who faced significant discrimination as a Black man and a new doctor in the 1950s, even said that though the proposal would end in an illogical conclusion, it was a novel idea.[73] Cameron cannot be credited, but the referendum for gay job rights was defeated by a nearly 4 to 1 margin.[74]

That Houston got a taste of Cameron's quarantine proposal was fortuitous; several months later in October 1985, the white male Texas state health commissioner, Robert Bernstein, put forth his own quarantine proposal that would have given state or local health officials the power to confine any person with AIDS who was deemed a public health threat because they would not stop engaging in risky activities.[75] Bernstein advanced this proposal after public calls for AIDS to be quarantinable by Haughton, Houston's health director.[76] Haughton, who would later say that breast cancer was a more serious public health threat than AIDS,[77] made this call in light of the infamous and tragic life of an alleged sex worker in Houston, Fabian K. Bridges.[78] The details of Bridges's life are contested. The gay press paints a radically different picture than the mainstream media. That the reports conflict is not surprising, as it speaks to the reason why marginalized communities have always created their own media to tell stories about themselves from their own perspectives.[79] The conflicting reports and a sensational documentary help to articulate how an "incorrigible" Black gay man, alleged to be a sex worker, ended up at the center of the AIDS quarantine debate.

According to the gay press, Bridges's story came to the attention of public health officials through a Minneapolis-based news crew from WCCO-TV that came to Houston in the summer of 1985 to learn about the gay community's struggles after the defeat of the employment referendum.[80] That story apparently did not prove to be very interesting, but producers learned about Bridges, a gay Black man with AIDS struggling with poverty and homelessness. Their recordings became a documentary that was then aired as part of a PBS *Frontline* episode, "AIDS: A National Inquiry," in 1986.

Before Bridges was diagnosed with AIDS, he worked a stable job earning $19,000 a year at the Harris County Flood Authority.[81] After his diagnosis, he got sick and entered a hospital, soon losing his housing and job. At the time the news crew arrived, Bridges was not even in Houston. After making his way to Indianapolis to try to seek help from his sister and brother-in-law who would not take him in but affectionately called him by his middle name, Kalvin, he ran into trouble with law enforcement for allegedly stealing a bicycle. Knowing he had AIDS, instead of filing charges against him, a judge and law enforcement officers purchased him a bus ticket to Cleveland, where his mother lived. The news crew went to locate him there, where they followed him as he tried to connect with his mother, whose husband would not let Bridges stay with her. Bridges struggled to find other housing since no shelters would take him. He eventually ended up in a hotel room paid for by the Red Cross as he waited for his Social Security disability payments to begin.

Houston's *Montrose Voice*, a gay publication bearing the name of Houston's "gayborhood," Montrose, reported that the news crew regularly paid for Bridges's lodging and food in order to continue filming. When Bridges told them he continued to have sex, the crew reported him to Cleveland public health officials.[82] Bridges eluded the film crew and returned to Houston, reportedly to pick up a van he owned to take back to Cleveland.[83] Eventually, Bridges needed money, so he contacted the film crew, which then followed him to Houston. While in Houston, he visited a doctor and told the doctor he continued to have sex, reportedly with at least twenty people. That doctor notified Haughton's office. In late September, Haughton placed Bridges under police monitoring and ordered him to quit having sex.[84] Apparently, Bridges initially said he refused the order, prompting an outcry over "incorrigible" AIDS victims and a two-day police hunt for Bridges, in which police tried to entrap him into having sex.[85] The tactic did not work, so they arrested him for public urination. An actual violation of his order would have been a third-degree felony, punishable by ten years in prison and a $5,000 fine.[86] Media relished the story.

On October 5, two doctors who had treated Bridges at different hospitals, one of whom had urged that he be given a quarantine warning, issued a statement defending their actions with Bridges and assuring that their actions were not "anti-homosexual" but "pro-health." The one who requested the quarantine warning, a white male physician, Robert Awe, stated, "I requested that this quarantine warning be served on Mr. Bridges because he was alone, confused, and frightened and obviously needed help. He had repeatedly refused the attempts by discharge planners, social workers, and myself to be placed in a boarding house or to contact the KS/AIDS Foundation. He preferred to be an independent 'street person.'"[87] The full text of the statement is not available, so it is impossible to contextualize the rest of their comments, but this excerpt is significant. Issued just days after a police manhunt for Bridges and the city health director's order to stop having sex, Awe suggested his call for quarantine emerged from his humanitarian pity and concern. Because Bridges was alone and in need of assistance, Awe called for his isolation. Awe juxtaposed his rational, pastoral care with Bridges's irrational desire to be independent and to remain on the street. Throughout his ordeal, Bridges ended up in *Time* magazine and repeatedly in Houston local media. In these depictions, as in the *Frontline* documentary, few even questioned whether Bridges was okay, instead insisting he was clearly demented and needed to be confined to a mental health institution. Diego Lopez, a clinical director for Gay Men's Health Crisis, and the only person of color or person living with AIDS on the *Frontline* expert panel, was the only one who expressed concern for Bridges, noting that the depiction of him was racist and homophobic and that Bridges was victimized by "all the systems that failed him."[88] As Judy Woodruff, the host of the documentary, noted, the gay community began protecting Bridges from all mainstream press.

On the advice of people from the gay community, including Houston's well-known white gay activist Ray Hill and the KS/AIDS Foundation Houston, Bridges voluntarily entered a hospital in early October, then lived with friends for a short time before dying in a hospital on November 17, 1985; he was buried in a pauper's grave because his family had no money for a funeral. That public health officials created hysteria over the need to quarantine Bridges just six weeks before he died is telling. Friends and supporters reported he was 6'2", 126 pounds, and suffering from genital and rectal herpes before he died. As one put it, "I feel he could not have given it away, let alone sold it."[89] The public affairs director at WCCO-TV, which followed Bridges for the documentary, admitted that his crew did not know whether Bridges lied about his sexual activity in order to get food and shelter from reporters. They also denied that Bridges was a prostitute.[90] For Bridges's part, he seemed to have little sense that his story would be taken up in the exploitative way that it was. The end of the documentary shows a clip of Bridges sitting in his Cleveland hotel room, wearing a black T-shirt and speaking in a soft voice. We do not know what the filmmakers ask him, but he responds, "Let me go down in history as being I am somebody, somebody that'll be respected, somebody who's appreciated and somebody who can be related to. There's a whole lot of people who just go, they're not even on the map, they just go."

Bridges's situation conjoined with one in San Antonio in which a man with AIDS (who may or may not have been a prostitute) told his physician he planned to keep having sex.[91] As reported in the *New York Times*, "When Dr. Courand Rothe, the San Antonio health director learned this, he threatened all 17 known AIDS victims in that city with felony charges if they engaged in irresponsible sexual behavior." Although Health Commissioner Bernstein was adamant that his proposal was "not an arrest and incarceration thing,"[92] that he was prompted by both fears about Bridges's sexual activity and Rothe's threat make his claim spurious. This was the first time in the United States that public health officials put forth a systematic quarantine proposal to manage people living with AIDS. In December 1985, in a 12 to 5 vote, Texas Board of Health approved Bernstein's proposal to add AIDS to the list of communicable diseases that could justify quarantine.[93] This vote sent the proposal into a thirty-day public comment period. After this period, Bernstein decided against the initial quarantine proposal thanks to lobbying efforts by the gay community and public health officials' belief that they needed the gay community as an ally if they were to successfully confront AIDS.[94]

Presumably, the influential gay community Bernstein imagined as his allies were middle-class, predominantly white organizations, people from different worlds than Fabian Bridges. They were likely the type of people who protested the *Frontline* special, not in defense of Bridges's dignity but because they "feared that Fabian would be seen by the general public as a metaphor for most AIDS victims, instead of as the aberration that he was. They feared that the visual impact of the documentary would overshadow the talking-heads panel discussion that followed, thus feeding a national homophobia that could increase calls for the quarantining of AIDS victims and carriers."[95] Bernstein reported that his organization would be turning its attention toward public education. Nevertheless, he stated of the quarantine, "We're not dropping it (concept). We're just going to try to do it in a less tumultuous way."[96] Here "less tumultuous" refers to the manner of doing—with less commotion, less disorder, and more peace—as opposed to the doing itself. Several states implemented proposals like the one Texas only proposed, including Connecticut in light of the uproar surrounding Carlotta Locklear.

Black men who were sex workers continued to be a concern for public health officials and police alike, prompting calls for quarantine and criminalization. The convergence between police and public health becomes even starker in the case of James Henry McIntyre, a twenty-eight-year old cross-dressing, gay, Black prostitute with AIDS.[97] McIntyre was known as "Miss Pocahontas" in the local gay community, perhaps a signaling of Indigenous heritage or for another reason unstated. In early 1987, the *New York Times* reported that McIntyre "passes his days in an isolated cell while officials of Jackson and Mississippi debate how to resolve the danger they fear he poses."[98] "Sometimes I'm lonely. Sometimes I cry. I wish I didn't have to be in here. The police don't like me," he told the *Advocate*.[99] Arrested for prostitution over sixty times, McIntyre was tested for HIV while serving a sentence for a misdemeanor the previous March.[100] A soft-spoken person, McIntyre reportedly asked an interviewer, "There's no way you can get rid of the virus? It just carries on? I always use condoms, so I couldn't transmit the virus, could I?"[101] We get no sense of how anyone may have answered his questions, but even in the moment of this encounter, it seems clear that while McIntyre may not have understood the gravity of his diagnosis, he took precautions that, if always taken, would have protected himself and others. Nevertheless, as with Bridges, some police bought him a bus ticket and sent him to California. With a sick mother in Mississippi, McIntyre returned in September. On December 11, 1986, after being picked up with a well-known white businessman in Jackson, police arrested McIntyre on a disorderly conduct charge, which they upgraded to a felony sodomy charge with a $20,000 bond so he would remain in jail, which he did for two months.

While incarcerated, news media learned of his situation as local officials were unsure of what to do, because as the white assistant district attorney Tommy Mayfield claimed, "This guy is obviously not going to quit doing what he does."[102] As in earlier cases, no one addressed the likely poverty McIntyre faced, having just returned to be with his sick mother after police used his illness as a reason to expel him to another state. Officials never mentioned that selling sex was his means of income. Mayfield looked to state health law for guidance. Under Mississippi law, public health officials had very strong quarantine powers, and state epidemiologist Ed Thompson stated that in the case of McIntyre, if prosecution did not work, he would use his quarantine powers to isolate him. In February, a grand jury decided not to indict McIntyre, and so state health officials decided to use their quarantine power, ordering him not to have sex without revealing his status, the first time such an order had been issued against a male prostitute, according to Dr. James Curran of the CDC.[103] The quarantine order was punishable by six months in jail and a $500 fine.[104] It also required him to refrain from donating blood and to receive counseling on sexually transmitted diseases.[105]

When interviewed by the media, McIntyre, like Locklear and Horton, realized what media had done to his reputation and job prospects even as he allegedly gave officials permission to talk about his case and insisted he was done with sex work. "I'm sure I can't get a job here. I'm sure everybody can recognize my face from TV."[106] With no options before him, McIntyre told the reporter, "I just plan to stay with my mother for about three months and then I'm going to California." There he planned to live with his grandmother. He continued with a sobering thought: "Sometimes I wish I had just contracted the disease and died. It would have been better all the way around." Though we have only traces of McIntyre's life, personality, and character, he had a clear understanding of his predicament and how widespread the problem of AIDS was on the streets of Jackson: "The police did me so dirty. I *would* have tried to help them, but I am not going to help them now."[107] No further information about McIntyre exists. His name occasionally shows up as a small anecdote in discussions of HIV criminalization, as his case is among the earliest,[108] but after February 1987, it is as if he disappeared. Disappearing him was always the point.

In each of these instances, when alienizing logic manifests as the need to quarantine Black prostitutes, a tension between casting out and capture looms large. On the one hand, these Black prostitutes living with AIDS were cast out by public health officials, police, and the courts—to other cities, to jails, to treatment centers. But when these individuals cast themselves out, they became fugitives in need of capture. These twin logics characterize the construction of a public health and police approach to quarantine on the backs of Black people. Yet as these stories also show, these individuals refused fungibility and wanted more for themselves. Unsurprisingly, the alienizing logic that animates the relationship between quarantine, criminalization, and Blackness will become the foundation for the exercise of the most egregious immigration quarantine in US history, which I address in chapter 5.

POLITICAL DISCOURSE

Beyond these high-profile stories involving the decision-making of public health officials in conjunction with police, lawyers, and courts, quarantine became firmly entrenched in the national political discussion on AIDS. As mentioned above, opinion polls related to AIDS regularly asked how respondents felt about quarantine. And right-wing politicians kept the issue germane. Although every state had some power to quarantine people to prevent the spread of communicable disease, between 1985 and 1987, nine states amended old laws or passed new ones empowering health officials to quarantine people with AIDS, and five states made knowingly transmitting AIDS a crime.[109] Some, even within the gay community, preferred the latter solution. Tom Stoddard, then of the ACLU and longtime executive director of Lambda Legal Defense and Education Fund in New York, said he "would far prefer the state dealing with these issues through criminal proceedings, because there is greater assurance of fairness and due process. There is much greater danger the state will abuse its power under the quarantine and commitment statutes."[110] As the previous section demonstrated, the line between criminal law and public health statutes is blurry at best, and the impacts of that blurriness is felt most by those already positioned as racialized outlaws within the citizenry: Black sex workers—but certainly many other groups could fall in that category as well. As Steven Thrasher has shown, the results of what we now call "HIV criminalization" has largely impacted Black men, especially gay men like Michael Johnson, known in the media as "Tiger Mandingo," a former college athlete arrested for sleeping with men without revealing his HIV-positive status.[111] As Trevor Hoppe explains, "The criminalization of HIV is but one of the more recent examples in public health history of an effort to control disease by coercion and punishment." He calls this phenomenon "punitive disease control."[112] Even as AIDS continued to be associated with white gay men in the US media, that association was only partial. Outside of the realm of public health, laws would be proposed and political decisions enacted on the backs of sexual and racialized outlaws.

In this section, I begin with California and the rhetoric surrounding Lyndon LaRouche and his two failed state ballot measures to mandate quarantine for people with AIDS. I then turn attention to Orange County Republican congressman William Dannemeyer, who made another proposal that operated within the alienizing logic of quarantine as he further legitimized the views of figures like Cameron. From there, I discuss Florida's quarantine law in contrast to what was proposed in California before turning briefly to the rhetoric of Senator Jesse Helms (R-NC). Together these pieces of the political puzzle reveal the prominence of quarantine rhetoric within the political sphere.

LaRouche was a fringe politician who gained various levels of notoriety and infamy throughout the 1970s and 80s for his lavish conspiracy theories and beliefs about well-known figures like Henry Kissinger and Queen Elizabeth. Originally a member of the Communist Party, LaRouche began turning to the right in the 1970s, running for president for the first time in 1976. In 1980, he and his followers founded the National Democratic Policy Committee.[113] The committee had no connection to the Democratic Party but would recruit candidates to run for local and national office as "LaRouche Democrats," lobby political entities such as legislatures and school boards, and put measures on state ballots. In October 1985, LaRouche's political machine began securing signatures for a ballot initiative designed to put many quarantine measures into effect. While health officials in other states considered various quarantine proposals, health officials and the California Medical Association denounced LaRouche's proposal, which would have redefined AIDS as "an infectious disease like measles or tuberculosis, and authorize[d] state and county health officers to use their quarantine powers to control the activities of victims and carriers."[114] The measure would also have prevented "suspected AIDS carriers from attending or teaching school or working in restaurants."[115] California Medical Association spokesman and former San Francisco director of public health Dr. Laurens White put the matter like this: "What you're talking about is concentration camps. If it becomes possible for a health officer to enforce blood tests and enforce quarantining, then the gay community is simply going to stop seeing anybody who might decide they're a threat."[116] As already evidenced, quarantine practices did not only or primarily target gay men, if they were not also prostitutes, but LaRouche's appeals rested significantly on homophobic beliefs about gay men's sexual practices and their connection with AIDS. Though the quarantine proposal was far-fetched and impossible to implement, LaRouche's supporters organized as the Prevent AIDS Now Initiative Committee (PANIC) and collected nearly 700,000 signatures with signs that said, "Sign here to help stop AIDS."[117] This number of signatures was nearly double the requirement to get on the ballot. It was the first time members of the US electorate were asked to vote on the rights of people with AIDS.

Virtually no major elected official supported the measure, which became Proposition 64. Most actively denounced it, with likely presidential candidate Gary Hart referring to it as fascist.[118] Even the state's Catholic bishops opposed it because of its civil rights implications and because they believed it would prevent the development of a cure.[119] San Francisco estimated that if Proposition 64 passed, it would cost the city roughly $69 million to track down people with AIDS and trace their contacts.[120] Nevertheless, organizers opposed to Proposition 64 scrambled, with polls showing an alarming amount of support for it and an even greater number of people uninformed or undecided as late as mid-October.[121] An ABC/*Washington Post* poll found 52 percent were opposed to Proposition 64, 31 percent in support, and 17 percent undecided—numbers that could legitimately swing toward affirming the proposition.[122] Although organizers opposed to the proposition still struggled to get the message out and to raise funds, in the end, they raised $2.3 million. The LaRouche measure failed in 1986 by a significant margin of roughly 71 percent to 29 percent.[123] Despite the wide margin, over two million Californians voted for it. Mostly white gay men and lesbians worked closely together to oppose the ballot measure, much like they had in 1978 against the Briggs Initiative, although there was reportedly less enthusiasm to do the wide-scale organizing of the decade before.[124] Still, organizers celebrated their win.

The celebration did not last long. By the spring of 1987, PANIC rebooted as Prevent AIDS Now In California and gathered signatures for an initiative for the June 1988 ballot described as a "mirror image" of the one that had just been defeated.[125] By December, supporters had collected over 500,000 signatures, more than 100,000 over the number needed to get on the ballot.[126] The new initiative became Proposition 69 and had all the same provisions as the previous one.[127] Once again, Californians voted against the quarantine initiative but with a narrower margin: 68 percent to 32 percent. In this instance, over 1.6 million Californians voted for it.[128] Almost immediately after the defeat of Proposition 69, Dannemeyer and others placed yet another initiative on the November 1988 ballot, Proposition 102, that would have achieved many of the provisions of the LaRouche initiatives; however, this proposition explicitly left quarantine language out.[129] It, too, was defeated by a roughly 3 to 1 margin. Although AIDS was never added to California's list of infectious diseases, California public health officials already had the right to quarantine people who presented a risk to the public health. LaRouche clearly wanted AIDS to be a unique target.

On the other side of the country, in January 1988, Florida considered expanding quarantine powers as first laid out in a Department of Health and Rehabilitative Services (HRS) policy paper. The proposal would put over $1 million toward a new "lock up" unit that would hold twenty-two adults and six juveniles with AIDS.[130] This was reportedly the first proposal of its kind. In presumably assuring the largest AIDS lobby group, one spokesperson commented, "It wasn't designed for gay people. The whole issue came up around prostitutes."[131] In April, the proposal grew more refined, and Governor Bob Martinez announced his support in his State of the State address: "The time has come to quarantine those whose character and conduct are a clear threat to society. AIDS carriers who refuse to stop spreading this fatal disease should no more be allowed to roam free than criminals armed with a deadly weapon."[132] Martinez's words need little interpretation as the alienizing logic is in full force, manifesting in a blend of quarantine and criminalization. But these words were not metaphorical. HRS spokesman Ray Wise explained that police would arrest people with AIDS and the courts would determine whether someone was a public health risk. First-time offenders would receive probation that would involve "limited activities and restricted associations." Second-time offenders would live in a halfway-house-style, twenty-four-hour supervised situation. "Incorrigibles" would be incarcerated "in a humane and dignified environment."[133] Florida's house of representatives and senate proposed different versions of the quarantine. For example, the senate version had up to a 180-day quarantine with little due process, whereas the house version maxed out at sixty days and included a court hearing before someone could be quarantined.[134] After months-long deliberations, Governor Martinez signed a large $18 million AIDS bill in July that included quarantine, alongside some important civil liberties protections for those afflicted, mandated education in public middle and high schools and state universities, and anti-discrimination provisions.[135]

Although, as stated before, a number of states introduced new quarantine laws or strengthened existing ones to deal with the problem of AIDS during the mid-1980s, by the late 1980s, there were few introductions of such proposals targeting the rights of citizens. This slow down can be attributed to several factors. First, with the exception of fringe figures, by the late 1980s, there was little confusion among public health officials about how HIV was spread, which meant that it was very hard to rationalize quarantine as a valid response to HIV. Second, calls for quarantine were slowly replaced with calls for criminalization of various behaviors associated with spreading HIV; criminal justice responses replaced public health responses as the preferred method for dealing with recalcitrant US citizens, including prostitutes and drug users. The impact of these laws cannot be understated, and like other criminal laws, they continue to largely target Black and other marginalized communities.[136] Third, the AIDS activist movement as captured most visibly in the work of groups like ACT UP was in full swing, and few actions related to AIDS could target US citizens without a significant public response that often embarrassed those making such proposals. Finally, those most committed to punishing people living with AIDS and making it a matter of moral rather than health concern had found another way to direct their homophobic, moralistic, and protectionist desires. To these people, AIDS had always come from the outside, along with so many of the other ills facing the United States, including subversive political identities like communism and anarchism and their related homosexuality.[137] When it was clear there would be no wholesale rounding up of homosexuals across the United States, that only a few prostitutes would ever be quarantined for spreading HIV, and that people cared about the civil liberties of most US citizens living with HIV/AIDS—if only because they would demand them publicly—then those who had been the loudest proponents of quarantine proposals would turn their agendas toward migrants.

For example, Dannemeyer was one of the only politicians in California that supported LaRouche's initiatives. Throughout his career, Dannemeyer had an intense focus on AIDS and male homosexuals, authoring a book about homosexuality and introducing numerous pieces of anti-gay and anti-AIDS legislation, including Proposition 102.[138] In the late summer of 1985, he hired Cameron to be his advisor on AIDS and homosexuality, calling him "a man of conscience."[139] Dannemeyer intimated that AIDS was a homosexual disease that could be contracted through casual contact long after this was completely disproved by science, yet at one point in 1988, Dannemeyer attended an event as a proxy for President Bush, with some noting that he was within "the mainstream" view on AIDS policy.[140] Dannemeyer, along with like-minded colleagues such as

Helms in the Senate, ended up with significant influence over AIDS policy in the United States. In June 1987, in the midst of a debate about the ban on HIV-positive migrants, Helms said to Lesley Stahl on *Face the Nation*, "I may be the most radical person you've talked to about AIDS, but I think somewhere along the line that we're going to have to quarantine if we are really going to contain this disease. We did it back with syphilis, did it with other diseases, and nobody even raised a question about it."[141] If they could not mass quarantine their fellow citizens, they could apply the same logic to those who were not citizens.

CONCLUSION

Thus, it was through the alienizing logic made manifest in quarantine that fringe politicians' and other public officials' ideas about AIDS and homosexuality began to garner mainstream appeal. As alien citizens, all US American homosexuals, including those with race and class privilege, ended up suffering because of problematic ideas from the right wing becoming dominant. US Black folks clearly withstood the worst of it. But a group that is rarely named in histories of HIV and AIDS—migrants—also endured dire consequences. In the fall of 1985, calls for quarantine and public concerns about AIDS reached a fever pitch. At the time, Acting Health and Human Services Secretary James O. Mason proposed an initial rule for the *Federal Register* that would change the definition of dangerous and contagious disease by adding AIDS for the purpose of immigration law, the subject of the next chapter. Thus, the targeting and isolating of people living with AIDS that, outside of prisons, never fully flourished in relation to US citizen communities was given new shape as a sound immigration policy.

CHAPTER 3

NATIONAL COMMON SENSE AND THE BAN ON HIV-POSITIVE MIGRANTS

"I am expected to disregard 12 years of my life, the years forming the bulk of my personal history as an adult," said a member of ACT UP who immigrated here from South America. "I am expected to give up the health insurance benefits and tax benefits I have paid into for 12 years—and still pay.

"All this because HIV, which I became infected with in the United States, turns me into a threat to my adopted country," he said. "All I have worked for is now threatened by bigotry, ignorance and political game playing."

—PRESS RELEASE, ACT UP SAN FRANCISCO
AND GOLDEN GATE, June 17, 1991

IN LATE 1987, THE UNITED STATES STARTED WHAT AIDS AND immigration activist Jorge Cortiñas described as the "worlds [*sic*] largest mandatory testing program."[1] Just months after approving the 1986 Immigration Reform and Control Act (IRCA), which opened a pathway to legalization for a number of undocumented people living in the United States, the US Congress passed a ban on HIV-positive migrants. Congress did this by adding HIV infection and AIDS to the list of the "dangerous contagious diseases" that barred someone from migrating to or regularizing their status in the United States. One of the results of this new law was that the millions of undocumented people eligible to regularize their immigration status under IRCA, as well as those already applying for permanent resident status through other channels, would be ineligible if their mandatory HIV test came back positive. As the South American migrant cited in the epigraph above notes, despite the fact that he undoubtedly contracted HIV in the United States and had made his life there, "bigotry, ignorance, and political game playing" turned him, and many more, into a national threat to be excluded.

Quarantine never made it into the law in a widespread way that impacted most US citizens, particularly not those who dominated in the rhetorical imaginary of AIDS. Instead, as mentioned in the previous chapter, alienizing logic catalyzed several state laws that criminalized HIV/AIDS. When it came to non-citizens, HIV/AIDS once again became an opportunity to enact alienizing logic, this time as politicians and public health officials alike rehashed long-standing racialized, xenophobic, and nativist fears about migrant health and sexuality. AIDS also generated new fears because HIV was imagined as a foreign disease, transmitted through the most deviant sexual practices, and it can be deadly. The first serious consideration that members of Congress gave to how to manage the spread of HIV or assist those afflicted was to pass the ban on HIV-positive migrants. A ban and a quarantine are not exactly the same practices, but they both emerge from alienizing logic. Furthermore, a ban that prevents some people from coming to the United States or regulating their status if they were already here can have similar effects as a quarantine: isolation, exclusion, and stigmatization.

Through an analysis of congressional debates about the ban and senators' reliance upon what I call a rhetoric of "national common sense," this chapter details how the law that defined HIV infection as a "dangerous contagious disease" and therefore grounds for immigration exclusion came to be. This history and the rhetorical grounds upon which elected officials made a case for, and agreed upon, the ban is important because they reveal the persistence of alienizing logic that manifests in interlocking rhetorics of public health, contagion, and immigration. This chapter also contributes to understanding of common sense and its many rhetorical manifestations, thus illuminating the logic of a significant source of rhetorical invention. Finally, this analysis furthers studies of public memory on HIV/AIDS by addressing an important, prolific site of rhetoric about HIV/AIDS that has hardly been mentioned in the scholarly record, even as it reveals the ways that AIDS structured the nation and its proper citizenry.[2]

The chapter begins with some context about what led to a ban even being considered in Congress. I then analyze the Senate debates about whether to exclude migrants with AIDS or HIV infection from the United States during the spring of 1987 as well as some media, activist, and medical discourse surrounding and sometimes influencing those debates. I center primarily on the predominant themes within the rhetoric of the key actors in the debate—Senator Jesse Helms (R-NC) and his self-described "nemesis," Senator Lowell Weicker (R-CT)—to show how seemingly irreconcilable differences between what Weicker described as "philosophy" and "science" are in fact reconciled through a rhetoric of "national common sense."[3] The discussion then turns to the normalization of this national common sense over and against medical science in the Department of Health and Human Service's (HHS) 1991 decision to leave HIV infection on the list of what by then was called "communicable diseases of public health significance." The chapter ends with the Senate and House debates over the 1993 National Institutes of Health Revitalization Act, in which amendments were put forth, and eventually approved, that codified the ban in law, removing regulatory power over the definitions of excludable conditions from the purview of the HHS.

PUBLIC HEALTH, HIV/AIDS, AND IMMIGRATION POLICY

By 1988, the United States had more reported AIDS cases than the entire rest of the world combined, totaling nearly 60 percent of known cases.[4] Fingers pointed from the United States to Africa and Haiti as the culprits. Surely cases in some countries were underreported, but by the available numbers, regardless of where HIV originated, the United States was a principal breeding ground for its spread. Most of the world regarded the United States as the primary exporter of HIV/AIDS. Nevertheless, key members of Ronald Reagan's administration and the US Congress supported and advocated passing laws to exclude those with HIV/AIDS from migrating to this country in order to supposedly stop the spread of HIV in the United States. In reading media, legal, and health news between 1985 and 1993, the years when the ban was first introduced, signed into law, and finally codified, only a few experts thought that excluding HIV-positive migrants was a good idea. Lawyers, public health officials, international diplomats, intelligence officials, and media pundits alike named the plethora of reasons why the HIV exclusion in immigration law was not only rash public health policy but also bad for human rights and international relations. For example, the World Health Organization maintained that travel bans due to HIV infection were against the International Health Regulations.[5] Physicians argued that exclusion would do little to stop the spread of HIV infection, and many legal experts and public health officials agreed.[6] One of the only expert bodies to support a ban was the US Public Health Service (PHS), an institution headed by a Reagan appointee.[7]

Before President Reagan had uttered the word "AIDS" publicly, his administration quietly worked on AIDS policy. Struggles over how to approach domestic AIDS policy were central to this secret flurry of policy development, yet immigration law was also set to be a prime target. On November 15, 1985, James O. Mason, the acting assistant secretary for health, Centers for Disease Control (CDC) director, and an eventual member of the general authority of the Church of Jesus Christ of Latter-day Saints, put forth a recommendation from the PHS to amend Title 42 of the Federal Code of Regulations by adding AIDS to the list of "dangerous contagious diseases" that render immigrants and refugees excludable under Section 212(a) of the Immigration and Nationality Act.[8] HHS secretary Otis R. Bowen, the former Republican governor of Indiana, approved this proposal on January 9, 1986, and it was opened for public comment in April.[9] By June of the following year, upon review of the comments received from 116 individuals and sixteen organizations, the HHS decided to add AIDS to the list and shortly thereafter amended the ruling to substitute "HIV infection" for AIDS "since individuals who are so infected, but do not actually have AIDS, are also contagious."[10] This rule, originally announced by PHS's Robert Windom, an internal medicine professor, in mid-May, would ensure that anyone seeking permanent residency in addition to those migrating for the first time would be tested.[11] The timing of this announcement was significant since applications for legalization through IRCA began to be processed on May 5. An HHS spokesperson told the *New York Times* that he did not know if this would impact those seeking legalization under IRCA.[12] Yet on July 6, 1987, the Immigration and Naturalization Service (INS) released a statement requiring all medical examinations to conform to the PHS guidelines, mandating that anyone with visible AIDS symptoms would be tested for HIV.[13] After Congress added HIV infection to the list of dangerous and contagious diseases, everyone applying for legalization between December 1, 1987, and the cut-off date of May 5, 1988, was HIV tested.[14]

Legal scholar Bettina Fernandez has suggested that there are reasons to pay attention to this timing. The State Department, which also opposed the exclusion of HIV-infected migrants due to the problems it would inevitably create for international relations and diplomacy, estimated that only 250 people annually would likely be excluded from immigrating to the United States under this rule. The roughly three million people eligible for legalization under IRCA had to reside in the United States continually since January 1, 1982—shortly after AIDS was discovered. Since people had to be continually present in the United States starting in 1982 in order to qualify, like the activist in the epigraph, anyone seeking legalization very likely contracted the disease in the United States. If it was likely that very few HIV-positive migrants would seek entry to the United States, and also the case that an infected undocumented person otherwise eligible for legalization contracted the disease in the United States, then the threat from outside would seem to be very minimal. This logic leads Fernandez to suggest that proposals for a ban on HIV-positive migrants primarily targeted the undocumented people already in the United States who wanted to legalize, regardless of their HIV status.[15]

This added step to legalization made the process challenging for applicants. Reports from California's Coalition for Immigrant and Refugee Rights and Services (CIRRS) found that the INS-designated civil surgeons tasked with testing applicants had limited knowledge of HIV/AIDS, provided no counseling or support for those who tested positive, and sometimes reported false positives.[16] Although those who tested positive could apply for waivers and continue their applications, the process was long, the standards were strict, and advocates worried most did not know about it. INS spokesman Duane Austin told the *New York Times*, "From the small number of waiver requests coming in, we can assume that the majority of people testing positive decided not to pursue their legalization applications."[17] Even people who had no fear of being HIV positive might have decided not to apply for legalization because of the possibility of taking an HIV test and no guarantee that their privacy would be protected. To this day, it is unclear how many people did not apply for legalization due to the HIV test, and I have not been able to locate any testimony or reports from anyone in this category. Whether motivated or incidental, the implementation of IRCA is part of a bigger frame of context for these debates, occurring amid the alienizing logic: in this instance, a confluence of fears about HIV/AIDS and fears about migrants and who could belong to the nation.

This ruling was published just a week after Reagan delivered his first public speech devoted entirely to AIDS on May 31, 1987. The ruling was simultaneous to Senate debates over the ban on HIV-positive migrants, which resulted in a final vote that implored the president to add HIV to the excludable list for immigration purposes.[18] By December 1 of that year, the exclusion was firmly in place. In the next section, I examine the contours of the Senate debate and the development of national common sense.

AIDS AND IMMIGRATION IN 1987 SENATE DEBATES

Obviously, Helms knew that this ruling from the PHS was in motion when he introduced an amendment to HR 1827, the Supplemental Appropriations Act of 1987 that included a ban on HIV-positive migrants. The Reagan administration was under increasing pressure to adopt a formal and systematic response to the AIDS crisis. Reagan's Domestic Policy Council met on April 1, 1987, to figure out how the president could have a more robust response to AIDS, framed within the positions of his most conservative advisors, Secretary of Education William Bennett and domestic policy advisor Gary Bauer, on how AIDS should be handled. From discussions in this meeting, Reagan launched his AIDS commission on May 1, 1987.[19] On May 7, 1987, amid this growing pressure, the US Senate began debate on the appropriations bill that had recently been sent to the Senate by the House of Representatives. Included in the act was an emergency provision to provide $30 million in funding to those with AIDS who had volunteered to participate in clinical trials for the drug AZT and who were too poor to afford to continue to take the medication now that it was approved and on the market. On May 21, 1987, Helms proposed Amendment 212 to the act, which attached a contingency to the emergency funds, namely that they could be released "provided, that none of the funds appropriated under this heading shall be available for use in any state, the District of Columbia, or any territory of the United States unless such state, district, or territory requires, as a condition for the granting of a marriage license, testing negatively for infection with the Human Immunodeficiency Virus: provided, further, that Section 212(a)(6) of the Immigration and Nationality Act is amended by inserting before the semicolon at the end thereof of the following: 'or who test positively for infection with the Human Immunodeficiency Virus.'"[20] This language in the second part mirrored that proposed by the PHS.

Helms's amendment sparked impassioned debate with senators from across the political spectrum offering their perspectives. The most notable challenger to Helms was Weicker, often regarded as the most liberal Republican in the Senate during the late 1980s. Weicker was generally considered an outlier in the Republican Party on issues of HIV/AIDS, and he was recognized as an important leader in bringing attention and funding to education, research, and prevention efforts. He disagreed strongly with those, like Helms and his allies in the Reagan administration such as Bennett and Bauer, who felt that testing was the only way to stop the spread of HIV. Just weeks before Helms introduced the amendment, the *New York Times* quoted Bennett and Bauer as advocating for premarital testing and testing of migrants. Also, on May 5, Reagan ally Representative William Dannemeyer (R-CA) introduced a piece of legislation in the House calling for mandatory testing of those seeking a marriage license, migrants, and select other groups.[21] Weicker, like Surgeon General C. Everett Koop, as well as most medical officials, regarded education on preventing infection as the best means of stopping its spread.[22] The CDC's consensus was in opposition to mandatory testing for those seeking marriage licenses or checked into hospitals, and even the PHS, which proposed the original HIV exclusion rule for migrants, held an official position against mandatory testing and in support of voluntary testing.[23] One way to explain this seeming contradiction is that the PHS opposed mandatory testing only for US citizens and likely only certain citizens at that.

COMMON SENSE

In addition to sharing opinions with the most conservative members of the Reagan administration, Helms drew from broader "commonsense" explanations put forth by the PHS, which centered only on immigration and not marriage licenses, and argued that given the existing list of excluded diseases, adding AIDS only made sense.[24] Helms located his commonsense approach in proximity to medical and scientific knowledge that affirmed his view. His rhetoric resonated with the PHS's justification of the original proposal in the supplementary information in the *Federal Register*, which stated, "It is proposed that AIDS be added to the list of dangerous contagious diseases since it would be anomalous to have diseases such as chancroid and lymphogranuloma venereum on such a list and not include AIDS. AIDS is added to the list because it is a recently defined sexually transmitted disease of significant public health importance."[25] By comparing AIDS with other diseases already in the exclusion list, Helms and the PHS's argument by analogy would seem only rational to many people due to existing fears about AIDS that people surely possessed in amounts far exceeding the ones they held for obscure diseases such as chancroid.

Within the context of political rhetoric, as Robert Ivie puts it, arguments make common sense when there is no other possible sense that can be made of evidence.[26] Helms worked diligently to ensure this would be the case.

Helms capitalized on existing discourses about migrants and disease as well as the cultural moment surrounding immigration resulting from the passage and implementation of IRCA. In his opening speech, Helms carefully maneuvered his commonsense rhetoric by selectively using scientific evidence and relying on guarded language so as not to make his common sense seem as if it was too aligned with particular moral or religious philosophies. For instance, he began, "The purpose of this amendment is to protect the general population against the spread of AIDS."[27] His use of the word "general" signals that his focus was not on those currently suffering from AIDS but rather on members of an imagined "general" population who were both innocent of the kinds of marginal lifestyles that presumably lead to contracting HIV/AIDS and at an abstracted risk of contracting it. Yet he kept his comments away from morally charged condemnations. In discussing the immigration amendment, he spoke only of the "citizenry" and the "American people" as a whole. This move shelters him from critics who might accuse him of turning AIDS into a moral concern.

Despite his frequent, virulent anti-gay rhetoric, in his speech, Helms did not directly mention homosexuality at all, only speaking of the increased rate of contraction among heterosexuals in contrast to the "established risk group," which he said everyone knew.[28] In addition to the shrouded homophobic rhetoric, as Jennifer Brier argues, "Neither Helms nor any of the amendment's supporters offered for the record stories of specific infected immigrants trying to enter the United States. Rather, they relied on descriptions of the African continent's ability to export the disease beyond its border to paint a picture of an imagined invasion threat for the nation."[29] The construction of "African AIDS" persisted during this time, rendering the entire continent "deviant."[30] To be sure, although Haitians were not visibly a part of the debates, their status as an original member of the "4-H" high-risk groups and long-standing fears of Haitian migration also informed Helms's claims.

Helms introduced both parts of his amendment and then noted that "there may be a great deal of argument about this amendment, but I cannot see why."[31] Here Helms began his strong appeal to common sense, focusing initially on the marriage component of his amendment. He stated, "Many States do not issue marriage licenses to individuals infected with rubella or syphilis. Common sense dictates that States should not do so for individuals who are infected with AIDS."[32] Drawing from a similar argument by analogy as used by the PHS in announcing the proposed ruling on immigration, Helms's claims of good and common sense could be seen as just that and in line with medical opinions. This point is affirmed as Helms cited statements and evidence from the PHS, the American Medical Association (AMA), and the CDC. None of these entities offered support for Helms's proposition in what he cited from them, as he cited statistics and projections about contraction of the disease only.[33] Nevertheless, Helms carefully located his argument in proximity to them to bolster his ethos. He then reminded the chamber that the American public was on his side. Citing several popular news polls about the beliefs on mandatory testing, Helms strengthened his claim of common sense for the marriage testing.

Helms used words like "simply," "fair enough," and "obvious" to describe his immigration proposal. He further compared AIDS to other excluded conditions, proclaiming, "I say again, what is the big deal? Why the opposition to adding AIDS to that already long list?"[34] Helms drew on a limited scientific and expert discourse to advocate his position as he cited the number of cases reported in the United States and worldwide as well as the number of infections predicted by Jonathan Mann, director of the World Health Organization's Special Program on AIDS. Helms followed the staggering statistics with a question: "Is this something to debate about?" He returned to the argument by analogy: "We are excluding individuals with infectious syphilis. This is in the law, and that is being done. In all candor, does it make any sense that we should not exclude—or, to put it more succinctly, forbid—the entry of individuals infected with the AIDS virus as well?"[35]

Ignoring the reality that most reported cases of HIV and AIDS existed in the United States, as well as the State Department predictions about the small number of people who would likely be excluded, Helms listed a series of facts that asked listeners to deduce their own conclusions about the obviousness of a need for exclusion. This point is best illustrated with the following: "It is only elementary that as the epidemic continues to spread abroad, immigrants in greater numbers will be bringing the AIDS virus to the United States. So my amendment, I think, simply makes common sense."[36] In referring to the statistical probability that with more infection abroad, more infected people will likely attempt to migrate, Helms's deductive argument was technically valid even if it ignored other important factors about the spread of HIV in the United States. Ignoring other factors is precisely the point, however, as he clearly aimed for his claim to be seen as the only possible conclusion. It is also possible that Helms referred to the increased likelihood of HIV-positive people migrating to the United States to take advantage of the US health care program, a claim that could not be corroborated.

The heated debate Helms initiated was the first major debate about AIDS to find its way to the full Senate floor.[37] Interestingly, none of the senators involved in the debate directly offered support for Helms's amendment. Several, including leading Republicans, stated their clear opposition to the amendment as proposed. Senators drew from a host of grounds for their arguments against the amendment, ranging from concerns over privacy, cost, and practical matters such as the reliability and feasibility of mandatory testing to concerns about the privileging of philosophy over science, discrimination, and driving at-risk people further underground. Several senators expressed worry, for instance, about how expensive mandatory testing would be both for garnering a marriage license and for immigration purposes.[38] More often than not, they primarily opposed the premarital testing, sometimes stating clearly their support for the immigration provision and other times implying such support.

Even for those who seemed most virulently opposed to this amendment, some important assumptions were present. Brier maintains, "Those who opposed the Helms amendment because of the marriage clause implicitly accepted and contributed to the idea that Africans posed the most serious risk to Americans, and in so doing imbued that risk with racial characteristics."[39] Moreover, those imagined as being entitled to the full benefits of legal US citizenship were included in the construct of the "American people" or the "public" that senators deployed as in need of protection. These claims actively participated in alienizing logic as others, whether "high-risk" groups, prisoners, or migrants, were not deemed part of the public that "public health" policies serve.[40] Thus, even when opponents such as Weicker insisted upon the problems with Helms's amendment, primarily on the basis of privileging science over philosophy, they shared certain parts of Helms's understanding of common sense—namely, a vision of who belongs to the nation-state and who should be protected.

NATIONAL COMMON SENSE

National common sense differs slightly from other more general conceptualizations of common sense. William F. Lewis articulates such a conceptualization, stating "reliance on a common understanding de-emphasizes objections based on claims to special knowledge or expertise. Common sense is so obvious to those who accept it that disagreement with its implications will often seem irrelevant, impractical, or unintelligible." Lewis continues, "Common sense establishes a transparent realism—a common sense statement is what everyone knows; a common sense judgment is what any sensible person would do."[41] Even in science controversies, John Lyne tells us, rhetors often make appeals to common sense.[42] Helms relied primarily on this traditional form of common sense to make his arguments. With national common sense, a rhetor appeals to and encourages judgments that "everyone" knows are best for the *nation*. As such, arguments relying upon and appealing to national common sense are deeply embedded in alienizing logic as they assume the two most important judgments that everyone will agree upon: the protection of national borders and the protection of the proper citizenry. National common sense is built from norms of racial, sexual, and cultural propriety.

During the debate, reliance on national common sense enabled an unlikely coalition with significant political impact. As I show, Weicker fundamentally disagreed with almost everything Helms rhetorically located in the realm of common sense, but their shared, though generally unstated, commitment to national common sense applied alienizing logic. In doing so, national common sense led to the scapegoating and exclusion of migrants and reinforced deeply conservative views about the importance of rigid national borders and the limits of belonging to a national community.

Weicker was the first senator to speak against Helms's amendment during the May 21 debates, and though he applauded Helms for bringing the issue to the floor, on the surface, the only thing Weicker shared with Helms was the following perspective: "Certainly, the threat of AIDS—the existence and the threat of AIDS—is the most severe crisis to be posed to this country in the lifetime of all of us, within and without this Chamber. I might add that that includes any armed conflict that occurred during that period of time."[43] Locating the AIDS crisis within national borders and making the comparison between AIDS and armed conflict (a metaphor common during this time period), Weicker implicitly equaled AIDS with a foreign enemy. Yet whereas he repeatedly characterized the positions of Reagan and Helms as "philosophical," meaning they argued from beliefs, not facts, he claimed his approach to containing and defeating that threat drew exclusively from the current science. Weicker indicted the divided approach of the Reagan administration as well as the amendment before the chamber when he stated, "Either we are going to go down the philosophical path or we are going to take the advice and the directions from the men and women of science."[44] Certainly, Helms emphasized popular opinion polls that strengthened his position, whereas Weicker stressed the scientific organizations. But Weicker clearly had no interest in completely separating the experts from the rest of the nation when he declared that "everyone in this Nation should take great pride in the rapidity of the discovery, isolating and cloning of the AIDS virus. Never before in the history of man [sic] has any Nation accomplished what was accomplished by our scientists and colleagues around the world in identifying, isolating, and cloning the AIDS virus."[45] Though mentioning "colleagues around the world," Weicker clearly imagined the advances made understanding the AIDS virus as US American accomplishments, with the pride belonging to all US Americans.

Reiterating that they were supposed to be debating an appropriations bill, Weicker then justified the original emergency funds, putting this expenditure in a long list of other expenditures already approved and crediting those monies and the fast response with prolonging and saving lives. He defended these responses as "traditional" and then proclaimed, "We have never asked people in the past, and we should not now ask, how did you get your disease. We never passed judgment on lifestyle or any other matter. If there has been a threat we have met it."[46] This utopian depiction of the US nation, as both heroic and traditional, partook in commonsense logic about the value of the nation and the valor of its inhabitants. Weicker also sought to confront the position of the most conservative wing of the Reagan administration that state and local governments should be the ones making decisions about AIDS policy. Weicker advocated for a unified national response to threats, no matter the content of those threats. Later in the speech, he extended the war metaphor, further locating AIDS as a foreign threat to the nation, explaining, "We faced that threat [World War II] as a nation. And we have to face this as a nation."[47]

One could argue that Weicker is the philosopher as he clearly did not provide an empirical account of the United States. His unspoken deployment of a national common sense that unifies the people through the language of tradition, and the invitation to the audience to imagine itself in the best light, only served as a premise with which to highlight how off-base and philosophical Helms and certain members of the Reagan administration really were. Weicker supported this through a return to science, insisting, "I do not rise to oppose the amendment of the distinguished Senator from North Carolina on the basis that I am a liberal and he is a conservative. That has absolutely no part in this debate. What has part in this debate is that every single credible scientific source opposes what the Senator from North Carolina is asking for."[48] Weicker's blending of a supposedly unified set of national values that engender the United States' traditional approach to threats with scientific discourse allowed him some important maneuverability. He could, on the one hand, utilize similar sources of invention as Helms and thereby connect with a general US American audience. On the other hand, he was still able to claim his primary grounding in science. The rhetorical maneuvering back and forth between these two lines of argument allowed an articulation with a version of "commonsense" discourse at the same time that Weicker disarticulated with the mere opinion and philosophy that he claimed informed Helms's amendment.

Although Weicker's appeals to this national common sense also manifested in the different ways he discussed the two specific components of Helms's amendment—marriage and immigration—he initially tried to ground his arguments only in scientific knowledge. In Weicker's discussion of the marriage license provision, he noted that one of the key concerns was that the tests available were not entirely accurate. This meant not only that some people would be given false positives but also that some would be given false negatives, which could give them a false sense of security. Weicker stated emphatically that no scientific or medical evidence existed to support mandatory testing for those seeking a marriage license. At first, Weicker stood firm in his position on the side of science.

When he came to the question of immigration, Weicker found himself unclear with how to reconcile the contradiction between the PHS's position and that of other scientific bodies. In fact, Weicker and other allies such as Senator Edward Kennedy (D-MA) repeatedly turned to testimony provided by CDC director Mason at a hearing of the Committee on Labor and Human Resources on May 15, 1987. Although Mason was unequivocally against testing for a marriage license and suggested "there are pluses and negatives" associated with the "terrible complexity" of whether to test migrants, it is important to remember that Mason was the PHS official who originally proposed making AIDS an excludable ground in 1985.[49] Because Helms aligned his commonsense argument with the PHS, this particular point made it hard for Weicker to stand so firm on the science as the PHS, a scientific entity, contradicted the position he took, even if others like the surgeon general did not.

In a back-and-forth with Senator John Danforth (R-MO), a conservative who was primarily concerned with the cost of providing money for medications and seemed to disbelieve scientific opinion about the accuracy of tests, Weicker returned to claims grounded in national common sense. Danforth called attention to the exorbitant costs of the $30 million emergency fund and wondered about the payoff, enacting a slippery slope argument that asked the Senate to imagine future costs that the government would be expected to incur once they make a commitment such as the one before them. Here Danforth signaled another dimension of national common sense that will be more significant in later debates: preserving the economic health of the nation. Danforth's insistent focus on costs, and his continual inflation of the numbers of infected people in order to lend credence to his claims, provoked Weicker to an impassioned discourse about the value of life and the problems with placing it in monetary terms. Here again, Weicker deployed a war metaphor, imploring his colleagues, "Yes, the business of life is expensive, not as expensive as the business of death. There are not many questions posed around here on that multibillion-dollar budget."[50] Weicker confronted the national commonsense argument about the importance of exercising economic prudence, showing how senators advocate economic restraint in selective ways. Several times over the course of this intense exchange, Weicker juxtaposed spending on HIV/AIDS with excessive spending on the military, naming it only as the "business of death." In building on his earlier claims about the United States' "traditional way" of affirming life, Weicker again drew on an unstated argument that articulated with a kind of national common sense. In this addition, spending on life should be more traditional than spending on death, particularly when the lives being debated were those imagined as a part of the US American citizenry.

Numerous senators, Republicans and Democrats alike, stated their opposition to Helms's amendment due to various concerns as mentioned above. After several senators offered their viewpoints, Danforth issued a point of order. He suggested that the original amendment to appropriate emergency funds for those who were on the clinical trial was legislation on an appropriations bill and therefore inappropriate. The presiding officer indicated that that point would lie. The effect of this would be that the point of order would also carry Helms's amendment, and as was revealed in debate, the original amendment would not be able to be reintroduced without substantial changes.[51] Killing both parts of the amendment together was a clear strategy on the part of Danforth who, as already shown, was skeptical about whether the original funds should be allocated. It is also possible, and both Helms and Weicker intimated, that Danforth issued the point of order to

protect senators from having to make a vote on either funding for HIV/
AIDS or mandatory testing, two polarizing issues among the US public.[52]

Weicker challenged the point of order, suggesting that the two parts
needed to be able to be treated separately. Others offered different suggestions for how to rectify the situation. Helms indicated he may very well
change his original amendment. When Weicker offered his closing statement, he repeatedly expressed his agreement with Helms to get a vote on
the amendment. This repeated agreement might seem like mere artifice,
but it foreshadowed the eventual agreement the two would share on issues
much bigger than whether a certain vote should take place or the importance of not tiptoeing away from the problem. Senator Don Nickles (R-OK)
intervened in Weicker's speech, asking him if he would agree to mandatory
testing for high-risk groups. Weicker responded, "Indeed, I have already
conceded part of the Senator's amendment is not that bad. The Public Health
Service itself feels that certain immigrants, the 530,000 that are asking for
permanent residence, should be tested."[53] Weicker followed his conditional
acceptance of the immigration exclusion with a procedural argument, stating, "But what we should not be doing, when all of this is in the works right
now, is taking this amendment on the whole, if you will, and sticking it on
the supplemental."[54] This statement was far from his earlier decrying of privileging philosophy over science. After conceding the point about immigration, Weicker concluded his speech with an impassioned plea to vote for the
$30 million in emergency funds for those in the nation. Weicker revealed
his ultimate concern, one that he shares with Helms and others: what makes
sense is protecting the nation's borders and the nation's proper citizenry—
even if their views on who is in the proper citizenry differ.

The entire debate on the amendment concluded with an agreement to
put aside the point of order and appeal in order to wait for the completion
of a private meeting between interested parties to see if an agreement
could be reached before returning to the Senate floor. The agreement had
already more or less been reached: Helms had indicated he was willing to
change his original amendment, which presumably meant dropping the
unpopular premarital testing piece, and Weicker had essentially conceded
the immigration exclusion, the provision his colleagues tacitly or overtly
supported.

After the closed-door meetings among interested parties, on May 29,
1987, Helms proposed a new amendment, number 248, which removed the
references to marriage licenses altogether. This new amendment read, "To
provide that none of the funds provided by the Act for the emergency

provision of drugs determined to prolong the life of individuals with Acquired Immune Deficiency Syndrome (AIDS) shall be obligated or expended after June 30, 1987, if on that date the President has not added human immunodeficiency virus infection to the list of dangerous contagious diseases contained in Title 42, Code of Federal Regulations."[55] The senator later changed the date to August 30 and then finally to August 31.

Just two days after Helms proposed this revised amendment, President Reagan delivered his first public address on his administration's policy on AIDS at a dinner on May 31 in honor of the American Foundation for AIDS Research (amfAR).[56] He gave the speech the night before the Third International AIDS Conference (IAC) opened in Washington, DC, at which Vice President George H. W. Bush was an opening speaker and booed by attendees for supporting Reagan's agenda.[57] More than three hundred people held a vigil for those who had died and protested the Reagan administration outside of the amfAR gathering. Jeff Levi, executive director of the National Gay and Lesbian Task Force (NGLTF) told the crowd, "I think it is more important to be memorializing all those who have died of AIDS . . . rather than validating a President who, so far at least, has failed to see the depth of this crisis."[58] The criticism carried inside the event too. Mathlide Krim, notable AIDS scientist and co-founder of amfAR, spoke before Reagan and called attention to the protestors: "Thousands of candles are flickering in the night outside this tent asking the question 'When?' The answer to those who stand outside depends on our national will."[59]

Despite Krim's veiled critique, Reagan started his speech focusing on money and much-needed medical science to advance research on HIV/AIDS, not mentioning that each year, Congress allocated more money for HIV/AIDS than the president requested.[60] He then talked about what needed to be done in the meantime before a vaccine would be found. The president stated his two-pronged approach: "Education is knowing how to adapt, to grow, to understand ourselves and the world around us. And values are how we guide ourselves through the decisions of life."[61] Reagan provided no concrete information about how the virus is spread, though he supplied extensive commentary on how society should treat people with AIDS and the obligations we have to ourselves and to others. He outlined the steps his administration had already taken or proposed at the federal level, including supporting some routine testing, adding AIDS to the list of contagious diseases in immigration law, and mandatory testing for federal prisoners. At the state level, he encouraged states to offer routine testing for those seeking a marriage license and those who visited an STD or drug abuse clinic.

He also encouraged mandatory testing in state and local prisons. The speech received criticism for failure to mention confidentiality among other concerns. An aid to California state senator David Roberti lamented the emphasis on the testing program "when, six years into the epidemic, we *still* don't have a massive education or prevention program in place."[62] Despite concerns, Reagan's speech paralleled the arguments presented in the May 21 Senate debate, including support for adding AIDS to the list of dangerous contagious diseases. With Reagan's public support, national common sense was codified in order to produce a seemingly unified position on the immigration ban.

With the marriage provision off the table, those proper US citizens seeking a marriage license were no longer targets for what Weicker viewed as unscientific, moralistic discrimination. Weicker had little ground upon which to defend against the immigration ban since his ultimate priority was the original $30 million emergency fund to help US citizens afford life-prolonging drugs, and continuing to argue against the ban might very well have led to those funds not being approved. His ground was further weakened since the science he trusted was conflicted on the point of the immigration ban. In the end, because Weicker premised so much of his argument on a rhetoric of national common sense he shared with conservatives like Reagan and Helms, even if he had hoped to protect migrant rights, it is clear that protecting migrant rights could not remain his concern. In alienizing logic, racialized migrants are an ultimate other to the nation.

Debate resumed in the Senate on June 2, as senators were then left to consider only the fate of migrants seeking to enter the United States and those who could pursue legalization through IRCA. Helms reintroduced his amendment, again noting its straightforwardness, and detailed how it was congruent with what the president outlined in his May 31 address. He also described it as "an incentive to help insure that the [PHS's] proposed rule adding HIV infection to the list of dangerous contagious diseases will be added to the list and will be added promptly."[63] Reinforcing the enduring nature of alienizing logic, he reminded the chamber that "The Federal Government has the obligation to protect its citizenry from foreigners emigrating [*sic*] to this country who carry deadly diseases which threaten the health and safety of U.S. citizens."[64] Helms repeatedly used words like "elementary," "logical," and "obvious" to describe his amendment.

Weicker began his response wondering why if the president has already indicated that AIDS will be added to the list of dangerous contagious diseases, an amendment of this sort should even be offered. He then again expressed his frustration that the appropriation of $30 million was still attached to whether the administration adds AIDS to the list of dangerous diseases. Helms quickly interrupted him, agreeing to detach the amendment from the emergency appropriations of $30 million to support those who participated in clinical trials. Weicker, in turn, agreed not to call a point of order against Helms's amendment for legislating on an appropriations bill, and thus Helms's new amendment read as follows: "On or before August 31, 1987, the President, pursuant to his existing power under section 212(a)(6) of the Immigration and Nationality Act, shall add human immunodeficiency virus infection to the list of dangerous contagious diseases contained in Title 42 of the Code of Federal Regulations."[65] Despite no connection to appropriations whatsoever, Danforth and others reluctantly agreed to allow the legislation on the appropriations bill even as some worried about the implications of doing so. Helms maintained the only reason he attached it to the emergency AIDS money in the first place was to make it appropriate in an appropriations bill. He also reiterated that he just wanted to provide support for what the PHS had recommended, to cajole the Senate into action, and to incentivize the president to follow through on his stated goals for AIDS policy.

Despite his impassioned opposition just over a week earlier, with the marriage license provisions and the appropriations contingency removed, Senator Weicker had little other than praise for Senator Helms's amendment and leadership. In his speech, he said, "In this Nation, when you hurt, we take care of you. If you are dying, we want you to live. We do not start making moral judgments or saying the judgment is up to God. The only judgment that we are concerned with on this floor is that which can bring relief to pain and from death, and that is something we have within our power with dollars going to science."[66] Turning completely away from the global significance of AIDS, the nation became the only unit worthy of protection, and the protection Weicker envisioned was the ultimate one: protection from certain death for which everyone held some responsibility.

In attempting to return to the values of the US American people, and the importance of letting the scientific voice reign, Weicker presumably imagined, at least in part, that he had been able to keep consistent with his original positions, seeming as if he had compromised rather than been compromised. Senator Bob Dole (R-KS) offered one of the few challenges to the new amendment on grounds of privacy and administrative bureaucracy.

This point was left to hang in the room as, in the end, a completely unified body of conservative and liberal senators approved the appropriations bill in a 96–0 vote, including Section 518, which added AIDS to the list of dangerous contagious diseases in immigration law.

A national common sense unified Weicker and Helms. This unity protects those already included in the bounds of citizenship and leaves those typically outside on the outside. As Antonio Gramsci has noted, common sense refers to the incoherent folklore and beliefs that characterize the conformity of a given people to the interests of the ruling class.[67] This understanding of common sense is useful because it locates it as a tool of hegemony and also recognizes its collective and contradictory dimensions.[68] As deployed by Weicker and affirmed by the Senate, national common sense that sets the bounds for who can belong and insists on protection of those who do is a classic example of a Gramscian understanding of common sense. No matter the international implications or the ethical concerns for non-citizens inside and outside the country, national common sense evades such considerations.

On June 30, in the House of Representatives, which assessed the conference report on the appropriations bill, only one representative, Representative Ted Weiss (D-NY), commented on Section 518, noting that it should apply only to those seeking entrance from the outside and not those currently eligible under IRCA.[69] No further comment was recorded. In June, the HHS published the final rule adopting its original proposal. By December 1987, the provision was in place, and it included those who sought legalization under IRCA. As N. Ordover argues, the impacts for already vulnerable people were devastating: HIV-positive undocumented people living in the United States could not regulate their status and were thus more likely to end up in detention. Ordover further contends that many did not seek health care due to fears of deportation and so often only showed up in emergency rooms once too sick to help. The ban affirmed alienizing logic as it "nurtured the age-old myth of the menacing, diseased alien." As Ordover claims, the ban promoted "a false sense of protection and of demarcation, suggesting that HIV is something 'outside' and we can keep it that way."[70]

Importantly, the bargain Weicker made with Helms opened the door for more coalescing with Helms that had dire consequences for all people in the United States, particularly the most impacted: queers and people of color. Just a few months later in October, Helms offered an amendment on another spending bill against funding any educational materials that promote homosexuality. That one, too, passed the Senate overwhelmingly. While there are no mentions of race or homosexuality in the debate over the immigration ban, as Helms upped his game, it became clear that the national common sense that animated Helms emerged not only from his concern about the spread of AIDS but also from his deeply held, conservative beliefs about sexuality, gender, and race. Importantly, the passage of the ban went virtually uncommented on in the gay press,[71] and I can find no record of any immediate protests of the ban. This would all change as the 1990 IAC approached, which is the subject of chapter 4.

THE 1990 IMMIGRATION ACT

In the years between the immigration ban and the passing of the Immigration Act of 1990, the federal government, now helmed by George H. W. Bush, faced pressure surrounding the ban and for its HIV/AIDS policies more generally. In the months following the approval of the ban, several public health officials lamented the decision as bad policy with some noting that there was no evidence to support mandatory testing as a preventative measure and others flat out calling it a "terrible idea."[72] In the summer of 1987, the presidential commission studied the issue. That summer Senator Kennedy also proposed the AIDS Federal Policy Act to create funds for counseling and testing and to protect the rights of those with HIV/AIDS, but a version of the bill was not passed until November 1988 in the Health Omnibus Programs Extension (HOPE) Act of 1988. This law instituted the National Commission on AIDS, which was designed to study, make recommendations for, and develop a national consensus on AIDS policy.[73]

As AIDS spread into the "general population" and new more palatable victims became visible, including Ryan White, a white, hemophiliac teenager from Indiana who contracted HIV from a blood transfusion, more people paid attention to the AIDS crisis as something impacting everyone. Organizers working on the immigration issue got occasional momentum. On February 9, 1990, a broad coalition of immigration, LGBTQ, and AIDS organizations coordinated by CIRRS in California was set to deliver testimony for a Senate Labor and Human Resources Committee hearing on INS HIV testing.[74] The hearing was eventually postponed and never rescheduled. The Bush administration was regularly under fire for inaction or improper action. In late February, police arrested a group of ACT UP members who protested INS offices after the agency denied the residency applications of two people living with HIV.[75] The same week, as international protests of US policy continued, the CDC told the Bush administration that only tuberculosis should remain on the list of diseases that could bar one from entering the United States.[76] Just two weeks later, the Food and Drug Administration (FDA) recommended that all Haitians be prevented from donating blood, a move prompting five thousand Haitians to protest outside an FDA office in Miami.[77]

Bush delivered his first address on AIDS to the National Leadership Coalition on AIDS on March 29, 1990, fourteen months into his presidency. In the speech, Bush insisted, "The transmission of HIV is as simple as it is deadly. In most cases, it's determined not by what you are but by what you do and by what you fail to do. Let me state clearly: People are placed at risk not by their demographics but by their deeds, by their behavior. And so, it is our duty to make certain that every American has the essential information needed to prevent the spread of HIV and AIDS, because while the ignorant may discriminate against AIDS, AIDS won't discriminate among the ignorant."[78] Bush avoided directly addressing race and sexuality and thereby ignored who was most impacted by HIV/AIDS. Race infused his speech, nonetheless. As Brier suggests, "While policy makers rarely spoke of race directly, images of people of color as sources of contagion suffused the public language spoken in Washington."[79] Bush praised the $3.5 billion that his administration asked Congress for to support research, treatment, and education and to protect civil rights. Despite his wordplay and seemingly anti-discriminatory stance, activists interrupted Bush wondering why he waited so long to talk about AIDS, and as media reported, activists were frustrated with the ongoing immigration ban. Police escorted out Urvashi Vaid of the NGLTF, an invited guest to the speech, after she disrupted Bush with a sign reading "Talk Is Cheap, AIDS Funding Is Not." She also lamented his failure to mention the immigration issue.[80] Other politicians like Representative Henry A. Waxman (D-CA) worried that his speech was nothing more than lip service.[81] One of the primary sources of pressure came from those wanting to attend the 1990 IAC, scheduled for San Francisco.[82]

Because Helms's amendment put the power of definition into the hands of Congress and not the HHS, activists and liberal politicians insisted that while the ban might not be immediately overturned, the power to define which diseases are grounds for exclusion needed to be shifted back into the hands of public health officials. As a concession to those protesting and boycotting the IAC, in April 1990, the Bush administration agreed to create a special "no-questions-asked" waiver and ten-day visas for those with HIV/AIDS attending relevant academic conferences in the United States, a move that replaced its previous waiver program announced in January that still required disclosure of HIV status.[83] Some advocates championed the new waiver, but others continued to decry it as divisive.[84] That same month, a group of AIDS activists with OUT! (Oppression Under Target!) chained themselves to the entrance of the INS headquarters in Washington in protest of the ongoing ban.[85] Two weeks later, activists from Stop AIDS Now or Else held simultaneous protests in Los Angeles and San Francisco by occupying INS offices to demand they "stop discrimination against people with AIDS or on the basis of sexual orientation."[86] Yet at the time, the Bush administration had not even supported a bill that would have given the HHS secretary the power to determine what should count as a dangerous contagious disease, even as the CDC already publicly recommended an end to the ban.[87] Also, in an internal memo from May 1990 to the HHS secretary, Louis Sullivan, Mason, assistant secretary for health, indicated that the department would propose legislation to repeal the law based on the opinions of medical experts, including two CDC committees, the AMA, the American Public Health Association, and seven national public health groups.[88]

Congress appeared to take up the question of the ban once and for all in the fall of 1990 as it passed the Immigration Act, and in the legislation, Congress returned the power to determine which diseases would be categorized as "communicable diseases of public health significance," the new category replacing "dangerous contagious disease," to the HHS secretary.[89] In the hearings and debates of the bill across 1989–90, there was little discussion of HIV/AIDS,[90] even though media reported that Republicans like Helms and Dannemeyer were "vocal opponents of moves to change the current policy."[91] Conservatives likely did not fight the legislation in Congress because the relevant provision only returned rightful power to the HHS and did not ask members to vote on whether they wanted HIV infection on the list.

Facing ongoing domestic and international pressure, in January of 1991, Secretary of HHS Sullivan announced that he would remove HIV infection from the list of excludable diseases, an action that was set to go into effect on the first of June.[92] The proposal was put into the Federal Register for a thirty-day public comment period, which was then extended for an additional sixty days.[93] AIDS, immigration, and gay and lesbian activists from around the country swung into action, urging supporters to participate in the public comment period.[94] The usual suspects expressed their dismay. Dannemeyer and sixty-six other Republican members of the House of Representatives sent a letter to Secretary Sullivan laying out their reasons for opposing the decision. The letter began, "We believe that the HIV carrier who is unaware of his infection poses the same public health risk as the carrier of an airborne communicable disease like tuberculosis."[95] This argument, premised on right-wing commonsense beliefs about homosexual sex, suggests that those engaging in unprotected gay sex (or sharing dirty needles) will spread their disease as if it is in the air.

The House Republicans were not worried about short-term visitors, which is curious since presumably people visiting the country might also engage in unprotected sex or drug use. The representatives addressed this point decrying the unfeasibility of testing tourists and visitors, noting that their interest was on migrants due to the economic cost, which they explained would be significant. Some medical officials like the AMA agreed that if there was a reason to ban HIV-positive migrants, it would be on economic grounds, but the AMA adamantly opposed restrictions on HIV-positive migrants.[96] This line of argument returned to the national commonsense idea of preserving the nation's economic health. The representatives drew on the AMA and premised this argument on future cost estimates based on the small number of migrants applying for legal status under the 1986 IRCA who tested positive for HIV and the average medical care cost of such a person over their lifetime.

The House Republicans' last argument against the proposal took a strange turn of logic. The letter stated, "The timing of the proposed change is curious in light of the acceptance by more and more medical organizations and public health officials of the importance of early diagnosis of HIV infection. They all agree that the earlier individuals know their serostatus, the better off we all are." This point is no doubt true, as medical officials insisted that managing HIV infection, for example, was easier than treating AIDS or opportunistic infections. However, they followed with this reasoning: "It goes without saying that those immigrants tested for the HIV infection and who are found positive should also be expelled. Because this proposed policy jettisons the requirements that immigrants be tested for HIV, it promotes ignorance rather than knowledge."[97] Clearly the "all" in "the better off we all are" does not include the well-being of migrants. The connection between the need for early diagnosis and the call to expel migrants who are HIV positive is unclear especially because it ignores the fact that by this time, public health officials virtually unanimously opposed all mandatory testing. The representatives further claimed that this action would then promote ignorance, presumably because migrants would not know if they were HIV positive. This claim, however, makes little sense given that Republicans like Dannemeyer repeatedly advocated against funding for education and focused only on the importance of mandatory testing and quarantine despite the best medical knowledge of the day consistently refuting the value of either.

Dannemeyer and his colleagues were not the only ones seeking to exert influence on the new policy. The PHS reportedly received between thirty-five thousand and forty thousand letters that opposed the proposal.[98] The *New York Times* stated that an anonymous health department official told the paper that an evangelical broadcaster apparently made this an issue on his program, particularly the issue of cost, and that because so many of the comments were so similar, he assumed they were generated from this call.[99] The NGLTF obtained a copy of a mailer from the Christian Action Network. The network, started by Martin Mawyer, a long-time affiliate of Jerry Falwell's Moral Majority, emerged upon the demise of the Moral Majority in 1990. It seeks "to protect America's religious and moral heritage through educational efforts."[100] The mailing, classic of the genre of anti-gay mailers throughout the 1980s and 90s, began, "Are there not enough homosexuals with AIDS in the United States that we now need to import more? That's exactly what's happening—more homosexuals, more AIDS, more death being brought to the United States—thanks to the liberals within the Department of Health and Human Services." The mailing went on to explain, in all capital letters, that the government is considering a proposal that would "ALLOW HOMOSEXUALS WITH AIDS TO FREELY ENTER OUR COUNTRY AND SPREAD THEIR DISEASE TO UNTOLD THOUSANDS MORE AMERICANS."[101] The language of the mailing echoed laments by other evangelicals within and outside of Congress.[102] It also reveals the pervasive logic that connects AIDS only with homosexuals and sees only "Americans," a category devoid of homosexuals, as worthy of protection from the dreaded disease. Although national commonsense arguments wane in the rhetoric of these debates, their presence remains in terms of which arguments would eventually win out—economic, anti-gay, and practicality.

Likely the most persuasive opponent of the new proposal was the Department of Justice (DOJ). The *New York Times* explained, "The Justice

Department says it is not trying to second-guess medical judgments by the Public Health Service. But it questions whether Dr. Sullivan adequately documented his conclusion that AIDS is not 'a communicable disease of public health significance.'"[103] Beyond this concern, apparently no one from the HHS consulted anyone from the DOJ even as that department was responsible for immigration laws. Although the White House encouraged Sullivan and Attorney General Dick Thornburgh to meet and come to a resolution, by the end of May, no such meeting had taken place. Sullivan defended his position and claimed that even without HIV infection on the list, many could still be barred if they were likely to become a "public charge" due to the high cost of their medical care. DOJ officials clapped back that it was not practical for an immigration officer to analyze a migrant's infection and health insurance and make a determination about whether they might become a public charge in the future. In late May, Sullivan announced the ban would remain for at least another sixty days while the HHS and DOJ worked out their differences.[104]

Again national organizers catalyzed their bases in order to win the end to the ban over the next sixty days. On May 30, 1991, ACT UP Golden Gate, CIRRS, San Francisco AIDS Foundation, Women's AIDS Network, and numerous other organizations held a press conference in front of INS offices denouncing the move and urging immediate action from the Bush administration.[105] On June 12, the AIDS Action Council issued a national action alert asking supporters to write to the CDC in support of Sullivan's original position to remove HIV from the list of excludable conditions.[106] Organizers planned several actions at INS offices throughout the country during June and July. In conjunction with Gay and Lesbian Freedom Day events around the country, ACT UP Golden Gate named June 26 a national day of action for protests at INS offices in different cities. A significant goal of these actions was to collect 150,000 postcards to send to the federal government in support of ending the ban.[107] Despite all of the efforts, in August, the Bush administration announced that while it would allow HIV-positive migrants who did not seek permanent residence to come to the United States, those who did would still be barred, clearly the best compromise the HHS and DOJ could reach. Those close to Sullivan shifted away from health-based arguments and toward an economic rationale. The move, and ongoing threats of boycott, prompted organizers of the Eighth IAC scheduled for Boston to announce they would move the conference to outside of the United States (see chapter 4).[108]

THE 1993 CODIFICATION

In September of 1991, Haitian's democratically elected president, Jean-Bertrand Aristide, was overthrown in a military coup, sending thousands of Haitians from Hispaniola into the sea fearing for their safety in the politically fraught and dangerous environment. The US Coast Guard began intercepting these people, sending most back to Haiti and sending many of those with a credible case as a political refugee to the US military base on Guantánamo Bay, Cuba, to be processed. While a small number of Haitians were processed and sent on to the United States to begin the process of filing for asylum, nearly three hundred of those who had a credible asylum case but who immigration officials claimed were HIV positive were kept on Guantánamo indefinitely as the US government tried to decide what to do with them due to the ban on HIV-positive migrants. Throughout the fall, attorneys for the detained Haitians began to file lawsuits against the government. Cheryl Little, an attorney for the Haitian Refugee Center, which filed a lawsuit, explained, "The Government is obliged to bring the Haitians quickly to shore after they are identified as potential refugees so that they can meet with their lawyers and begin their asylum claims. Asylum laws provide no mandate for HIV screening."[109] As the lawsuits made their way through the courts and more Haitians were processed, it seemed clear that no matter the legal precedent that Little mentioned, the HIV-positive Haitians were going to be stuck. Pundits and politicians regularly debated different dimensions of the Haitian migrant crisis, especially what to do with those who were HIV positive.[110] Congressional Democrats put forth a plan to issue a six-month moratorium on returning any Haitians to Haiti.[111] In late February 1992, the Bush administration told immigration authorities on Guantánamo that the Haitians would be required to file their asylum claims and go through the entire process while detained there, a moved denounced by asylum advocates.[112]

Around this time, AIDS activists who already had connections with the Haitian community, such as Black AIDS Mobilization (BAM!) in New York, began to focus serious attention on the Haitians' plight. Coalitions in defense of the Haitians began to emerge. Others in San Francisco, who were already utilizing the upcoming IAC as a reason to continue to push the immigration issue, also started publicly addressing the Haitians' plight. At a March 23, 1992, Resistance Haiti demonstration, Jorge Cortiñas explained why lesbians and gays were in solidarity with the detained Haitians, noting that immigration law has always been "stridently racist" and "staunchly homophobic."[113] Attorneys in New York City also reached out to ACT UP New York, encouraging them to draw attention to their cause. Thus, throughout 1992, various groups in the United States continued to keep the pressure on the immigration issue, pressure which is discussed more fully in chapters 4 and 5. The issue came up numerous times on the presidential campaign trail, and candidate Bill Clinton promised he would end the HIV ban.[114] This promise gave detained Haitians hope. Twenty-two-year-old Marie Jo Jeudy told a reporter, "I still believe he can change it. . . . A promise is a debt . . . and he's the one that made the promise . . . so if he doesn't change his mind, I'm staying here and dying."[115]

By early 1993, the issue was coming to a serious head in the United States. Pundits, politicians, lawyers, activists, and ordinary people decried the inhumanity of indefinitely imprisoning people seemingly for no reason other than their health status. Given the history of Haiti's successful slave rebellion and US-Haitian relations, their status as Black Haitians served as the unspoken grounds for their detention. The detained Haitians stated this plainly. In a letter to Jesse Jackson, detainee Elma Verdieu wrote, "We know the reason why we have been spending all this time here in this hell, Guantanamo. . . . Because we are Haitians and we are blacks."[116] Verdieu signaled the commonsense racism and economic arguments that always accompanied conversations about Haitians in the US public sphere. An editorial in the *Washington Post*, for example, lamented the ban but reminded readers of the stakes: "Immigrants, refugees and those granted political asylum become a permanent part of the American community and must be cared for. If, for example, the hundreds of HIV-positive Haitians now being detained at Guantanamo Bay are to be admitted, steps must be taken by the federal government—not the City of Miami, Dade County or the State of Florida, where they will probably reside—to provide for them. An assumption of this responsibility should be part of the president's new initiative."[117] Because by this time the medical and public health establishment's overwhelming agreement that the ban was bad public health policy was indisputable, the public had a better understanding of HIV/AIDS, and the increasing visibility and acceptance of gays and lesbians, the fear-based appeals and commonsense arguments that carried so much weight even two years earlier seemed to carry less weight at the dawn of the Clinton administration. Yet the *Washington Post* editorial reiterated the national commonsense argument about the economy: HIV-positive migrants will financially burden the US American people, and so Clinton must create a plan to support the Haitian migrants when he overturns the ban.

Debates raged on in the United States, but the Haitians trapped at Guantánamo Bay had already begun a hunger strike as a desperate but calculated effort to urge the US government to relieve their suffering. The camp president, twenty-seven-year-old Michel Vilsaint explained, "Even if the lawyers set a date for us to leave, we will not stop the strike. The immigration people have lied to us in the past."[118] Nevertheless, as the Haitians further languished, and the day after President Clinton's first State of the Union address, with a Democratic majority in the Senate, the US Senate voted to maintain the HIV ban, 76–23, including thirty-four Democrats. The Senate added the provision to the National Institutes of Health reauthorization bill, which was approved 93–4.[119] In March, the House followed suit, voting to accept the Senate's vote on the ban 356–58.[120] With a veto proof majority, Clinton's plans to overturn the ban were foiled, and it made bad political sense to pursue it further in his first months in office. One Haitian, Yolande Jean, responded directly: "Everything he says is a lie."[121] Furthermore, some claimed that many gay rights activists who had been among those pressing hardest for the overturn were no longer as prominent in their opposition, "preferring to concentrate on efforts to lift the ban on homosexuals in the armed forces."[122] Still, ACT UP chapters continued to work with Haitian solidarity committees, participating in a Haiti Solidarity Week in early February and a demonstration at the State Department later in the month.[123] Moreover, well-known activists such as Jesse Jackson and actress Susan Sarandon joined the cause.[124]

The Senate debate leading up to the vote on the ban featured different key players than the one six years earlier, but several of the same themes came to the fore. To be sure, it was not that Helms had forgotten the issue. Wary of Clinton's more liberal approach to AIDS, on January 20, 1993, the day of Clinton's inauguration, Helms introduced the "AIDS Control Act of 1993" in order "to control the spread of AIDS." Though Helms was the only sponsor, no media reported on it, and the bill never made it out of committee, pieces of the bill would show up in other legislation, including the provision that would have mandated that the president, regardless of the HHS secretary's view, return HIV infection to the list of "dangerous contagious diseases [sic]."[125] On February 16, the Senate began debate on S.1—The National Institutes of Health Revitalization Act, which included an extensive section on AIDS-related research that provoked broad discussion. Senator Alan Simpson (R-WY) spoke first on the HIV ban, and he provided the framing for the debate about the ban: "Is HIV infection a communicable disease of public health significance? And second, is a person who will develop AIDS likely to become a public charge?"[126] Simpson believed that the answer to both questions was "yes." He noted the incredible cost associated with AIDS over a lifetime and that while the US policy for waivers should be generous in terms of family reunification and conference attendance, the ban should remain.

The "public charge" exclusion has existed in immigration law since 1875 and is premised on the national commonsense idea that the US citizen taxpayer should not bear any economic responsibility for migrant health or welfare. This typically excluded those migrants who did not have traditional family support networks, especially women; those from "undesirable" countries of origin; and those in poor mental or physical health. Such a commonsense idea emerges from the deep structures and logics of capitalism that form the United States and the role of the family and traditional morality that uphold it. As Grace Kyungwon Hong writes in a slightly different context, "Family is a category of normativization for the citizen-as-capitalist, but *only* insofar as it is simultaneously a category of exploitation for the noncitizen immigrant and the racialized poor."[127] In this way, long before the turn to "family values" as an overt discourse during the first Bush administration, US citizens with a good nuclear family and strong moral values were central to the operation of capitalism. The dependence of men's productive labor in the paid workforce on women's unpaid reproductive and domestic labor, and the twin citizen responsibilities of protecting and reproducing the nation, put the good moral (white, citizen) family at the center of the capitalist formation and maintenance of the United States. The citizen-capitalist family has also long been the rationale for excluding and exploiting racialized and "immoral" alien citizens and migrant others on moral and economic grounds. Thus, in this debate, the deep alienizing logic coupled with the national common sense of protecting economic and moral health come to the fore.

Early in the discussions on February 17, Senator Nickles introduced Amendment 37 in order to define HIV as "a communicable disease of public health significance," have waivers for non-migrant travelers, and, outside of HIV, not limit the HHS to make regulations about communicable diseases.[128] Thus, Nickles's amendment, though less restrictive than Helms's amendment before it, similarly sought to put the power to define HIV as a significant communicable disease in the hands of Congress. Senator Kennedy immediately offered an amendment on the amendment. His would have kept the current list in place for sixty days (and later amended to ninety) in order to make time for a review of costs to the US health care system before letting the president and HHS secretary render a permanent decision, thus still participating in national commonsense rhetoric. Like Helms and Weicker in 1987, Nickles and Kennedy rose as the key antagonists in this debate. Although the two also seemingly disagreed on much and Kennedy directly questioned Nickles's motives throughout the debate, as Kennedy's amendment shows, the two actually shared the same primary concern: economic burden. Nickles just wanted to act quickly, whereas Kennedy advocated a delay in order to study the problem to assess the costs.

Nickles and his allies overtly supported the ban by arguing that the removal of the ban would come with an exorbitant price tag, and it would lead to more US Americans getting HIV. The worries beneath these arguments, however, absolutely reflected antipathy toward Haitian (and other Black) migrants, fears about the "homosexual agenda," and a concern about the further spread of HIV into the heterosexual community. Although Kennedy and his allies did not directly oppose the ban, their opposition to the amendment put them in the position of making arguments against the ban and its logic. Kennedy and his supporters questioned the inconsistency in ban supporters' positions on cost (e.g., why push people underground who will end up in emergency rooms?), threats to the public (e.g., why not ban visitors, too?), what it means to support the public (e.g., why not support comprehensive sex education?), and the necessity for the ban in the first place (e.g., the public charge provision already exists in immigration law; there is no public health rationale).[129]

Nickles introduced his amendment noting that lifting the ban would "cost lives." He then said, "It will cost hundreds of millions of dollars. It will overburden an already overburdened health care system, one we are having a very difficult time affording today."[130] Throughout the debate, Republican senators offered support for Nickles's amendment based on the question about costs. Senator Nancy Kassebaum (R-KS), a co-sponsor, noted that even though experts all agreed that there was not a public health reason to have such a ban, the potential costs justified why HIV-positive migrants should be banned via legislation. At different points, Senators Simpson, Orrin Hatch (R-UT), and Herb Kohl (D-WI) also offered support for Nickles's amendment, primarily on economic grounds. Simpson proclaimed, "At a time when health care costs are one of the most significant elements in our current economic crisis, a disease, which has such high medical costs, has to be of public health significance."[131] Near the end of the debate on February 18, Kohl asked, "Do we want to let people into this country who have illnesses that are prohibitively costly to our health care system—whether covered by medical assistance programs, or employer provided insurance?"[132] Kohl's reasoning faltered here, revealing that while costs are part of the rationale, there was something more significant motivating support for the ban. Why would one need to worry about banning people with employer-provided insurance given that they would likely not cost the government anything, and if a person lost their job and were not a US citizen, that person could be removed using the public charge provision? Clearly, cost concerns provided cover for the alienizing logic found in what must be a xenophobic position.

Because the ban supporters spent so much of their time on the question of cost, Kennedy insisted that fully understanding the cost implications required research. He also questioned why, if the issue was only cost and protecting the US American taxpayer, people with renal failure and cancer are allowed to migrate. Kennedy then offered a rationale for the seeming contradiction in the logic of the ban's supporters, remarking, "That is hogwash. All of us know what is happening out here. It is a similar kind of effort we saw last week in terms of gay bashing. We understand that."[133] Kennedy lambasted what he viewed as the political theatre of the Republicans advocating for the ban, noting that despite Republican alarm about "opening the floodgates" or sending "an invitation" to HIV-positive people globally, in general "one-tenth of 1 percent" of people who applied for immigration to the United States in previous years were found to be HIV positive. Kennedy proclaimed, "What the supporters of the Nickles amendment are saying— and we all know what they are saying here today—is you have 268 black Haitians in Guantanamo Bay. . . . The proponents of this amendment say, 'Send them back. Send them back. We do not care.'"[134] Kennedy shared concerns about costs, but here he pointed to the unstated premise beneath the Republicans' worry: the potential immigration of Black Haitian migrants with a deadly disease, without economic security, and some with child. The common sense of anti-Blackness that undergirds both US capitalism and the founding of the nation-state holds no space for Black welfare, only for the exploitation of Black labor.[135] Furthermore, Adam Geary notes "the absolute centrality of antiblack racism in structuring the conditions of emergence and mechanisms of dispersion of the AIDS epidemic," which heightens the stakes even more in applying this common sense.[136]

Despite his overt charge of racism against his Republican colleagues, Kennedy affirmed the importance of keeping certain people out. He reminded his interlocutors that the attorney general already had the power to exclude or return migrants deemed likely to become a public charge.

Although refugees would not be subject to public charge provisions since they flee political violence, Kennedy, whether intentionally, lumped the Haitian refugees into this category, subtly reinscribing the popular idea that only economic migrants flee Haiti. Furthermore, Kennedy insisted that the real threats to the health of the US American people are those illegally crossing the Mexico-US border.[137] Although Kennedy trafficked in racism, on its face, Kennedy was not participating in the same anti-Blackness of his colleagues. After submitting several letters from numerous experts, service providers, and activists against the HIV ban, Kennedy restated the problems with taking "an action that flies in the face of the best scientific information, as a means of responding to cost concerns."[138] Nickles, of course, refuted Kennedy: "I resent almost the undertone that this is a racist amendment because it is not." He continued, "This amendment is written because we want to protect the health of Americans. This amendment is written because we want to protect the taxpayers. It was not written to discriminate against any race."[139] Although twice in the debate Nickles compared people with HIV to diseased fruits and vegetables, Nickles insisted he had not paid attention to race at all with regard to his proposal, despite the presence of the Haitian crisis in the media.

Haiti was on the mind of others and continued to inform every aspect of the debate. Helms went on a screed against Haitians insisting that nearly 15 percent of the Haitian population was said to be HIV positive at the time and that Haitians refused to use normal immigration channels.[140] Senator Connie Mack (R-FL) was more measured, but in the final debate on February 18, he expressed concern about his home state and the Haitians' future: "Where will these people go once they achieve permanent resident status? According to the Congressional Research Service, some 64 percent of all Haitians who received permanent resident status in fiscal year 1991 expressed the intent to live in Florida."[141] Mack voiced worry about the economic burden without questioning the refugee status of the Haitians. But near the end of the debate on February 17, in a comment directed at Kennedy, Simpson supplied just such a concern:

> The Haitians at Guantanamo are awaiting admission as refugees. A refugee is a person fleeing persecution. . . . A person is not a refugee who simply does not like their country anymore, does not want to be drafted, does not like the economy but just wants out, or is frightened by something that happened in the political government within their district. That is not a refugee. Either we keep and stick with the UN

definition of refugee and the US definition—and that is what it is, but let us not make economic refugees political refugees. There is a difference.[142]

Almost uniformly, the United States government has refused refugee status to Haitians, long insisting—no matter the political conditions on its part of the island—that Haitians are all economic migrants.[143] Fashioning the Haitians imprisoned at Guantánamo as such then participates in this history in a way that offers a robust rationale for keeping the ban.

Other than Kennedy, Senator Dianne Feinstein (D-CA) was the only one to offer any defense of the imprisoned Haitians. During the February 18 debate, Feinstein lamented, "I never believed that I would find myself, standing on the floor, debating a policy which would keep in existence a detention camp, where people, who would otherwise be free, are kept behind barbed wire, quarantined without adequate health care until they die, solely because they have an incurable disease, which is not casually transmitted."[144] Senator Barbara Boxer (D-CA) also insisted that a politics of fear, division, and hate should not be the basis for health decisions.[145]

Although Congress writ large had repeatedly showed a lack of concern for US Americans with HIV as the primary victims were homosexuals and drug users—many Black and of color—the infamous "general population" was, in Nickles's view, increasingly at risk with the migration of HIV-positive people. Nickles explained the different strains of HIV that predominate in the United States versus in other countries. He was concerned about HIV 2 "being transmitted throughout the heterosexual community."[146] Although in 1987, homosexuality only operated enthymematically—as an unstated premise for claims—in the debates with the presence of popularized, presumably heterosexual victims such as Ryan White, Nickles could name his worries overtly. Others, including Dole, Trent Lott (R-MS), and Helms, echoed this concern about the heterosexual population. Lott was the first in the debate to comment in ways very reminiscent of Helms's use of national commonsense arguments in 1987. Referring to the fears his constituents expressed to him, Lott summarized, "'Are you serious? You are talking about opening up the floodgates and allowing people to come in as immigrants with a problem, a disease that is sexually communicable?' They do not understand that. I do not understand that."[147] A little bit later, Lott bolstered these justifications for the ban, proclaiming plainly the common sense of it: "The President stated the other night directly that what we need more of in Washington is common sense. Certainly I agree with that. The current policy which excludes people who have a communicable disease, of public health significance, is the most commonsense policy I have ever heard."[148] Part of what was up for debate was whether HIV/AIDS is a communicable disease of public health significance, but Lott took it as fact, which became the basis for his commonsense argument. This argument was all the more urgent because those who are part of the commons, the "general population," were visibly and palpably at risk.

In these debates, although heterosexual members of citizen-capitalist families were at risk, the risk still came from the recklessness of the badly behaved. Nickles repeatedly reminded other senators of the role of behavior in comments such as, "It is spread by having multiple sex partners, and it is spread through IV, or intravenous, use of drugs. This is in 90-some percent of the cases who are HIV positive."[149] Thus, while Nickles expressed worry about the health of heterosexual citizens, he once again showed that his real concern was about the morality of the nation. Helms made such a concern plain as he sounded off at the activists who by 1993 had been agitating against the government, cultural institutions, and pharmaceutical companies for years: "These AIDS activists are not satisfied with receiving merely fair treatment. They are constantly demanding special legal privileges and priority funding for their own specific programs."[150] The stakes were then laid out. Nickles and colleagues were concerned about the health *and morality* of heterosexual US American taxpayers, and Kennedy and others were concerned with fairness of policy, both in terms of who should be able to make health regulations and with regard to immigration policy. Other Democrats such as Feinstein expressed concern about driving people currently in the United States underground, and those people being the most affected. They also emphasized the need for more education. These feeble efforts opposing the ban aside, as in 1987, the alienizing logic of national commonsense arguments related to protecting the proper heterosexual citizenry and US borders, related to the health of the economy and anti-Blackness, won the day.

The Haitians on Guantánamo, many of whom still participated in the hunger strike while senators debated, would have no political chance to be released. They only found freedom when their legal cases resulted in their court-ordered release.

CONCLUSION

National common sense can easily be the grounds to render seemingly incommensurable positions commensurate in the name of the national interest. This chapter shows how alienizing logic became embedded in national common sense in ways that led to scapegoating and exclusion of migrants. This chapter implores us to discover a richer understanding of common sense to confront it in its multiple and subtle manifestations. Undoubtedly, the logic that rationalized the exclusion of one non-citizen group was already being simultaneously deployed to exclude and punish those that ostensibly should have been protected as citizens, as the previous chapter evidences. Although senators such as Weicker and Kennedy were less willing to sacrifice US citizens than were others such as Helms, they, too, relied on alienizing logic that had already long been used to exclude both citizens and non-citizens, revealing the risks of this national common sense. But as the next two chapters will show more clearly, migrants and citizens alike fought alienizing logic as it manifested in immigration law.

PART TWO

RESISTING ALIENIZING LOGIC

BOYCOTTS AND PROTESTS OF THE INTERNATIONAL AIDS CONFERENCES

HANS-PAUL VERHOEF, A DUTCH AIDS PREVENTION WORKER LIVING WITH AIDS, flew from Amsterdam to the United States on April 2, 1989, on his way to the National Lesbian and Gay Health Conference in San Francisco.[1] Customs officials at the Minneapolis–Saint Paul International Airport discovered the drug AZT in his baggage. When questioned about his possession of the antiretroviral medication, Verhoef admitted he had AIDS and was taken into Immigration and Naturalization Service (INS) custody. Verhoef was the first person to be detained under the then two-year-old regulation. INS spokesman Duke Austin noted that Verhoef should have applied for a waiver, but according to the *Washington Post*, Verhoef's doctor contacted the US embassy only to be told that the HIV ban was unenforced. Austin went on, "The fact is that he admitted to us that he is a carrier. Once he did that, we had no choice."[2] Although Austin does not say it directly, he implies that when it came to tourists and AIDS, INS used a version of a "don't ask, don't tell" policy. Presumably, if not for the presence of AZT in his bag, Verhoef would not have prompted questions, even though he came to the United States for an AIDS conference. Austin also seems to imply that if Verhoef had just lied, he could have avoided detention. But once engaged in a speech act of truth-telling, the INS's hands were tied. Verhoef remained in detention for five days, and INS denied him a waiver. AIDS activists from the AIDS Coalition to Unleash Power (ACT UP) as well as local groups in the twin cities protested and drew attention to the case. Immigration judge Robert Vinikoor overrode INS's denial and released

Verhoef under the following conditions: post a $10,000 bond (which he did thanks to the Minnesota AIDS Project), promise to leave within three weeks, and abstain from sex during his US stay.[3] Verhoef refused to promise abstinence but assured the judge he would practice "safe sex."[4] Verhoef made the conference in San Francisco, and he also used his new and brief fame to lobby elected officials about the problems with the law.

In the interim, lawmakers who overwhelmingly approved the HIV ban in 1987 now lamented the reach of the law. "At no time during the debate was there any discussion indicating that this policy was intended to bar entry of individuals visiting the United States," wrote Senator Alan Cranston (D-CA) in letters to Attorney General Dick Thornburgh and Secretary of State James Baker.[5] Scientists and AIDS activists worried about what would happen with the Fifth International AIDS Conference (IAC) in Montreal in June. Many would fly through the United States, and if the ban was now being enforced, those travelers could be detained. HIV-positive migrants living in the United States who wanted to attend the conference in Canada would also be at risk of not being able to return home. Scientists discussed introducing a resolution at the IAC to get the 1990 conference, scheduled for San Francisco, moved in accordance with the policy of the World Health Organization, which refused meetings in countries with HIV screening for travelers.[6] In May, INS officials announced that those HIV-positive people traveling to the United States for conferences, to visit relatives, or for medical treatment could be permitted with a thirty-day waiver.[7] Those in the AIDS community noted that this move was a step in the right direction but demanded the entire policy be thrown out, for travelers and migrants alike.

This chapter considers the rhetoric of boycotts and protests of the IACs between 1989 and 1992. The 1990 and 1992 conferences were scheduled to be held in the United States despite it banning the travel of HIV-positive people. The boycotts and protests of these conferences are important sites of rhetorical investigation because they represent a key instance of transnational coalition building that resisted the codification of alienizing logic in US immigration law. AIDS activists and other supporters who had focused extensive energies on the rights and needs of US citizens inside US borders turned their attention to international matters and building sustained transnational connections in order to fight HIV/AIDS and repressive governmental policies and save lives. This is a story of how a global coalition catalyzed the world to ban the United States. At the same time, an examination of the boycotts, threats of boycott, and subsequent protests reveals unique characteristics of boycott rhetoric and how boycotts connect with and compel other kinds of rhetorical movement strategies. In this chapter, I first discuss boycott as a rhetorical strategy and consider the dearth of scholarship about boycotts in the fields of rhetoric and communication. Next, I provide some context on the IACs and why boycotts were proposed and carried out by international public health officials, scientists, and government bodies. I then consider how the rhetoric of the boycotts catalyzed activist protests, particularly by groups such as ACT UP San Francisco/Golden Gate, the AIDS Coalition to Network, Organize and Win (ACT NOW), and the Coalition for Immigrant and Refugee Rights and Services (CIRRS).[8] The boycotts and protests opened space for scientists to move into the political realm as well as illuminated the significant differences in the ways people experienced HIV/AIDS across cultural and national contexts.

BOYCOTT AS STRATEGY

Phaedra C. Pezzullo notes the paucity of attention to boycotts within the fields of communication and cultural studies.[9] This dearth is somewhat surprising because boycotts, an example of what James C. Scott calls "weapons of the weak," hold such a significant place in US American protest history, and scholars have been immensely preoccupied with protests and movements.[10] A psychologist and leading social scientific thinker on consumer boycotts, Monroe Friedman notes, "It can be argued that the boycott has been used more than any other organizational technique to promote and protect the rights of the powerless and disenfranchised segments of society."[11] One reason for the lack of attention to the intricacies of boycotts as a rhetorical strategy has to do with a view of boycotts as primarily an economic activity. Even Pezzullo, who draws from Friedman, defines a boycott *campaign* as "a concerted refusal to spend money as well as to convince others to refuse to spend money on a product or service in the hopes of changing specific condition(s) or practice(s) of an institution."[12] Despite the emphasis on the economic, Pezzullo maintains that the importance of looking at these kinds of protest as rhetoric and communication scholars lies in how boycotts reveal the blurry lines between the economic and the cultural in order to effect political change.[13]

Some boycotts do not involve economic campaigns but may issue a call to action against particular kinds of non-economic participation. For example, oppositional parties who view an election as unfair may boycott that election in order to render it illegitimate.[14] Marginalized people may boycott practices of the powerful when they suspect that the aims of those in power are against the marginalized people's own interests, such as a 2003 boycott of the polio vaccine by numerous people in northern Nigeria. In that instance, not only did rumors exist that the vaccine would spread other disease, but many also wondered why Western doctors were so eager to vaccinate a population when routine health care was otherwise scarce.[15] They thus boycotted the vaccination. Scientific and academic boycotts involve researchers simply refusing to collaborate with scientists or institutions from a particular country due to the policies of that country's government.[16] Such boycotts have economic implications, but a lack of intellectual progress and humiliation are the main methods to incite change in policy or action. This last kind of boycott in particular raises another long-standing concern around boycotts as a strategy—the question of boycotts and freedom of speech—which has likely prevented rhetoric scholars from spending significant time with boycotts as a subject of study.

Some critics have argued that boycotts are inherently violators of free speech even though the 1982 Supreme Court case *NAACP v. Clairborne Hardware Co.* suggested that boycotts are protected by the First Amendment in that states cannot prohibit a peaceful boycott that has as its end goal political reform and not merely economic hardship.[17] Legal scholar Gordon M. Orloff vehemently disagrees with this view, arguing, "A political boycott is a coercive *mode* of expression that, regardless of its goals, deprives its victims of their freedom to speak and to associate as they please."[18] Orloff's definition of a political boycott here is actually economic as he describes it as the use of "economic coercion to force its victims to speak or act politically in a way that furthers the goals, not necessarily of the speaker, but of the boycotter."[19] His view is thus that boycotts are coercive, not expressive conduct, and in this way they not only limit free speech, but as coercive and not merely persuasive, boycotts become hard to categorize as communication or rhetoric.

Philosopher Claudia Mills defines a political boycott slightly differently than Orloff, noting that they may have economic implications, but they are primarily actions "targeted against a political entity, e.g., a nation or a state."[20] Although she understands there are very good strategic and even moral reasons to justify political boycotts, she notes that there is a risk that "boycotts not only fail to produce persuasion but actually work against the possibility of its production."[21] The American Association of University Professors has long held a position against academic boycotts for similar reasons, namely on the grounds that they "strike directly at the free exchange of ideas."[22] This position has been hotly debated since the 2005 call from members of Palestinian civil society for a boycott, divestment, and sanctions movement against the state of Israel. Opponents of the cultural and academic boycott of Israel offer arguments that are relevant to contextualizing the boycotts proposed in 1990 and 1992 against the IACs.

In making a case for the value of a universal principle of academic freedom, perhaps especially in relation to international politics, Ernst Benjamin writes, "The use of academic freedom to identify, publicize, and condemn human rights is a better course [than the tactic of boycott]. We believe that academic freedom is given us not so that we may deny it to some but so that we may encourage it for all."[23] Like Mills's view of all political boycotts, for Benjamin, an academic boycott denies others their right to academic freedom and therefore should be avoided because a proliferation of discourse is preferable. Such analysis does not fully take into account power differentials between those compelled to boycott and those who are its subjects. This view also holds the free exchange of ideas above all other values. Nick Reimer agrees with critics of boycotts on the grounds of free speech and academic freedom in one sense. He claims that all academic boycotts do "curtail the free flow of ideas by withdrawing from certain arenas of collaboration," but they do so usually with a goal of expanding academic freedom in the long run and in the name of a higher order of justice.[24]

On the other end of the spectrum are those who maintain that boycotts are central to democracy. Therese J. Lee insists that "the political boycott is a critical tool of petition."[25] Lee refers primarily to the political consumer boycott and says the case for boycott as a protected right is especially keen as money has been defined by the US Supreme Court as speech. For Lee, the boycott has a leveling effect by which consumers are put on more of a balanced playing field with producers.

The case of Palestine/Israel is again instructive when speaking particularly about academic and cultural boycotts. Steven Salaita, a former university professor fired from a tenured position at the University of Illinois for his pro-Palestinian activism and social media messages, also brings forth the question of power. He notes that while boycotts are undoubtedly protected forms of speech, "It is impossible to speak, or be heard, with a set of impartial senses. Free speech, in both philosophy and practice, is attached to structures of power (seen and unseen, discernible and oblique, steady and unstable). Despite the state's professions of fairness and benevolence, free speech is never fixed or disinterested."[26] In other words, despite best attempts to apply freedom of speech or academic freedom universally, this application is always selective. Salaita uses the case of the Palestine academy to illustrate his point: "Palestinian students and professors experience forms of institutional repression that on US campuses are virtually unimaginable. For decades, universities in the West Bank and Gaza Strip have been bombed, invaded, looted, and closed for extended periods. Students, staff, and professors often can't make it to campus because of checkpoints and unexpected curfews. Their political activity is closely monitored."[27] Salaita and others like him thus note the double standard that undergirds blanket calls to academic freedom. Palestinians do not experience academic freedom because of the repressive government and military occupation of the state of Israel, thus calls against boycott in the name of free speech or academic freedom already function to uphold repression for some people who do not presently have access to such freedoms. Salaita's points also suggest that whether boycotts coercively suppress free speech or academic freedom in the name of a higher order of justice, or whether they are actually protected forms of expressive conduct, they are a site of rhetorical production: the calls to boycott, the discourse that surrounds such calls, the opposition to such calls, and rhetoric that results from boycott activity.

The boycott of the 1990 IAC and the threat to boycott the 1992 conference help illustrate some of the rhetorical dimensions of boycotts. These boycotts did not rely on economic pressure to incite change; instead, they relied on moral and political pressure, making rhetoric their central mechanism. Boycotters did not necessarily seek to hit program organizers or host cities in the pocketbooks; they withdrew their attendance and encouraged others to do so in order to pressure the United States to change its immigration laws. Moreover, in exploring activist rhetoric that questioned a boycott, encouraged one, and otherwise considered a boycott's merits, a fuller picture of what is at stake in a boycott and also what kinds of rhetoric a boycott can engender and inspire also becomes clearer.

LEADING TO BOYCOTT OF THE INTERNATIONAL AIDS CONFERENCE

The first IAC, hosted by the World Health Organization, the US Department of Health and Human Services (HHS), and other collaborators, drew two thousand participants to Atlanta, Georgia, in 1985. Just four years after public health and medical professionals first recognized the new disease, this collection, primarily composed of scientists and public health officials, dedicated itself to understanding HIV from a biomedical perspective and to finding a cure. In 1988, after three conferences and an increased complexity to the perspectives present at the conference, including sociologists, behaviorists, and people living with HIV, the International AIDS Society (IAS) was founded and tasked with running the conferences thereafter. In the midst of this time, and as discussed in the previous chapter, the US federal government also passed a ban on HIV-positive migrants wishing to come to the United States. AIDS activists in the United States also became increasingly organized and agitational in their approach. The IAS found itself in the middle of controversy as early as 1987 when activists expressed frustration with a lack of political leadership at the conference in Washington, DC.[28]

Before turning attention to the 1990 conference, it is important to briefly discuss what happened at the conference the year before because it helps to lay out what the stakes were, the positions taken, and some of the key actors. At the Montreal conference in 1989, the theme was "The Scientific and Social Challenge," which set the stage for how the event would transpire.[29] Twelve thousand people reportedly attended, and it was the first conference not just to address but emphasize the psychological impacts of HIV/AIDS, ethical and legal issues, economic concerns, and other social dimensions of the disease.[30] Some scientists cautiously embraced the new breadth of the conference. Prior to the conference, Anthony Fauci, head of the National Institute of Allergy and Infectious Diseases, reportedly said, "Social issues are very important and they should be an important part of the way we look at the meeting. My own concern is the size of the meeting."[31] While he and others worried about the feasibility of meaningful conversations given the number of people and breadth of topics at the conference, they also felt it was important for scientists to be face-to-face with people living with AIDS. Others such as Robert Gallo, a controversial figure and one of the scientists credited with discovering HIV, held very different views.[32] Gallo quipped, "I heard that one of the speaker topics here was women's rights. Well, if I want to go to a meeting on women's rights, I'll go."[33] Clearly, even the inclusion of a social perspective on the official agenda was off-putting to some. This comment is especially troubling given the ways that women were long excluded from AIDS research, including the ways AIDS often manifested in women being excluded from the definition of the disease.

Activists were not content with social issues simply being on the agenda. During the conference opening ceremony, between 150 and 300 activists primarily from ACT UP New York, but also AIDS ACTION NOW! of Toronto and Reaction SIDA of Montreal, occupied the stage and rows reserved for VIPs in order to protest inaction by their respective governments as well as the ban on HIV-positive travelers to the United States. Although Canada did not have a blanket ban like the United States—that is, people with HIV could enter—the Canadian government could legally exclude people sick with AIDS just like it could exclude other sick people.[34] Protestors chanted "shame," carried signs proclaiming, "The world is sick," and read a manifesto against discrimination and inaction, delaying the ceremony by more than an hour.[35] Activists planned alternative events during the entire week of the conference.[36] Several others infiltrated the conference throughout the week. Even though it cost $500 to attend, activists made several copies of the badge of one "Mr. Gestos," so they could freely move about the conference.[37] Some simply attended the sessions, while others heckled prominent speakers, including Canadian prime minister Brian Mulroney, Zambian president Kenneth Kaunda, and New York City commissioner of health Stephen Joseph.[38] As one reporter put it, activists, particularly with ACT UP NY, "shifted the entire focus of the event to the trials and tribulations of people with AIDS."[39]

Although the HIV ban was not the only issue of concern for activists and other people living with AIDS, it was prominent. By the Friday of the conference, members passed a resolution calling on governments to end travel restrictions for HIV-positive people.[40] Politics had clearly infiltrated the conference. Still, for Fauci and others, the disruptions were too much, and there was an important line between social issues on the agenda and political activists disrupting it. By the end of the conference, Fauci told reporters, "If next year's AIDS conference is so intermingled like this one, with social aspects mixed in with pure science, you'll have a political convention, not a scientific meeting. Scientists simply won't come."[41] Fauci's comments reflect the tensions between scientists and activists that would characterize the late 1980s and early 1990s. Whether Fauci meant his comments as a threat, a challenge, or simply an expression of his frustration, most scientists did not stop coming because of the political nature of the IAC. In fact, the events at the Montreal conference ensured that political perspectives would always be part of the conversation.

THE 1990 SAN FRANCISCO INTERNATIONAL AIDS CONFERENCE

Due to continued pressure from activists and, in this instance, the fact that they generally agreed with activists on the problems with the HIV bans, physicians and scientists were also developing political savvy. For example, Robert M. Wachter, who was then an assistant professor of medicine at the University of California, San Francisco, and San Francisco General Hospital and the program director of the 1990 conference, wrote in his 1991 memoir, *The Fragile Coalition: Scientists, Activists, and AIDS*, about the kinds of decisions scientists found themselves making in order to respond to, accommodate, or sometimes placate activists.[42] Such decisions included carefully planning the order of events at the conference in order to manage disruptions and calculating the manner in which they issued invitations to speakers and then publicizing rejections before the conference to minimize activist ire.

Yet it was clear that the scientists and public health officials organizing these events did not always fully grasp the importance of including political perspectives and those of people living with HIV. This lack of understanding extended far beyond the question in relation to the IACs. As Deborah B. Gould shows in her extensive history of ACT UP, the failures of scientists and politicians to act on behalf of the humanity of people living with AIDS was a significant catalyst to the creation of ACT UP and the necessity for a confrontational, spectacular approach to making demands.[43] Ordinary democratic means of change-making were not only largely unavailable to the people most impacted by AIDS, but the rapid rate in which people were dying required a more immediate response than such channels generally provide, even under the best of circumstances. And as a general rule, scientists rarely if ever consulted the people impacted by their research. So even as it was becoming clear that politics and the voices of people impacted by research would be present from this point on, activists would have to insist upon the meaning that presence would have.

At the 1986 conference in Paris, San Francisco was chosen as the host for the 1990 conference.[44] Given both the city's role as epicenter for the disease and also its unique community-based approach to responding to the disease, San Francisco was a seemingly ideal choice to host. Because HIV-positive, non-US citizens would no longer be allowed to travel to the United States to attend the conference, this severely limited who would be able to participate in the important conversations scheduled. The question of the ban apparently did not come up quickly enough, or perhaps organizers believed that the ban would be lifted beforehand. As a result, the IAS did not move the 1990 conference on the grounds that there was too little time to do so.[45]

Because of the ban, immigration officials regularly questioned people about their HIV status upon entering the United States, although doing so inconsistently. If an HIV-positive person applied for a visa to travel to the United States, they had to declare their HIV status and apply for a waiver. If they were to receive a thirty-day waiver (which was not guaranteed), then their status would be indicated on their passport, and the details would be filed at the US embassy in their home country.[46] In April 1989, San Francisco health commissioner James Foster announced that he would be asking the commission to withdraw its sponsorship of the conference.[47] Due to this policy, in November, more organizations began announcing their intent to boycott the conference. The Geneva-based League of Red Cross and Red Crescent Societies was one of the first to call for a boycott of the conference due to US immigration law.[48] Others announced around the same time. The UK AIDS Consortium for the Third World advised all of its thirty-two member organizations not to attend.[49] It is important to note that these first calls did not come from activists in the United States but rather from an international cadre of service providers, public health officials, and scientists. This fact is significant because their calls to boycott were not intended to be political; instead, because the importance of including people living with HIV/AIDS had already been established, they withdrew attendance in order to advocate for those most impacted by HIV/AIDS.

This overarching intention is clear in the variety of stated reasons organizations offered for their support of the boycott and opposition to the US policy. The National Commission on AIDS argued that the policy "unfairly discriminates against people who know they have AIDS, while thousands who may be ignorant of their infection are permitted to enter without question."[50] The commission chair, June E. Osborn, went on that the policy also implies that HIV and AIDS are "a general threat" as opposed to an infection with restricted modes of transmission. Sue Lucas, the UK AIDS consortium's secretary, noted that the procedure people would be required to follow if they wanted to come to the United States for the conference "clearly compromises the confidentiality of HIV positive people and people with Aids [sic], and could be particularly serious for nationals of countries where the Government suppresses the rights of people who are HIV positive. By offering sponsorship to help people to attend the conference, the agency may be putting an individual into the position of either identifying his or herself as HIV positive or breaking the law."[51] The National Association of People With AIDS also withdrew its participation based on concerns about confidentiality.[52] The Canadian AIDS Society echoed this critique noting that the policy could lead to discriminatory treatment for anyone whose name was entered into such a database.[53] At least initially, these boycotters were concerned only or primarily with the travel restrictions and said little about the broader immigration ban.[54]

The threat of boycott put additional pressure on the IAS, which, at least rhetorically, actively opposed the entire ban. The IAS campaigned President George H. W. Bush to overturn the ban. In return for its efforts, in April, just two months before the conference, the IAS secured ten-day waivers for all HIV-positive delegates to attend this conference and all subsequent "White House-approved scientific or professional" AIDS-related conferences to be held in the United States. This visa differed from the thirty-day waiver in that it was shorter, specific to professional meetings, and did not require a passport stamp.[55] The administration charged HHS secretary Louis Sullivan with determining which conferences were "in the public interest" and therefore qualified for the special visas. The ban on HIV-positive migrants stood. The IAS's decision to continue with the conference anyway signaled to many its complicity with flawed US laws. In the eyes of many would-be participants, the government's waivers did not address the larger problem with the restrictions, which stigmatized and discriminated and could function to drive HIV-positive people underground.[56] Furthermore, the waivers created a distinction between temporary travelers and individuals seeking long-term immigration status, and many accused the government of making that distinction in order to weaken the links among all those opposed to US policy. Others accused organizers of the IAC of being similarly complicit in this governmental concession by willfully separating the "travel" and "immigration" issues.

IAC organizers likely did lack political will in tackling the issue of the immigration ban. In the conference program, organizers noted their "extensive" work with the US government "to eliminate all restrictions on travel by HIV-infected individuals" and promised continuing steps toward eliminating them. Conference organizers also stated, "The conference believes that US policy restricting entry of HIV-infected individuals is discriminatory, unjustified by medical knowledge regarding transmission of HIV, and counterproductive to the goal of identifying solutions to the AIDS pandemic. HIV-infected persons have important contributions to make to the success of the Sixth International Conference on AIDS. Accordingly, the Conference has established many programs to encourage the participation of HIV-infected individuals in all aspects of its program."[57] This statement is telling in a number of ways. First, the statement repeatedly emphasizes the word "travel," avoiding the word "immigration." Travel is, of course, the dimension that most directly impacts the ability of the conference to happen, but it was also what the US government was willing to compromise on. Second, while lauding the conference's abstract efforts to change US law, the only specific action the conference claimed to have taken in reaction to the controversy was to include more HIV-infected people on its program. No doubt activists had demanded this step for years, but it was not a direct response to the present controversy around the immigration ban.

Although the responsibility was not solely with the IAC organizers to pressure the US government, others felt left with little other choice. Thus, numerous countries and individuals as well as 130 groups and organizations from around the world chose to boycott the conference.[58] While some conference organizers suggested that attendance and registration at the conference was not much affected by the boycott, others maintained that up to one thousand possible delegates participated in the boycott.[59] Some put the numbers as high as two thousand to three thousand people not registering who otherwise would have.[60] Regardless of the actual number of participants in attendance, significant organizations and actors in global discussions on HIV/AIDS boycotted the conference, including the countries of France, Canada, Great Britain, Norway, Sweden, and Switzerland; the European Parliament; the international League of Red Cross and Red Crescent Societies; the British Medical Association; Oxfam; the Canadian AIDS Society; and the British, Canadian, French, and Norwegian Red Cross societies.[61] Boycotters did not make this decision lightly given that they were left with a terrible choice: either tacitly support or endorse the US law that had potentially deadly implications for HIV-positive people or risk the lives of people living with HIV and AIDS by not participating in this crucial exchange of scientific ideas about the disease. In taking the principled stance to boycott the conference, boycotters hoped to send a strong enough message to the United States and other governments that it was the governments and not the boycotters who would have blood on their hands. Life and death, after all, was the currency boycotters hoped would be persuasive.

As already suggested, many of the original boycotters were physicians, scientists, and service providers and so not readily identifiable as activists.

In fact, several activist groups did not join the boycott until the spring of 1990, but they were able to use the energy and media attention generated by the boycott to draw attention to the immigration issue, as well as others. Those involved in San Francisco's AIDS and immigration activist community with organizations like ACT UP San Francisco, ACT NOW, and CIRRS had a first protest in relation to the HIV ban in February 1990.[62] ACT UP announced a protest at the INS office for February 27 due to "the agency's denial of the applications for legal residence of two people with HIV infection."[63] The press release went on to explain that those HIV-positive people wanting to regularize their status under the 1986 Immigration Reform and Control Act had to apply for a waiver, and while three had been granted before, INS had now denied two for what ACT UP describes as "racist" and "ignorant" reasons. They thus organized the protest in which six members were arrested.[64] At the protest, a gay Mexican man named Jesus Reyes gave a speech, announcing he was under deportation proceedings because he had AIDS. In his speech, Reyes noted his presence was to show support for "this struggle against death,"[65] which was what was at stake with the immigration policy. The protest highlighted the inhumanity of INS policies, though it is unclear how much attention focused on the upcoming IAC.

By late March, activists had the conference on their radar and planned a nationwide phone zap for the national INS office in Washington, DC, in early April. The call to action proclaimed that people with AIDS were under attack by the INS. It also said that the current law and policies made the upcoming conference inaccessible. Among the demands on activists' list was an end to mandatory testing and waivers for all those migrants with HIV in the United States so that they could remain on humanitarian grounds.[66] National activists were encouraged to call the office, whereas local activists were asked to be present, with the call to action exclaiming, "While you harass inside, we'll harass outside!" Although activists had different demands impacting visitors and migrants, the call refused to divide the two into separate issues.

The first national zap against the INS paved the way for activist organizing for actions to take place at the conference itself. Throughout the spring, ACT UP SF and partners sent letters to announce the major INS protest to occur the day before the conference began on June 19, 1990. In English- and Spanish-language letters to national organizers, ACT UP SF publicized the protest and demands and asked for financial and physical support. They let recipients know of the widespread support already in place, including several national chapters of ACT NOW and AIDS activist groups in Amsterdam, Paris, London, Sydney, and Rio de Janeiro holding solidarity protests.[67] Furthermore, throughout the spring, partners such as the NAMES Project, which sponsors the AIDS Quilt, the National Gay and Lesbian Task Force, High Tech Gays, the People With AIDS (PWA) Health Group, and others joined the boycott. The NAMES Project said of its withdrawal, "We cannot in good conscience display the International AIDS Memorial Quilt at this very important international meeting knowing that memorial panels for those who died of AIDS may enter this country but those living with HIV/AIDS may not."[68] This statement is important because it shows the far reach of the boycott: the NAMES Project had far less radical politics than groups like ACT UP or ACT NOW.

Activists organized a series of events during the week of the conference, culminating in the Lesbian and Gay Freedom Day Parade on June 24. These events included workshops and a forum in the days leading up to the conference and marches and demonstrations during the conference targeting different issues each day.[69] On June 17, several key actors in the community spoke in a forum called "Speaking Across Borders." The speakers included communities directly targeted by alienizing logic, such as injection drug users, sex workers, migrants, prisoners, women, and people of color. The forum designed for both education and mobilization brought together a diverse group to bring a national and global perspective, with a specific focus on exclusionary border and immigration policies.[70] On June 18, community organizations held a press conference outside of the INS office to demand that the Bush administration "remove all travel and immigration restrictions against people with HIV infections."[71] The groups charged that despite Bush's longtime insistence that his office's hands were tied on this matter due to the conditions of the 1987 Helms amendment, the Office of the Comptroller General had, two weeks earlier, concluded that the president has complete control over which diseases are grounds for exclusion. They demanded that the INS stop denying waivers and the Bush administration take action. In addition to the press conference, ACT UP SF initiated an open letter to President Bush, co-signed by fourteen other organizations. The letter used the occasion of the conference as well as the widely held views of the public health community, including the Centers for Disease Control (CDC), against the restrictions to demand an end to the ban and an overturn of the thirty-five permanent residency application denials already made by the INS.[72]

On the day the conference kicked off, local activists again held massive protests. Protestors marched and chanted outside the Moscone building in San Francisco and staged media spectacles. The ban ignited these protests, but they also focused on issues like the speed of drug trials; homophobia and perceived arrogance among those in the scientific community; lack of attention to people of color, women, and injection drug users; and a US law that prevented homosexuals as well as HIV-positive people from legally migrating to the country.[73] The Immigration Act of 1990 overturned the ban on gay and lesbian migration later that year. Some international activists also planned protests during the conference. For example, a group of activists in Australia staged a demonstration at the US consulate in Sydney in order to draw attention to discriminatory US law and to show solidarity with the boycott and protest of the conference in San Francisco.[74] The significance of the boycott and the media coverage it attracted for several months helped to make the protests and actions more visible. Several official delegates of the conference reportedly gave their passes away to protestors who would then be able to get through security in order to attend (and disrupt) the closing session, specifically the speech of HHS secretary Sullivan, scheduled to be the last of the conference. What is interesting about activists' attendance at the conference is that some reports indicated that if you count the infiltrators inside and protestors outside the conference, several thousand more people participated in the conference than would have otherwise. While such participation cannot be attributed solely to the boycotts, the boycotts undoubtedly created rhetorical space and perhaps more importantly media attention that fostered activist participation.

Secretary Sullivan's closing ceremony speech is certainly reflective of increased participation. Sullivan, an African American biomedical researcher from Atlanta, served as president of Morehouse College's medical school prior to his post in the Bush administration as Bush's only Black appointee.[75] Like Bush had done for Reagan in 1987, Sullivan spoke as Bush's proxy at the conference. Sullivan's record on AIDS, like that of his boss, often drew ire, a fact that conference organizers acknowledged. Scheduled intentionally at the end because organizers knew Sullivan would be disrupted, his speech drew a huge crowd and was also one of the most widely covered actions that activists staged. In preparing for the conference, ACT UP LA called on people to "stand and turn your back on Sullivan and his meaningless rhetoric."[76] Targeting Sullivan was not without risk. A Sullivan aide allegedly informed activist and photojournalist Sheldon Ramsdell that "if Sullivan's speech would be disrupted, that ACT UP would be denounced as a 'racist group.'"[77]

Paul Volberding, a physician at San Francisco General Hospital who created there the first inpatient ward for people living with AIDS and Chair of the IAC, came to the stage to introduce the closing ceremony's last speaker, Secretary Sullivan. In his introduction, Volberding used the word "honorable" to describe Sullivan. Whether the official cue, activists immediately began groaning, and the sound steadily increased. Volberding waited for the audience to quiet, but it never did. Sullivan took the stage and calmly began his speech as planned. Protestors rushed the stage and played sirens, whistles, and horns. Protestors held signs and started chanting. For several minutes the proceedings were stalled as activists interrupted. Eventually the chants erupted into activists screaming "Shame! Shame!" and shaking their fists in unison at the stage. Others chanted slogans demanding action and threw crumpled paper and paper airplanes toward the stage.

Sullivan never lost his composure and only once addressed the protest in general stating, "Let us not turn our frustrations into theatre. . . . We cannot become symbols driven by slogans. Using the media as a proxy to provide high drama. We must find the compassion and the humanity to transcend misunderstanding, and yes even transcend hatred and violence. The truth of the matter is that we need each other, and that will always be so."[78] Sullivan's address to his angry audience reflected precisely the reasons for their anger. Speaking at a time when tens of thousands of people had already died in the United States while the government provided only minimal funds and moralistic recommendations for individual behavior changes and widespread testing, Sullivan reduced the coordinated protests to mere "theatre" and "high drama." His call for "compassion" and "humanity" in the face of the material conditions that literally plagued the United States and large parts of the world lacked compassion and ignored the humanity before him. His words remained largely inaudible over the crowd, and he continued his speech lauding the advancements and financial resources that the Bush administration was putting forth in the fight against AIDS.

Protestors clearly had an impact and brought scientists, even those who were unwilling, into political space. After the events, some scientists were quoted saying that they agreed that Sullivan deserved such treatment due to the discriminatory policies he supported and represented.[79] But backlash also ensued. As Gould shows, after the disruption, Sullivan referred to ACT UP members as "un-American," a "fringe group," and "adolescent" and said he would never meet with them.[80] Mainstream media also chastised activists for this action. The *New York Times* lead editorial on June 26, 1990, argued, "But for all their righteous rage, it's important for them to see that shouting down Dr. Sullivan is counterproductive. If ACT UP's members would only keep their faith in education and hard lobbying and put down their bullhorns, they might find their rage surprisingly well understood, and effective when focused in the right way on the right targets."[81] The *San Francisco Chronicle* followed suit in disparaging activists' lack of civility, paying little mind to the fact that civil democratic processes had achieved little for people living with AIDS.[82]

It is also important to mention that not all the activists involved shared beliefs about which strategies should be implemented. ACT UP NY's Larry Kramer wanted to riot.[83] ACT UP NY as a whole decided not to boycott and only protest. ACT UP NY member Tom Cunningham noted, "Not joining the boycott was a painful decision for us. . . . But we do need the opportunity to challenge AIDS researchers and the pharmaceutical companies. We will not be silent."[84] In this way, ACT UP NY members adopted a viewpoint similar to those who believe boycotts infringe on free speech. Despite disagreements, the boycott and disruptive protests clearly opened space for scientists to express political views they might not have otherwise expressed.

Many of those who chose to attend the conference wore red armbands, as recommended by the Bay Area Physicians for Human Rights to indicate solidarity with those who boycotted and in opposition to discriminatory laws. Other delegates prepared protest statements to be read before or during their scientific presentations.[85] Lars Olaf Kallings, a Swedish physician and founding president of the IAS, spoke in the closing ceremony. Kallings used his powerful platform to express frustration with discriminatory policy and showed at least superficial support for protestors.[86] In the middle of his speech, Kallings stated forcefully, "The IAS has concerned itself with the needs of infected persons and the protection of human rights, a corner stone for successful prevention of HIV infection. Prejudice and discrimination are hindrances to implementing intervention programs. It is shameful when unfounded discrimination is ennobled to law as is the case with travel restrictions instituted by several countries."[87] The crowd erupted in loud applause for several seconds at the frankness of Kallings's words. He went on, "The symbolic impact is even greater than the practical. How can we expect the private person to behave in a rational and responsible way to prevent HIV infection and/or to reject prejudice when states first set a bad example by instituting irrational laws and then, even worse, after realizing that the laws are unscientific and useless, through political bigotry, do not change them?" It is unclear whether Kallings meant to subtly chastise protestors or people who have contracted HIV for irrational and irresponsible behavior or both. But the crowd again erupted in applause for Kallings's words, which while not naming the US government directly, clearly targeted it.

Like some other scientific speakers, Kallings lamented the way that he believed politics obstructed scientific advancement and research. For example, Fauci, who just a month earlier was subject to a raucous protest by AIDS activists who stormed the Bethesda, Maryland, campus of the NIH with signs reading "NIH—Negligence, Incompetence, and Horror," made no mention of the ban or discriminatory governmental policy in his closing ceremony address.[88] In his brief political comments during an otherwise dense scientific speech, he instead insisted that while activists and scientists could and had worked together, it was unfair for activists to charge scientists and doctors with being uncaring or to call them names. Undoubtedly activists found it unfair that they had to resort to such tactics in order to influence conversations that were, for them, a matter of life and death. Unlike scientists such as Fauci, Kallings seemed more outraged by the politics being played by governments than those of activists. Kallings finished the political section of his speech, interwoven with applause and support from the audience:

> It is in this context that we so much regret the atmosphere, which has colored the preparation for this conference when the free exchange of scientific information is obstructed due to political reasons. However, at this moment, we should look forward and continue to push for travel restrictions to be rejected in all countries. I understand that due to the remarkable political changes towards openness and freedom in Eastern Europe, we may expect that the current travel restrictions for HIV infected persons will be discarded in some of these countries. Let us hope that such good examples will promote changes in other countries as well.[89]

The audience chuckled together at this point of the speech, recognizing the irony of countries that were recently part of the Soviet bloc now having freer and less discriminatory policies than the United States and Canada. Kallings again did not mention any country by name.

As Kallings went on, he became more explicit in his indictments:

> And let us hope that it will be possible to sponsor future International
> AIDS Conferences in North America. For the moment though, this is
> very uncertain. IAS has resolved that further IAS sponsored conferences
> will not be held in countries that restrict the entry of HIV-infected
> travelers. Therefore, IAS resolves to withdraw its sponsorship of the AIDS
> International Conference on AIDS in Boston if US immigration policy
> continues to restrict the travel of HIV-infected persons. And to discour-
> age IAS members and other concerned individuals from attending AIDS
> conferences in any foreign country whose official policies restrict the
> travel of HIV infected persons. This is also in accordance with the views
> expressed by the Boston organizers.

Although Kallings stuck to the more neutral term "travel," mentioning immigration only once and immigrants not at all, this forceful statement finally explicitly called out the United States. Kallings's careful maneuvering to this final indictment reflected the unease that scientists had with the influence of politics in public health matters, whether activist or governmental. Notably, Kallings did not directly mention the protestors or praise any of their actions for pushing the conversation about the ban or any other issue. Nevertheless, at least the immediate audience responded affirmatively to his message. And perhaps against his own intentions, Kallings's overt blending of science and politics by announcing the future intentions of the IAS not only affirmed the legitimacy of the boycott and protests of the Sixth IAC in the eyes of the major sponsoring organization, but it also indicated the legitimacy of further boycott should travel laws not change.

THREAT OF BOYCOTT AND PROTEST OF THE 1992
INTERNATIONAL AIDS CONFERENCE

Evidence of the impacts of the boycott and looming protests can be seen by looking at the fallout at the 1991 conference in Florence, Italy. Although Italy did not have restrictive HIV immigration policies, the occasion of the conference still highlighted that even though a smaller number, US and other HIV-positive immigrant delegates from countries with bans may not be able to attend for fear they may not be able to return home.[90] Furthermore, the 1992 conference was still set for Boston, sponsored by Harvard University's AIDS Institute, and activists and other boycotters alike wanted to either ensure that the US law would be changed or that the conference be moved once again. Thus, protests continued in Florence.[91]

Reports from the time suggest that conference organizers had given the US government until November 1, 1990, to overturn the ban on HIV-positive immigration.[92] President Bush did sign a new and far-reaching immigration bill into law in late November, and it includes a provision that shifted the decision for whether to exclude people from the hands of Congress (where it had been since 1987 thanks to an amendment by Senator Jesse Helms attached to the 1987 Supplemental Appropriations Bill; see chapter 3) to the HHS secretary. By this time, Secretary Sullivan, still a regular target of AIDS activists' efforts, had publicly stated that there was no public health reason to exclude HIV-positive people from immigrating to the United States. The Bush administration then planned to lift the ban on June 1, 1991, just weeks before the Florence conference began. As activists awaited the decision, they ignited a national phone zap for late May, asking supporters to contact Roger Porter, assistant to the president for economic and domestic policy, demanding that the administration "Keep partisan politics out of public health decisions."[93]

On May 30, 1991, a broad coalition of activists, public health officials, and service providers again held a protest in front of INS offices, reacting to news reports that the president was going to renege on his promise to overturn the ban. The coalition also issued another open letter to President Bush. In it, they called on Bush not to heed "the misguided hysteria of extremist demagogues" such as Jesse Helms and William Dannemeyer and to follow the guidance of all national public health leaders.[94] Over twenty diverse actors signed the letter, including Volberding, two California assemblymen, Catholic Charities, and community organizations supporting Latinos, Asian Pacific Islanders, American Indians, and others. In a fiery speech spoken directly to President Bush, activist Jorge Cortiñas insisted:

> Last year, community based organizations from around the world reacted to special visas giving HIV+ attendees of the AIDS conference permission to enter the US with disdain and continued their boycott. They recognized that it isn't about one conference anymore. It's about codified and legalized harassment and persecution of people with HIV. . . . Ten years into this epidemic and your administration still behaves like cavemen when it comes to public health policy. If your [sic] so goddamn interested in the cost to our medical system, then start distributing condoms in schools and prison and start exchanging dirty needles for clean ones and stop new infections and stop harassing immigrants.[95]

The anger and desperation in Cortiñas's speech is palpable. He called direct attention to the hypocrisy of continuing the ban on the grounds of public health and costs. But the efforts of such a diverse coalition would be for naught. Since the announcement in January that Bush would listen to public health officials and overturn the policy, conservatives around the country, influenced by Dannemcyer, galvanized a massive letter-writing campaign in support of the ban. The administration received over forty thousand mostly negative letters, which led Bush to decide to keep the ban in place, at least for another sixty days.[96]

On June 17, 1991, ACT UP SF, ACT UP Golden Gate, and Queer Nation released that sixteen AIDS activists were arrested that morning at the local INS office where they congregated to present a list of demands regarding immigration policy. They decried federal agents' donning of rubber gloves to take protestors away and that officers not only treated protestors brutally physically but also made AIDS-phobic and homophobic remarks. The action coincided with two days of global actions surrounding the Florence conference (June 16–21, 1991), threatening that if the next conference was not moved, "it would not be allowed to open."[97] This threat and the Bush administration's decision, even if only temporary, prompted Harvard's Max Essex, the chair of the Eighth IAC, to give his closing speech in Florence with the announcement that "there will be no conference in Boston unless all American travel and immigration restrictions against HIV-infected people are lifted by August 3rd." Finally, activists had compelled conference organizers to address both travel and immigration restrictions together. Still, Essex expressed his frustration with activists for threatening to close down the Boston conference if only the travel restrictions were lifted. He also chastised them: "I am grieved that the crass, domestic, American political agenda and the ultimatums I have received from activists have conspired in a bizarre alliance to deny the free exchange of information necessary to fight AIDS." Essex highlighted that uncomfortable position boycotters found themselves in electing to adopt this strategy. Furthermore, Essex reminded his audience that 95 percent of all new HIV infections are in the "third world"; thus, "We must not be so preoccupied by our own domestic policy problems that we close our minds to their pain and suffering."[98]

Although Essex reluctantly agreed to move the conference, assuming that activists would make good on their threats, he was clearly angry about being put in this position. He also, on the one hand, suggested here that his priority was the conference and the exchange of information over and against immigration restrictions while, on the other hand, showing concern for victims in the "third world." Essex's indictment of activists for essentially being privileged Americans seemed impervious to the fact that while ACT UP might have been the loudest voice, many of the activists of ACT UP who cared about this issue were migrants and, furthermore, that it was mostly migrants of color from those same "third world" places who were impacted by the US policy. Nevertheless, Essex drew a line in the sand, one that catalyzed activists into further action.

Keeping the pressure on, and continuing to use the occasion of the Florence conference, a broad coalition of activists again protested at INS on June 26.[99] The coalition also announced it would be working on its own postcard campaign, asking supporters to send in comments to the CDC by August 1.[100] A wide swath of people spoke at the rally, including Bob Nelson, chair of the San Francisco Interreligious Coalition on AIDS. In his speech, Nelson explained that since December 1989, most major religious groups in the United States as well as President Bush's bishop, the Right Reverend Edmond Browning, had signed on to a declaration that "included an article calling for non-discrimination in regards to HIV infection for anyone wishing to travel or establish residency in the United States." He went on to read from a statement of the AIDS National Interfaith Network from April 1990 decrying the policy, adding at the end, "Any such limitation of travel may be easily seen as racially motivated."[101] It is widely known that ACT UP chapters, perhaps most famously ACT UP NY, had antagonistic relationships with religious institutions. That the Bay Area groups readily included mainstream religious organizations in their coalitions, and that Cortiñas saw Nelson's speech important enough to include in his archives, is at least a small testament to the importance of religious groups in supporting this issue, particularly because religious groups had a call to support the stranger, often interpreted in contemporary times as migrants. Including religious groups in these actions likely reflected the long-standing relationship that many ACT UP members in the Bay Area had with religious people through organizing around Central American solidarity and sanctuary, which is what former ACT UP member Kate Raphael told me in a conversation we had in March 2018. In fact, according to Raphael, Central American solidarity work brought some to AIDS activism in the first place.

In response to the outpouring of public support for the existing law generated by the conservative campaign, and the Bush administration's June 1 decision, staff of the Harvard AIDS Institute issued statements urging people to contact the CDC to express outrage at the current law.[102] Throughout the summer, ACT UP also urged letters and postcards, hosted another phone zap on July 7, and held an additional speak-out event on July 20, 1991. By July 20, ACT UP reported having collected more than sixty-five thousand postcards against the restrictions to be delivered to Charles McCance, director of the Quarantine Division of the CDC.[103] In this comment period, AIDS activists far surpassed the number of postcards and letters that conservatives sent during the last comment period.[104] Still, in early August, the Bush administration announced that it was essentially keeping the ban: it would allow people to enter the country as long as they did not apply for permanent residence.[105]

After the announcement, activists penned a letter to the organizers of the Eighth IAC indicating that a Boston conference would be subject to direct action in order to stop the conference, "including a boycott (both physical and financial), non-participation and disruptive protests."[106] They invited other organizations to sign on, and within weeks, many did, including several international ACT UPs, the San Francisco AIDS Foundation, CIRRS, and the Gay Asian Pacific Alliance. In August, Britain threatened to again boycott the Eighth IAC if the HIV ban was not lifted, according to a letter sent by Secretary of State for Health William Waldegrave.[107] Organizers decided that the 1992 conference would not be held in Harvard but abroad. By September 1991, they decided to hold the conference in Amsterdam. Activists continued their efforts targeting the conference for while it was no longer held in the United States, HIV-positive migrants living in the United States still could face detention or deportation upon their return from traveling abroad to attend.

As the conference approached, the Immigration Working Group (IWG) of ACT UP Golden Gate and ACT UP SF led the international charge, using the attention focused on the Amsterdam conference as an opportunity to further put pressure on the US government. The IWG called July 19, 1992, a "Day Against Travel and Immigration Restrictions" to draw attention to the US policy.[108] Urging organizations to stage appropriate "high visibility actions" that the media could not ignore, the IWG suggested sites like INS offices but also "symbolic and real borders." In addition, members spent all spring writing letters to celebrities, world leaders, and global ACT UP chapters to gain more support and attention. These letters were addressed to leaders such as French president François Mitterrand and European member of Parliament Juan María Bandrés Molet and celebrities including Magic Johnson and Elizabeth Taylor.

Activists also sent letters to conference organizers, demanding time at the podium to focus specific attention on the US policy. Most specifically, they requested that Tomás Fábregas, an HIV-positive legal permanent resident in the United States from Spain, be the person with AIDS selected to speak at the opening ceremony, a request the conference organizers repeatedly did not approve. In a letter endorsed by more than forty-five international organizations, the IWG argued to the conference chair Jonathan Mann that activists felt stonewalled as they had no say in who was allowed to speak at the opening ceremony and were told that the decision to exclude Fábregas was due to time constraints.[109] The IWG insisted on the necessity of speakers selected by activists in order to represent people living with AIDS and the political perspective. Presumably, this letter also functioned as a threat to disrupt the ceremony, similar to how ACT UP disrupted the closing ceremony at the San Francisco conference and the opening ceremony at Montreal.

In typical ACT UP fashion, activists and organizers used creative, aesthetic, and outrageous means to draw international attention. One strategy involved showing copies of French citizen Fernand Beauval's passport. The HIV-positive Beauval had applied for a visa and a waiver for the 1990 conference, and so his passport included the special stamp US immigration officials used to designate HIV-positive status, a practice that later changed—most travelers had their HIV-positive waivers stamped on their passports until the 2000s.[110] In a March 25, 1992, letter, the IWG's Fábregas asked Beauval for his passport in order to visually compare the stamp required by the US government with red "J" stamps that Nazi Germany required on the passports of European Jewish people before and during WWII.[111] As with all Holocaust analogies, the comparison of HIV-positive people with victims of the Holocaust was to evidence the severity of the US law. This tactic was a familiar one, as ACT UP frequently deployed the "AIDS as genocide" frame.[112]

The centerpiece of the protest strategy in Amsterdam involved ACT UP's media work and its press conference to denounce US policy. These media events created one of the most memorable moments of the entire protest and opened up possibilities for hearers to make connections among and between countries, policies, and treatment of HIV-positive people. Before, during, and after the July conference, Fábregas dared US immigration authorities to detain and deport him as he sought to reenter US territory after attending the conference in Amsterdam. Fábregas played a crucial part in activism drawing attention to the US policy, building links between queer direct-action groups like ACT UP, predominantly gay non-profits like the San Francisco AIDS Foundation, and immigration advocacy groups such as CIRRS. Furthermore, he and the IWG, for which he was a leader, worked tirelessly to build international awareness of the US ban and, as mentioned, to gain support from major world leaders and celebrities through an extensive letter-writing campaign. Fábregas had a special fondness for actress and gay icon Elizabeth Taylor, who was an early supporter of the rights of HIV-positive people. Taylor eventually responded to his requests and spoke alongside him at a press conference that he encouraged her organization, the American Foundation for AIDS Research (amfAR), to host in Amsterdam during the 1992 conference. Taylor became a willing advocate for the cause, and at one point, she held up her passport for the camera to see and stated, "Imagine if I tested positive for HIV. . . . I'm sure the immigration people would be very courteous, and my travel arrangements back to England would be very comfortable. But back to England I would go. You see, I carry a British passport. . . . Would Mr. Bush really prevent me from returning to the US? Would he really keep me from my children?"[113] Taylor was a household name and a beloved star to many ordinary US Americans. Her whiteness, beautiful appearance, celebrity, and way of speaking English positioned her as an insider. Yet, in this statement, she uses her privileged position of belonging to challenge the contours of alienizing logic. She not only announces herself as migrant, but she also further locates herself on the outside, taking the subject position of someone with HIV and requiring her audience to imagine her as such.

Fábregas's remarks both at the press conference he coordinated along with Taylor on July 23, 1992, and upon his return to the United States on July 25 help to illustrate the way that the previous two years of boycott, protest, and threat of boycott enabled the possibility for transnational coalition building to resist alienizing logic. In his statements, Fábregas used the US national border both as a literal site and a metaphor for all borders, as a theatre in which to call for transnational coalition. In his Amsterdam statement, Fábregas began by suggesting he was merely there to offer his personal experience as "a person trapped by the dangerous and discriminatory HIV and immigration travel restrictions."[114] He personally spoke of those in the United States and how stressful the policy had been for him and his partner, but he did not look to make the occasion about him:

> We are joined by over four and one half million people of every national-
> ity who have been forced by the U.S. government to submit to HIV testing

when applying for residency in the United States of America. And we are joined by the seventeen million foreign born currently living throughout the U.S. who need to be reached, and can be reached, but are not being reached with the education and support of services we know are effective in preventing the transmission of HIV. I am one of them, and I can assure you that those seventeen million will not seek an HIV test if the result means possible deportation.

Here Fábregas noted the connection between all those who suffer under such policies, calling out the irony that these policies actually enable rather than prevent the spread of HIV, for people who can and should be reached are not being reached due to the policy.

But Fábregas did not intend to make his experience a stand-in for all others. He recognized his relative privilege: "I am here today. But I left many friends at home who cannot risk making their story known." Fábregas began by telling the story of another member of the ACT UP IWG, a Brazilian national who could not get his permanent residency approved because he contracted HIV (in the United States). Fábregas described the negative health impacts his friend experienced under the stress, but he again stopped, wishing not to make the experience of people in the United States a stand-in for all others. He explained, "African students who have earned the opportunity to pursue a university education in Europe are required by Belgium to be HIV tested and may be denied entry if they are HIV positive. Burma offers a harrowing example of the consequences of these restrictions. Young Burmese girls are working in the brothels of Thailand. They work until they contract HIV, at which point they are deported. In April of this year, 25 of these HIV positive women were turned over to the Burmese military who then injected them with cyanide. I wear this black arm band for them." One can and should point out the exoticism and orientalism that potentially undergirds Fábregas's Burma/Thailand example. It is the one that receives the most specific detail as a history and will likely strike listeners as the most horrific and unbelievable. In this way, one could, with relative ease, let Belgium and the United States off the hook for merely testing and banning. But an additional reading is also required here as Fábregas's use of this example functions in other ways. First, so-called first world countries like the United States and Belgium are implicated in the extreme example of Burma and Thailand as they are each presented as manifestations of similar policies and logics. Second, the example is not unreflexively harrowing—that is Fábregas's framing after all—and as a result it reveals the potential scale of the problem of fear of and discrimination against HIV-positive people, especially those already alienized: homosexuals and sex workers the world round. Although some in the United States may not feel bad for supposedly over-sexed US American homosexuals, the flipside of orientalism is a first world desire to save, as Gayatri Chakravorty Spivak famously put it, brown women from brown men. But in blurring the experiences and subjectivities among and between migrant gays in the United States, African students in Belgium, and Burmese sex workers in Thailand, Fábregas called those who heard his speech to understand the complex interrelatedness and impacts of HIV/AIDS for a transnational community.

Fábregas ended his Amsterdam statement by telling President Bush when and where his flight arrived back to the United States. Upon his arrival and wearing a "No Borders" T-shirt, Fábregas denounced US policy, even as he reentered the country without major incident. While his arrival speech focused entirely on the US policy, he repeated many of the same points from his speech two days prior. The US border became a site at which a broader coalition was possible, especially since the Bush administration refused to rise to Fábregas's challenge, evidencing not only what Fábregas referred to as the "moral repugnance" of the law but also the arbitrariness in which it was applied, an arbitrariness that in its constant threat likely led to the death of many.[115] In emphasizing this point, Fábregas signaled the need for a transnational coalition to fight AIDS but also to fight global discrimination since AIDS truly knows no borders, even as AIDS functions as a mechanism that determines which bodies can cross which borders when, why, and how.

CONCLUSION

In this chapter, I have emphasized boycott as a legitimate rhetorical strategy, one that both catalyzes other kinds of protest and rhetorical action and enables transnational coalitional possibilities. This chapter has shown not only the rich rhetorical life of boycotts themselves but also how boycotts work so forcefully to create rhetorical space that would not otherwise exist. This chapter also reveals the necessity for examining boycott campaigns that are not primarily asking consumers to use their economic power as a mode of persuasion. In this instance, a boycott that highlighted the threat of possible death through the withdrawal of participation in scientific and public health discourse aimed to send a powerful message.

By the early 1990s, boycott and other actions, as well as the global reach of the AIDS pandemic, had certainly led to many transnational networks, coalitions, and other kinds of relationships built out of necessity and fear in order to save and sustain lives. Both the boycott of the Sixth IAC and the onslaught of national policies that banned HIV-positive immigration leading up to it required nothing less than transnational cooperation not only among scientists but also among activists and others living with HIV/AIDS who demanded the human right to migration. Cooperation between activists and scientists also became essential. To be sure, this cooperation was always fraught, and the confrontational strategies of ACT UP and other direct-action AIDS activists were by this time under regular derision from all corners.[116] Nevertheless, this extended campaign evidences the ways that boycotts move people across national borders, political beliefs, and health status.

Still, while such actions facilitated transnational coalitions, the original boycott and the subsequent protests, zaps, letter-writing campaigns, and actions as well as the threat of a second boycott of the Eighth IAC did not persuade the US government to change its position on HIV-positive migrants. As discussed in chapter 3, by 1993, despite campaign promises to the contrary, President Bill Clinton signed the ban permanently into law, a law that stood until 2010. The IAC only returned to the United States in 2012, after a twenty-two-year hiatus due to US policy. This "failure" must be contextualized though, for as Gould maintains, movements are about more than their political objectives. She argues that ACT UP "was a place to elaborate critiques of the status quo, to imagine alternative worlds, to express anger, to defy authority, to form sexual and other intimacies, to practice non-hierarchical governance and self-determination, to argue with one another, to refashion identities, to experience new feelings, to be changed."[117] These results cannot easily be studied rhetorically, but their significance should not be ignored. For example, in June 2015, several AIDS activists in San Francisco celebrated the twenty-fifth anniversary of the protests of the Sixth IAC. They brought back several who participated in and orchestrated the protests in order to commemorate the important events and educate a younger generation of queers about this significant time period.[118] So while the immediate impacts may have been mixed, the legacy of AIDS activism lives on.

Furthermore, the original boycotts and the related protests certainly inspired the movement created in the mid-2000s that eventually secured the law change. The Coalition to Lift the Bar started in 2006 by HIV, queer, and immigration advocates and activists to change the law. Many of the same arguments that boycotters and AIDS activists used twenty years earlier remained central to the coalition's work, which eventually, through tireless effort, succeeded.[119] N. Ordover, one of the founders of the coalition, reiterates one lesson activists learned well in the early years: "As queers set out a progressive agenda, our project must be about the reshuffling and restructuring of power. This won't happen unless we act to expand human rights, ensure the mobility of people and ideas (the kind of globalization the left can get behind), and expose the lunacy and treachery of borders. We cannot afford to be less ambitious than this." This is certainly a point AIDS activism on immigration reiterates over and over and one that remains relevant in thinking about globalization, transnationalism, and power.

CHAPTER 5

AIDS ACTIVIST MEDIA AND THE "HAITIAN CONNECTION"

> One thing I have noticed since the beginning of history is that white people have been trying to create another planet where they can put us in order to separate us. . . . I think they are trying to create that planet now, and they are starting with the Haitians.
>
> —TWENTY-EIGHT-YEAR-OLD ELMA VERDIEU,
> detained at Guantánamo Bay

JUST OUTSIDE THE FRONT DOORS OF THE IMMIGRATION AND Naturalization Service (INS) Varick Street Detention Center in Manhattan, a diverse group of twenty-five to thirty activists marched in a circle. They demanded the release of two HIV-positive Haitian migrants, Rigaud Milenette and Silieses Success, who, due to ailing health, had been sent from the US HIV detention camp on Guantánamo Bay, Cuba, to the INS detention center on Varick Street. Success's three-month-old son, Ricardo, had developed pneumonia on the base, which prompted officials to send Success and her son to the Walter Reed Military Hospital in the United States. After tiny Ricardo died, authorities promptly sent Success to Varick Street.[1] INS had determined that Milenette and Success qualified as political refugees, but due to discriminatory US policy, they remained detained. Opposing this indefinite detention, activists marched with homemade signs declaring, "Don't Jail People for Their HIV Status," "ACT UP lucha contra HIV borders," and "INS = Koupab."[2] They chanted in a cacophony of accents, "2-4-6-8 INS Discriminates" and "Hey hey, ho ho, send Bush to Guantánamo." Someone brought an effigy of President George H. W. Bush and placed it amid the protestors with a sign strapped to its neck: "Vote for me. I'm the concentration camp president. This self determination thing will not stand. (That's a promise—Ask Barb)."[3] Damned Interfering Video

Activists (DIVA) TV, an affinity group of the AIDS Coalition to Unleash Power (ACT UP), captured this October 30, 1992, protest and others like it in which US-based activists participated between late 1992 and mid-1993.[4] These agitations and actions in the United States amplified the ongoing protests of nearly three hundred Haitian refugees the US government detained on Guantánamo Bay after the September 1991 ousting of Haiti's democratically elected president Jean-Bertrand Aristide. The United States indefinitely detained the Haitians, who had credible fears of persecution in Haiti, on the basis of their alleged HIV-positive status.

Like so many of the protests against the ill treatment of people living with AIDS during the late 1980s and early 1990s, this one would have been lost in history if not for the efforts of AIDS activist media makers. Alternative media that emerges from marginalized groups about those groups have historically served many important functions, including as a voice for social movements.[5] This alternative media, produced largely by queer people about queer people, served numerous important functions at the time, specifically, as Roger Hallas puts it, "*contesting* the dominant representation of AIDS and *attesting* to the experience of people living with AIDS in the midst of this trauma."[6] AIDS activist media thus actively challenged alienizing logic that manifested in dominant media representations of people living with AIDS. As the protest documented above shows, even if most AIDS activist media makers were queer, what they produced had important implications for alienized communities who were not targeted for gay and lesbian identities, including Haitians. Within the US history of HIV/AIDS, the twin manifestations of alienizing logic in ban and quarantine converge in the treatment of Haitians. AIDS activist media makers resisted and documented this convergence.

AIDS activist media that extended beyond queer representation did not begin with the videos made as a result of the spectacular politics of groups like ACT UP. Well before ACT UP or the Guantánamo Bay detention, queer print media, particularly the *New York Native*, provided some of the most comprehensive reporting on AIDS issues available during the early years of the pandemic, arguably defining the genre of AIDS activist print media.[7] Such a characterization is not without controversy. For example, as the Black gay writer Melvin Dixon charged, "Few men of color will ever be found on the covers of the *Advocate* or *New York Native*."[8] Few writers of color wrote for the *Native*, for which I provide no excuse. Their reporters and representation reflect a broader problem in US news that scholars have called "the racialization of news," which describes the complex relationship between racism and news content.[9] Perhaps these facts about the paper make it even more surprising that the *Native* devoted extensive coverage to the so-called Haitian connection: Why were Haitians seemingly more susceptible to AIDS than other groups? Why was Haiti targeted as the origin of the disease? Unlike most mainstream publications, the *Native* relied heavily on Haitian voices and provided long-form reporting on the issues.

How mostly white, AIDS activist media makers challenged the alienizing logic of AIDS as it impacted Haitian communities is important for two key reasons. First, this activism was both complicit with and resistant to US policy and dominant representations of Haitians; thus, it ultimately offers an important example of the strengths and shortcomings of media as a mechanism for solidarity and coalition building among differently empowered people. Second, relying on the materials these activists produced allows us to tell a story about how alienizing logic impacted Haitians and how people resisted when few other primary source materials exist that can do so. AIDS activists like ACT UP, and their alternative media arms like DIVA TV, kept detailed records that other activists and groups who may have been involved in similar actions apparently did not, just like the *Native* reporters told stories from perspectives that other gay and English-language publications generally did not.[10]

In order to understand how AIDS activist media challenged the alienizing of Haitians from the beginning of AIDS in the United States through the release of the last of the Haitian migrants imprisoned on Guantánamo, I first discuss the connections explicitly made between Haitians and HIV/AIDS in the US public sphere during this time period and how the *Native* challenged dominant views. The second part of the chapter turns to six segments of James Wentzy's AIDS Community TV, which documented how AIDS activists protested the Haitian imprisonment at Guantánamo in ways that highlighted the voices of the detained migrants, pressured the US government, and assisted the team of lawyers who eventually argued the case and won the remaining detainees' release.

HAITI IN THE *NEW YORK NATIVE*

As stated in the introduction to this book, in 1982, the US Centers for Disease Control (CDC) first designated those at high risk for contracting AIDS. Those groups were colloquially called the "4-H Club": homosexual men, Haitians, hemophiliacs, and heroin users. The separate designation of Haitians proved highly controversial because they were the only national group originally marked at risk,[11] and Haiti was already maligned in the US public sphere as the supposed origin of AIDS, a claim disputed by experts such as Paul Farmer.[12] With the CDC designation, Haitian community and political groups, although acknowledging Haitians had been affected, denounced their singling out.[13] Haitians in both countries felt the impact of the stigmatization. Those in the United States faced rampant discrimination by employers, landlords, the media, and general public.[14] In Haiti, the once flourishing tourist industry was decimated by 1983.[15]

Although mainstream newspapers such as the *New York Times* occasionally reported on the plight of Haitians in relation to AIDS or the linkages among Haitians, Haiti, and the origins of the disease in the early years, the gay press, particularly the *New York Native* provided more comprehensive and consistent reporting. In his memoir, the *Native*'s controversial editor, Charles Ortleb, notes that he was willing to publish virtually anyone's perspective on the disease if he thought it might be helpful in finding a solution.[16] This permissive approach to information meant that in addition to publishing cutting-edge views, the *Native* also grated against the opinions of mainstream science and, in some cases, of radical activist groups like ACT UP, who tentatively trusted the scientific establishment's claims on AIDS. For example, the *Native* published controversial pieces questioning the links between HIV and AIDS, suggesting a cover up of the relationships between AIDS and chronic fatigue syndrome, and describing the early AIDS drug AZT as poison. Ortleb, an author and filmmaker, was also the publisher of *Christopher Street* and *TheaterWeek*, and to this day, he continues to challenge the establishment on AIDS and write screeds against people like National Institute of Allergy and Infectious Diseases director Anthony Fauci. Cultural critic Douglas Crimp noted that the *Native* was "perhaps the most acclaimed" information source on AIDS during the early years, but eventually, "Rather than performing a political analysis of the ideology of science, Ortleb merely touts the crackpot theory of the week, championing whoever is the latest outcast from the world of academic and government research."[17] Steven Epstein echoes this point, insisting that "Ortleb and his staff's efforts not only got New York state health officials to investigate the connection between ASFV and AIDS, but Ortleb's influence was such that James Mason flew to New York in early 1984 to try to reason with the *Native*'s publisher. Mason even gave Ortleb a scoop—two weeks before he spoke with the *New York Times*—about LAV being the probable cause of AIDS."[18] Although Ortleb did publish about

LAV and HTLV (the two names for the virus that was eventually called HIV), he did not want to be co-opted by government scientists. Such reporting eventually prompted ACT UP to boycott the *Native*; a loss of readers led the paper to fold in 1997.[19]

Nevertheless, when it came to Haiti, Haitian issues, and AIDS, this bimonthly gay paper published around twenty full-length pieces from 1982 to 1987, about the same number of pieces on these issues that the daily *New York Times* published in that time frame. The *Native* is important because it shows the connections that members of a mostly white US American gay community made with regard to another maligned group from the earliest days of the epidemic, even when overlaps between the groups were not always clear. This reporting also reveals the complexity of advocacy or activist journalism.[20] No other paper was more committed to putting out every bit of information regarding AIDS in the early years in an avowed effort to save lives, and even people who disliked the *Native*'s approach praised its diligence.[21] When it came to Haiti, that information was far more comprehensive than what mainstream papers produced, regularly featuring the voices of Haitian doctors and telling stories from ordinary Haitians in the United States and Haiti. Other times, and undoubtedly unintentionally, that information trafficked in some of the worst stereotypes about Haiti and Haitian people. The *Native*'s complex and affirmative reporting on Haiti is actually more surprising than its problematic reports for, as Robert Lawless argues, "most of the works on Haiti that the public reads are based on myths, most of which are, at best, uninformed and plagiaristic and, at worst, mean-spirited and narrow-minded. These myths are intimately connected with broader forms of racism against blacks by whites."[22] With this reality in mind, I now turn to the *Native*'s reporting on the "Haitian connection" to AIDS in the 1980s.

THE HAITIAN CONNECTION

The *Native* first reported about the so-called Haitian connection in July 1982, around the same time other publications covered this supposed connection. Dr. Lawrence Mass, a co-founder of the Gay Men's Health Crisis, who authored the first US report on AIDS in the *Native* on May 18, 1981, also wrote a short piece on the Haitian connection. Mass's report differed from the one offered a week earlier in the *New York Times*, which focused on the number of cases and quotations from CDC epidemiologist Dr. James W. Curran.[23] Mass reported that thirty-four cases had been found in Haitians in the United States, including men and women, none with reports of drug use or homosexual sex.[24] He also reported on eleven cases of Kaposi's sarcoma in Port-au-Prince, the Haitian capital. He explained that while many questions remained unanswered, these cases suggested an infectious agent and that either AID (one of AIDS's previous names) traveled from Haiti to the United States or vice versa. He also wondered whether earlier reports of gynecomastia or breast enlargement in Haitian male refugees had any connection with the new disease. In his report, Mass mentions neither Haitian culture nor any direct connection with gay men in the United States. The tone of the article is matter of fact.

Such inquiries emerge in the second piece the *Native* ran, which indicates how the maligning of Haitians was never far from fears about gay male sexual practices. In an article attempting to explain to a gay audience what was then known about AID, Mass interviewed Dr. Dan William, a private physician who treated numerous gay men in his practice. Mass asked William questions about AID, including spending considerable time on why Haitians were afflicted. William offered one explanation for the incidence of AID in Haitians, which tracks with the epidemiology of hepatitis B: that Haitians are part of an "environmentally disadvantaged community" "who live in close quarters and unsanitary conditions."[25] Although this paints a negative picture of Haitians in part, it simultaneously points to the structural conditions that create the worlds in which Haitians live. In Mass's next piece, also an interview, the New York City Health Department commissioner, David J. Sencer, corroborated this claim, pointing to "malnutrition" and living conditions of "extreme poverty."[26] When asked further whether Haitians brought AID to the United States, William replied, "Perhaps yes. Haiti has been a popular tourist resort for many, including gay men. One possibility is that gay men vacationing in Haiti acquired AID through sexual contacts with Haitians. Another possibility is that Haitians brought this disease to the US during recent immigrations."[27] William's matter-of-fact explanations of his view of the living conditions for Haitians due to poverty and sexual tourism offered little judgment. Yet he supplied the links between gay sex tourism in Haiti and AID as a central hypothesis about the disease's origin, and unlike Mass's previous report, William suggests only Haiti as origin. This kind of sense-making—marking Haiti as origin and linking the spread of AID with Haitian poverty and sex tourism, which also thrives due to poverty—became more fleshed out as *Native* reporters began a sustained focus on the African swine fever virus (ASFV) and its connections to AIDS.

For years, the *Native* reported on possible links between ASFV and AIDS, with particular focus on the relationship to Haiti.[28] Harvard pathobiologist Dr. Jane Teas originally put forth the ASFV theory. In a letter to *The Lancet*, Teas posited "that ASFV, which was discovered in Haitian pigs in 1979, may somehow mutate and be transmitted to humans who eat pork and who are already immune-suppressed (a common condition in malnourished populations). It is further postulated that gay men vacationing in Haiti—prone to immune-suppression themselves—had sex with virus-carrying Haitians and carried it back to the US."[29] Teas's view was that ASFV, which had been found in multiple countries over the years with a 60 percent to 90 percent death rate, manifested differently in Haiti because at points in its existence there, ASFV only had about a 3 percent death rate. This lower death rate possibly meant that ASFV had transformed, and perhaps one of the ways it transformed was through an ability to jump from one species to another. The *New York Times* reported on this theory a day later but did so without mention of the Haitian connection and only to note that two other scientific groups found no evidence to support the theory.[30]

From the start, the ASFV-to-AIDS theory was highly controversial. Haitian and US doctors clapped back at Teas's hypothesis. Ronald K. St. John of the Pan American Health Organization called the theory "unwarranted speculation," charging that "allegations, without strong supporting epidemiological evidence, that one country is responsible for introducing an illness are reminiscent of syphilis in the Middle Ages, when the French worried about the 'Italian disease,' and vice versa."[31] Haitian researcher Emmanuel Arnoux and colleagues were more direct, proclaiming, "Such speculation is damaging to Haiti and to Haitian communities abroad."[32]

Native reporter Anne-christine d'Adesky, a white woman, activist, and journalist with strong connections to Haiti (her father was born there, and she spent summers there growing up), produced several of the *Native*'s long-form stories on the "Haitian connection." d'Adesky acknowledged that Teas's theory was racist and harmful.[33] Yet, the *Native* editor and reporters felt that, despite the controversy, the theory was worth pursuing in order to find an origin and thus a solution to AIDS. The pursuit was especially important because, as editor Ortleb suggested, the US government had an investment in not pursuing links between ASFV and AIDS.[34] Thus, the paper continued to run stories that kept the theory alive, questioning CDC and health officials about their unwillingness to pursue it.[35] Their reporting continued long after the scientific community accepted HIV as the cause of AIDS.[36]

A FULLER VIEW OF HAITI

Although the *New York Native*'s activist journalists occasionally trafficked in the usual myths about Haiti and Haitians in their pursuit to find the truth about AIDS, the reporting refused narratives commonly taken up in mainstream venues that exoticized voodoo practices and other spiritual/cultural beliefs as the explanations for why Haitians were afflicted with AIDS.[37] The *Native* took a different approach, providing its readers with a deeper understanding of the Haitian context and US-Haitian relations as well as making links between Haitian and gay communities in ways that were not damning or judgmental.

For instance, the *Native* reported on fragile coalitions among Haitian and gay groups in the United States. An illustrative piece explained how in the early 1980s, after the designation of Haitians and homosexuals as two of the high-risk groups, the Gay Men's Health Crisis, one of the first organizations to provide direct services to people with AIDS, reached out to the Haitian Centers Council offering "to help set up clinics and translate brochures into Creole."[38] The "cordial, but cool" response refused assistance and signaled the fears that shaped Haitians' existence in the United States. Nevertheless, Haitian physicians and community leaders recognized the need to deal more directly with the taboo issue of homosexuality in Haitian culture and to build connections with the gay community. As one Haitian former school principal turned US taxi driver told *Native* reporter Joe Dolce, "Gay people and Haitians have one thing in common: in some people's eyes, neither of us are very desirable."[39] Certainly, as with all of humanity, heterosexual Haitians, non-Haitian gays, and gay Haitians had more in common than their alienized, undesirable position, but those commonalities were rarely mentioned in mainstream media. A 1983 report on Haitians' protest of their designation notes both Haitian reticence to collaborate with gay activists about AIDS and some Haitians' sense-making about the Haitian-AIDS connection, which many attached to homosexual Haitians. The *Native* reported that one woman held a sign reading, "American homosexuals have AIDS. Canadian homosexuals have AIDS. Why don't you say Haitian homosexuals have AIDS. Instead of Haitians have AIDS."[40] This sign asks a legitimate question about the politics of stigmatization and potentially reflects homophobic beliefs. Yet Haitian Coalition on AIDS doctor Jean-Claude Compas noted collaborations between his group and the Gay Men's Health Crisis to lobby for funding.

Additionally, the *Native* relied on Haitian voices to contextualize not just homophobia in Haiti and within Haitian communities in the United States but also to help explain why, even in the face of being isolated as a national group at high risk for AIDS, Haitians would not admit to homosexual sex. As Compas put it, "No Haitian would admit to homosexuality or IV-drug use to a non-Creole-speaking person. Those are two very taboo subjects. It took an AIDS patient of mine three months before he finally admitted that he had sex with men."[41] In these cases, Haitians understood gay male sexuality and beliefs about it to be central to their own predicament.

The *Native* kept this connection fresh in its readers' minds in other ways by reporting on gay politics and politics more broadly in Haiti. This reporting is remarkable because it removed the conversation about AIDS from one about targeted identities (e.g., Haitian or homosexual) toward supplying readers with an understanding of the cultural, political, economic, and historical logics and institutions that created the AIDS crisis in Haiti, how the United States was implicated, and what that might mean for all people with AIDS in the United States. A 1983 article explained that Haitian and foreign gays were the target of raids under President Jean-Claude Duvalier's regime as part of a "campaign against AIDS."[42] The article challenged the "there are no homosexuals in Haiti" hypothesis proffered by the Haitian government and elicited empathy from US gays about AIDS as a gay rights concern in Haiti.

The importance of understanding Haitian culture and politics in the United States and Haiti remained central to the *Native*'s approach to challenging the alienizing logic that maligned Haitians. d'Adesky wrote two sets of stories on Haiti and Haitians in 1985 and 1986. In late 1985, she wrote about the plight of Haitians living with AIDS in the United States and Haiti. In mid-1986, right after the overthrow of Duvalier, she focused on his regime's cover-up of AIDS in Haiti and, in the second piece, the cover-up of the links between ASFV and AIDS. These reports dug deep into dimensions of the Haitian context that exacerbated the AIDS crisis there and implicated the United States for its foreign policy on Haiti and domestic immigration policy. In general, these pieces had little if anything to do with gay sexuality, making this coverage in a gay paper especially striking.

d'Adesky's first report in December 1985 offered an exploration into how AIDS afflicted Haitians in the United States societally and medically. The article also showed that despite the stigma, Haitians were at a lower risk than others designated as high-risk groups, and it relied on the testimony of Haitian physicians to contextualize the unique problem for Haitians in the United States. The report quoted Dr. Compas explaining, "The average patient has no coverage, is not legally documented, and therefore cannot benefit from many health services. They have a problem finding housing and are discriminated against in employment."[43] As with previous reports, Compas observed that while many Haitian men did not admit homosexuality or show physical evidence of anal sex, eventually some admitted to having been prostitutes in order to pay their way to the United States, further implicating poverty as a leading cause of AIDS. d'Adesky's second report turned attention to the problem in Haiti itself, continuing the themes of poverty and lack of education. Here d'Adesky covered what was known about AIDS in Haiti, how physicians tried to combat the disease, and the serious obstacles they faced.

The first piece in 1986 appeared four months after d'Adesky's previous reports and Duvalier's overthrow. d'Adesky provided a comprehensive look at how AIDS had been denied under the Duvalier regime based on a series of interviews with Haitian physicians working on AIDS. Since the government denied the existence of AIDS, and physicians did not have access to labs or funding for AIDS research, their knowledge of the disease was based on their experiences treating people, trying to address the issue of blood donations, and confronting societal stigma and lack of knowledge.[44] d'Adesky also supplied an overview of poverty in Haiti, incidence of tropical diseases that complicated treatments, and the inability of doctors, even after Duvalier's fall, to roll out a nationwide education campaign to inform people about risks. These issues were compounded by a 98 percent illiteracy rate in Haiti. d'Adesky asked about homosexuality, and the physicians were conflicted about how to respond. Dr. Jean-Michel Guerin commented, "We do not have homosexuals here, but we have men who are bisexual and promiscuous." He went on, "In that sense, we have a more serious problem than in the US, since if it was a homosexual group the disease would be contained to one group and might be traceable."[45] Although the physicians said that they did not have enough information to speak definitively about the role of homosexual sex and prostitution in transmitting the disease in Haiti, Guerin insisted, "We do know that AIDS in Haiti is not a homosexual disease, nor is AIDS a Haitian disease."[46] These comments on homosexuality signal that there was a strong taboo against homosexuality, and Haitian physicians seem to have been careful not to let their personal views enter into their assessments. Their commentary though did indicate that the AIDS crisis in Haiti was not simply due to homophobia even as that prejudice may have contributed to its spread, as it did in the United States. These grounded and nuanced interviews thereby complicate stereotypes about Haitians, homosexuality, and homophobia. Instead they emphasized poverty, government inaction, and serious need for more scientific and medical resources. Such detailed analysis turned attention away from the stigmatization of a particular group of people or an entire culture toward the structural reasons that Haitians contracted AIDS, which was rare in US media reporting.

In the second part of 1986, d'Adesky's report took up the vexed question of the connection between ASFV and pigs in Haiti. Once again, d'Adesky centered the voices of Haitians when offering a detailed exploration on how the theory of an ASFV/AIDS connection played out in Haiti. Although such reporting kept alive a theory the scientific establishment discounted, and potentially further maligned Haitians via their relationship to pigs, the emphasis on Haitians' experiences of having their pigs slaughtered as a result of the ASFV outbreak in the 1970s and Haitian scientists such as Guerin's interest in the possible links offered a perspective seen nowhere else in non-Haitian media in the United States.

Not without controversy, the *Native* avidly reported on Haiti, the links between gays and Haitians, and the Haitian connection to AIDS in ways that contributed to the stigmatization of Haitians but also in ways that attempted to build solidarity with Haitian communities afflicted by AIDS and provide political economic contextualization of Haiti and Haitians. These journalistic efforts are a vital part of the story in the gay activist community's readiness to participate in efforts against US Haitian refugee policy and the imprisonment of HIV-positive Haitians at Guantánamo Bay in the early 1990s.

THE HAITIAN PRISON CAMP

After the military coup that overthrew Aristide in September 1991, thousands of mostly young, politically active Haitians fled their country seeking refuge and, shortly thereafter, the Bush administration realized that many headed for the United States. In response, the Bush administration began erecting an emergency camp and processing center at Guantánamo Bay to process and detain refugees and, in so doing, circumvented international law. The United States has a long history of applying alienizing logic to Haitians, including using the Coast Guard to intercept and return Haitians who flee to the United States, labeling nearly all Haitians "economic migrants" as opposed to political refugees or asylum seekers (see also chapter 3).[47] In this instance, the Bush administration claimed it feared a crisis if Haitians set foot on US soil because international refugee law includes a policy of non-refoulement, which means that countries must hear an asylum seeker's case once a person requests refuge at or from within its borders. Due to the political gravity of the situation following the coup, the US solution was once again to intercept Haitians and, this time, to deposit them in the liminal political zone of the Guantánamo Bay naval base.[48] The US government claimed Guantánamo was not in fact the United States, but it was also clearly not *not* the United States, making it an ideal site—both internal and extra-legal—for determining if the Haitians had a credible fear of persecution while bypassing questions of non-refoulement. If the United States accepted that a person had a credible case, they would be permitted to enter the United States proper. The vast majority of Haitian claimants, however, were returned to Haiti.

Around three hundred Haitians whose fears of persecution the United States deemed credible still found themselves detained on Guantánamo because the US government said they, or an accompanying family member, had tested HIV positive.[49] This health status was a problem because, as addressed in the previous chapters, in 1987, the US Congress passed legislation that defined HIV infection as a "dangerous and contagious disease" for the purposes of immigration law, effectively barring anyone with HIV or AIDS from immigrating to the United States or regularizing/naturalizing if already in the country. President Bush upheld this policy, and President Bill Clinton later codified it. Although during this time, the Department of Justice made exceptions for some HIV-positive refugees and asylum seekers, Haitians were not afforded this exemption.[50] Instead, the US government forcibly quarantined HIV-positive Haitians in a military-run, open-air detention center called "Camp Bulkeley," some for more than a year and a half, in conditions that included inadequate food and medical treatment, insufficient shelter, no freedom to leave the camp unsupervised, and infestations of pests.[51] As Bob Brutus, who was detained at Camp Bulkeley for twenty months, put it, "That ain't no camp. That's a jail."[52] Haitian detainee Elma Verdieu insisted, "Just because someone has been diagnosed HIV-positive, does that give them the right to create a living hell for those people? The living conditions here, instead of helping us to live, are killing us quicker."[53]

The US Public Health Service (PHS) knew these conditions created a potential health crisis at the camp. CDC director James O. Mason wrote a letter to the INS commissioner in March 1992 expressing his concerns about the health conditions and reportedly never received a response.[54] INS representatives did not apparently see a problem as spokesman Duke Austin defended the conditions, claiming they compared "very, very favorably" to refugee camps around the globe.[55] Although PHS officials were allegedly "frustrated" and "outraged" that INS did little to nothing to improve conditions at the camp, there is no indication that they did much to press the issue. This response reveals what the camp represented, for as Neel Ahuja writes, "The twin specters of invasion (the mass of the dispossessed who could theoretically arrive from the world over) and contagion (the absolute refusal of HIV-tainted bodies) coalesce in the ambivalent figuration of a humanitarian camp."[56] The INS was tasked with the care of the detained Haitians as well as their containment. Furthermore, it is no accident that the United States put Haitians in these conditions as opposed to other refugee groups. As A. Naomi Paik argues, "Understanding why these HIV-positive Haitian refugees were imprisoned requires recognizing not only Haiti's history as an imperial possession but also the long-standing conception of black bodies, particularly Haitian bodies, as carriers of contagion."[57] Indeed, as already shown, such a conception plagued Haitians from the earliest days of the AIDS pandemic, manifesting in the most extreme way on Guantánamo Bay.

The imprisoned Haitians vigorously challenged their situation using a variety of methods including letter writing, appeals to celebrities and media, negotiations with facility officials, property destruction, and hunger strikes. They formed the Association des Réfugiés Politiques Haïtiens and continually demanded their rights, grounding their claims in international law.[58] A handful of scholars have addressed the existence of this concentration camp and the resistance to it.[59] Legal scholars and one popular book, Brandt Goldstein's *Storming the Court*, offer accounts centering the strategies, risks, and even heroism of a coalition of attorneys from the Haitian Centers Council, Yale University, and the Center for Constitutional Rights (CCR).[60] Paik's book *Rightlessness* gives a detailed account of the resistance efforts of the imprisoned Haitians, based on their testimony in three court cases and their family and press communications. Although Paik briefly discusses—and attorney on the case, Michael Ratner, explicates more fully—the political struggle in the United States, scholars have hardly taken up the support supplied by US activists across a wide spectrum: Haitians, gays, celebrities, students, people living with AIDS, and their allies.[61] Perhaps the absence of an inclusive account is because outside of media reports, few historical sources documenting this activism exist. For example, when it comes to AIDS activism, the only physical remnants of ACT UP New York's work on this issue include a small archive in the New York Public Library consisting of segments of about six episodes of Wentzy's AIDS Community TV, minutes from meetings, newspaper clippings and fliers, and two interviews in the ACT UP Oral History Project, which feature activists speaking about the Haitian actions. As far as I can tell from extant archival materials, books on AIDS activism, and conversations with a handful of AIDS activists from the time, most other ACT UP chapters did not focus on the Haitian detention, or if they did, they failed to document it.[62]

Similarly, existing collections centered on Haitian-US relations and Haitian refugees in the United States, such as the Ira Gollobin Haitian Refugee Collection 1972–2004 or the Assotto Saint archives at the New York Public Library, do not appear to include any significant information on this detention. Saint (1957–1994), a queer Haitian-American, HIV-positive activist, and artist living in New York City, wrote briefly in his book *Spells of a Voodoo Doll* about his own efforts to support the detained Haitians.[63] Götz-Dietrich Opitz offers an explanation for why some members of the Haitian diaspora in the United States may have been reticent to publicly focus on the detained refugees even while working on issues surrounding the overthrow of Aristide. Opitz explains that the detention

affected the Haitian public in the US and contributed to the "waning of mobilization" in the community. Haitians' traumatic experience in the US during the 1980s of being collectively stigmatized as HIV-carriers led many of them to shun the refugee issue in public for fear of reoccurring AIDS-related accusations. Whereas in the 1980s *all* Haitians in the diaspora were victimized regardless of class and color, AIDS-related discrimination on Guantanamo was limited to "black, poor" Aristide-supporters from Haiti. In addition, Haitian HIV-infected refugees on Guantanamo were in conflict with the public relations campaign to rehabilitate Aristide's exile government. In the Haitian community, the US Guantanamo policy resulted in a vigilant passivity toward the refugee issue.[64]

Opitz's comments help to explain the dearth of materials in extant Haitian archives, but US Haitians were not entirely inactive on the Guantánamo detention. For example, in April 1993 during a march of thousands of Haitians from Congress to the White House in order to challenge US policy on capturing and returning Haitians to Haiti, they also criticized the government for continuing to hold the HIV-positive Haitians on Guantánamo.[65] Later that same month, twenty-six-year-old Joel Saintil, a first-year medical student when he fled Haiti, died only eight days after being released from Guantánamo. Two hundred rageful Haitian protesters took his body to the INS office in Miami to vividly show his death was the government's fault.[66] Haitians were also active on AIDS in general, regularly challenging the US ban on Haitians donating blood until it was finally lifted for good in 1991. For instance, on September 24, 1983, roughly eight hundred Haitians marched through Brooklyn to protest the CDC high risk designation.[67] The most notable action took place on April 20, 1990, when between fifty thousand and one hundred thousand Haitians and their allies in New York shut down the Brooklyn Bridge for several hours to protest the blood donation policy.[68] Despite these examples, issues related to race, class, homophobia, and HIV stigma may have turned some US Haitians away from much overt activism on behalf of those detained on Guantánamo Bay.[69]

AIDS COMMUNITY TV: "QUARANTINED BY THE USA"

Numerous groups filed lawsuits against the government to challenge the detention and deplorable conditions of the camp.[70] Ultimately, in February 1992, after the INS indicated that the detained Haitians would be allowed into the United States to file their asylum claims,[71] Harold Hongju Koh and Ratner, who were co-teaching a class at the Yale Law School's Lowenstein Human Rights Clinic, took the case with their students and a few other attorneys, arguing it from multiple directions and eventually succeeding in getting Haitians released to the United States in June 1993.[72] The legal battle has been well documented and, in fact, serves as a case study for human rights legal advocacy at its best.[73]

Undoubtedly, the complex and creative legal maneuvering of the attorneys is laudable. It is a case study of the need for political-legal coalitions, even if strategies and approaches are not only very different but also a source of dis-ease for lawyers. For example, in an article for *Harvard Human Rights Journal*, Ratner notes that because he and the other attorneys believed that a newly elected President Clinton would overturn the Bush-era policy on the detained Haitians, they advised that the detainees should wait on Clinton before taking extreme actions of any sort. When Clinton changed course upon his election, the Haitian detainees began a hunger strike. As one of the detainees, thirty-six-year-old Jean Benedic explained, "I can't live in this hell anymore. If they want 10 or 15 of us to die for the rest of them to live, then 10 or 15 of us will die."[74] Despite the strikers' resolve, the attorneys had mixed feelings about it. But Ratner writes, "The hunger strike gave them a semblance of control over their situation and made the lawyers work harder. It forced us to send delegations to the camp. It gave us a reason for pushing public figures such as Jesse Jackson to go to the camp. The hunger strike turned out to be very successful, and it is an example of outside organizing around a legal proceeding, beyond the legal team's grand plan."[75] Ratner clearly shows the significance of the "self-directed" protests of people most directly impacted by abuse or injustice.[76] Their bodies are already imperiled, and when they further imperil themselves to make a political point, this very often can catalyze more decisive action.

Solidarity or "other-directed" protests will not have the same effect as the self-directed protests, but they are still significant. In addition to the pressure the Haitians applied, Ratner explains that AIDS activists were one of the most important constituencies in the coalition. Although the legal team approached ACT UP initially to keep the media attention on the issue, they knew that ACT UP would not be under their control. Ratner recalls:

> We also learned not to hold back an activist strategy for fear it would backfire and cause the politicians to get upset. The politicians had already factored in the negative; we did not have to do it for them. Taking aggressive political action also yielded unanticipated, positive results. For example, while we approached ACT-UP solely to enlist their political support and their militant public presence, its members subsequently were key in locating service providers for the Haitians, a critical requirement for their release. These unexpected benefits cannot be overemphasized. Thoughtful activism is necessary to win legal battles and can achieve multiple and unforeseen objectives in struggles that are in essence political. Silence, on the other hand, achieves nothing.[77]

In the remainder of this chapter, I provide texture to Ratner's recollections and his brief timeline and description of actions that US-based activists took in support of the detained Haitians and to keep the spotlight on legal efforts. Specifically, I analyze the rhetoric of the actions DIVA TV documented and Wentzy produced in six episodes of AIDS Community TV related to the Haitian detention. I flesh out the episodes with contextual material taken from letters, posters, and other documents pertaining to solidarity actions from the ACT UP NY archives. The public displays found in AIDS Community TV highlight the kinds of actions people engaged in and the rationales they provided for their activism. The multicultural, multiracial constitution of the actions and the people interviewed for AIDS Community TV also points to the complex coalitional nature of this work. Furthermore, this analysis indicates the absolute vital importance of alternative media to achieving movement objectives and recording the history of those achievements.

PROTESTING THE HAITIAN DETENTION

As shown in the minutes of the regular membership meeting and coordinating committee meeting, ACT UP NY was first asked to be involved with the issue of the Haitian detention in late March 1992.[78] Beginning in the fall of that year, reports about detained Haitians and ACT UP's involvement regularly showed up in ACT UP meeting agendas. ACT UP members including Walt Wilder, Betty Williams, and Esther Kaplan offered reports and announcements as a part of the Emergency Coalition for Haitian Refugees (ECHR) and the Shut Down Guantanamo Coalition NY, which resisted the quarantine of the Haitians. In her interview with Sarah Schulman and Jim Hubbard's ACT UP Oral History Project, ACT UP member Betty Williams, a white, heterosexual Quaker, detailed her and Bro Broberg's involvement in helping to resettle Haitians released from the camp into the United States. Williams depicts the extreme lack of resources they had available as they attempted to resettle refugees. Eventually Housing Works and AIDS housing organizations could no longer accept more refugees, which meant the US government could have returned those refugees to Haiti. Williams recalled, "And Bro and I took a really deep breath and we lied. We lied to the Justice Department. We lied to the military and said, yes, we had housing." In the end, they resettled more than one hundred Haitians. Furthermore, she described her and Broberg's trip to Guantánamo to interview the refugees and learn the gravity of their situation in order to figure out how to help.[79] The two HIV-positive Haitian political refugees mentioned at the start of this chapter, Rigaud Milenette and Silieses Success, were sent to the Varick Street Detention Center after being released from Guantánamo, prompting one of the first public protests DIVA TV documented about the Haitian issue in New York on October 16, 1992.[80]

The original collective known as DIVA TV started in 1989 with a mission to do police countersurveillance. It was no longer producing videos by 1990.[81] Wentzy joined ACT UP in 1990 upon his HIV diagnosis and brought an almost obsessive work ethic to documenting the work of AIDS activists through what Alexandra Juhasz calls the revitalization of DIVA TV 2. His labor resulted in a weekly cable access program, AIDS Community TV. Wentzy's style is typical of alternative media producers of the time, focusing less on high-quality production and more on documenting the words and actions of activists in order to inform an audience primarily made up of other AIDS activists and people living with AIDS. From the archives of AIDS Community TV, there are three full episodes and three shorter segments on the Haitian refugees between the fall of 1992 and the summer of 1993, usually under the headline "Quarantined by the USA." These segments and episodes depict the protests and acts of civil disobedience outside of INS and other federal buildings, including footage of an action that resulted in the arrest of more than twenty people on February 23, 1993.[82] They also feature speeches, interviews, and letters from experts and people impacted by the crisis, which offer insight into some coalition members' rhetorical perspective.[83] For example, some of the speakers in the videos are survivors of Guantánamo who denounce the deplorable conditions, offering details about their treatment at the hands of US military officials. Others are Haitian activists living in the United States who describe the inconsistency of the medical information provided to the refugees or who read letters from refugees pleading for assistance. Some are attorneys working on the various cases. Still others are white gay men outraged by the criminalization of HIV and who stand in solidarity with the Haitians.

The grainy videos rarely include name keys for speakers, and the location of the actions are only knowable based on what people say or visual context cues. Although the person behind the camera, presumably Wentzy, sometimes asks questions the audience can hear, other times the answers are edited and so the prompt is unclear. Sometimes a clip starts in the middle of a speech or action with little context, and often these actions are spliced with clips from mainstream news reports that tell a very different story. The juxtaposition is an important part of the political work the episodes do because it evidences how other media outlets marginalized the perspectives that Wentzy centers.

From these episodes and segments, which comprise no more than 120 minutes of video, we get a surprisingly comprehensive understanding of the rhetorical appeals that activists used to make their case for the release of the Haitian refugees, the closing of the camp at Guantánamo, their critique of the government's general policy on HIV-positive migrants, and its racist double standards, among other points. In this section, I identify how activists identify contradictions and double standards in three primary ways: the racist isolation of Haitians for differential treatment, the contradictory application of US law and policy, and the militarization and criminalization of health care.

THE RACIST ISOLATION OF HAITIANS

The most prominent theme across the videos is participants' outrage at the racism inherent in the ongoing detention and the differential treatment of Haitians. Several of the speakers interviewed at protests note that the treatment of the Haitians is a manifestation of anti-Black, anti-Haitian racism. For example, in the first episode, a Black woman from Black AIDS Mobilization (BAM!), one of the coalitional partners, proclaimed, "We think that what's happening is really racist and very homophobic in the sense that Haitian refugees are being tested to see whether or not they're positive for the HIV virus [sic], and other people who would like to come to this country are not tested in the same way. Cubans aren't tested, Eastern Europeans aren't tested for HIV virus [sic], and why are the Haitian refugees marginalized in this way and left in horrible conditions?"[84] Although she framed the critique as a question, the answer is meant to be clear. As shown in her statement, which mentions homophobia, activists note that racism does not occur in isolation from other kinds of oppression. The analysis is intersectional.

Activists insisted that classist views about Haitians also inform policy, with one white man noting, "These are not people that are fleeing here for quote unquote economic reasons, the false brush that has painted the refugees by the George Bush administration."[85] Although such critiques set up a damaging dichotomy between "legitimate" political refugees and "illegitimate" economic migrants, they simultaneously call out the US government's anti-Haitian position because it returned people whose claims to a credible fear of persecution it deemed legitimate. The analysis did not stop at race, country of origin, and class because ultimately, the question of the detainees' HIV status loomed. A white lawyer on the case added, "They were targeted because they are or were in the government's mind, testing HIV positive and this special procedure was developed just for HIV-positive Haitians at Guantánamo. It doesn't exist anywhere else in the world; it does not exist for any other group of people."[86] In this comment, the lawyer named plainly the US state's actions, ensuring that there was no ambiguity about what the state was doing and to whom.

The activists insisted on keeping attention on anti-Black racism and how it intersected with economic and health discrimination. They provided a longer historical context on US-Haitian relations that revealed enduring alienizing logic that has long isolated the first free Black republic in the Western Hemisphere and deemed Haiti as a unique threat.[87] One white gay male activist explained, "As those who understand the history of US-Haitian relations throughout the last two centuries, it's been one of domination and control by the United States. We occupied Haiti for nineteen years and physically destroyed their resistance movement during that occupation and set up a counterinsurgency army which is ruling Haiti today."[88] This historical context is important to understand because without it, the isolation of Haitians in that moment might itself seem like an isolated action of the US government. In actuality, there is significant historical precedent of contradictions in the application of US law when it comes to Haiti and Haitians, which is the second line of argument that activists use.

CONTRADICTORY APPLICATION OF US LAW

Activists name numerous contradictions in the US approach to the Haitians. In the first episode of AIDS Community TV featuring one of the protests at the Varick Street Detention Center, a white gay male activist explained why they are there and then lays out the contradictions in the US application of law. On paper, the United States abides by international refugee law, which requires that it allow people with a credible case to go through a full and fair asylum process. The activist insisted, "These refugees have won the right to an asylum hearing; in other words, they have convinced INS officials, who are very hard to convince, that they deserve an asylum hearing and have got a fear of persecution. . . . These are legitimate political refugees and we demand their release into the community now."[89] This same activist later elaborated on a deeper contradiction in the US position on the Haitian refugees: "Today it's the United States government that's trying to boost up that military regime [in Haiti], all their hypocritical doubletalk as supporting democracy to the contrary is worthless. The entire world understands that the Bush administration is not supporting Jean-Bertrand Aristide who was the choice of the Haitian people in 1990 and remains the choice of the Haitian people. So that there is a very clear connection between US foreign policy and the racist policy toward Haitian refugees."[90]

Several activists reiterated the anti-democratic role the United States had in creating the situation that led the Haitians to flee while publicly pronouncing its belief in democracy. But contradictions abound in the way the United States applied the law to Haitians. A lawyer defending the Haitians described the US government's legal position to ensure the refugees had no legal rights on Guantánamo and could be kept in inhumane conditions. She explains:

> The point is that it's a place of absolute military and governmental power, and the people who live there literally have no rights, that's the government's whole position in our lawsuit. "You can't come into court and challenge what we're doing to these people." "Why?" "Because they have no rights." "Why do they have no rights?" "Because they are aliens on a military base which is outside of the United States." Ok, if you point out why they are on a military base outside the United States except that you went and put them there, they're like, "yea, that's true, but people, aliens in that position have no rights."[91]

International and US law endow asylum seekers with certain rights but because these asylum seekers were on a military base that, as stated above, is and is not the United States, the US government saw no reason to reconcile this contradiction over the lack of rights that would normally be a given. These people are essentially rightless, not only without rights but without the right to rights.[92] This point leads to the final contradiction activists identify: the militarization and criminalization of health care.

THE MILITARIZATION AND CRIMINALIZATION OF HEALTH CARE

Despite the government's framing of its policy banning HIV-positive migrants as, at least in part, a matter of concern for public health, the exclusion of all migrants and detention of the Haitians defied the commonly held views of public health officials. These policies were not only detrimental to health but also led to the treatment of HIV-positive people through militarizing and criminalizing their bodies as a mode of "care." In a video clip of one middle-aged white man, likely a doctor or scientist giving a speech at what is probably the International AIDS Conference in Berlin, he explained:

> Duke Austin, a spokesperson for the Immigration and Naturalization Service, is quoted as arguing that the quarantine is necessary to protect

the health of INS and military personnel. . . . To state the obvious, it is only if INS staff are having sex, sharing drugs, or beating immigrants so violently that their victim's blood enters the batterer's body that there is in fact a risk of infection. Moreover, all three activities that would lead to staff being infected are already illegal, and the only reason INS staff and detainees are in the same place is because of INS policy. So on its face, a public health rationale is absurd. But I think there's another, an underlying rationale for the exclusion of HIV-infected immigrants, and that's that the United States doesn't want to bear the cost of caring for people with HIV infection.[93]

This speaker identifies one of the rationales for US policy, the cost of care, and reiterates that there is no public health protocol for detention unless horrific treatment is happening at the prison. As chapter 3 shows, he was not off base. A young white woman who had just returned from the camp explained in one video, "The words 'concentration camp' immediately came to mind when we walked in and saw these 280 people, kids, families gathered under military supervision in an airplane hangar."[94]

At an event denouncing US policy, one activist read a letter written by detainees: "Here they humiliate us and treat us like animals. Our peaceful protests are brutally repressed by helicopters, planes, hundreds of soldiers, and dogs. We are hand-cuffed, beaten, and forced to sleep outdoors. Lizards, rats, snakes, scorpions, and flies attack all of us, from infants to adults."[95] Text in the most comprehensive episode on the issue in May of 1993 reported that because of the Haitians' ongoing protests over their treatment, "Over 300 Marines in full riot gear descended on the sleeping refugees in a military operation more brutal than that of July 18, 1992." The next screen added, "The soldiers arrested 31 refugees, including a seven year old boy. Several women were subjected to vaginal searches."[96] In another episode, a woman who just returned from the camp explained what the detained Haitians say about their situation: "If we were really sick, we would be in hospitals, we wouldn't be treated this way as prisoners. You can see they're not being treated as sick people. They've been assaulted, they've been harassed the whole time they've been in there. They've been thrown in jail within the jail. And mistreated in several ways. And when they are sick and they bring it to the attention of the doctors, they don't get the medical attention that they need."[97]

Obviously, none of these criminalized and militarized conditions are conducive to preserving health and in fact might be described as processes of "slow death." As Lauren Berlant puts it, "Slow death refers to the physical wearing out of a population and the deterioration of people in that population that is very nearly a defining condition of their experience and historical existence."[98] Some attempted suicide, and several others were only sent to the United States when their health condition became so dire that death was imminent.[99] The contradictions these activists identified and the media attention they kept on the issue intervened in processes begetting death. The videos reflect a coalition of voices, each speaking about a different dimension of the impacts of US policies grounded in contradictions. These videos not only helped inform audiences and keep the pressure on the US government, but they also provide an important historical record.

CONCLUSION

Upon finally being released into the United States, twenty-two-year-old Wesner Derosier told a *Stonewall News* reporter that he often wondered if he should have stayed in Haiti even though he and his brother were involved in Aristide's presidential campaign and were no longer safe. He said that while he was incarcerated, "I used to think of an old Haitian proverb. 'It is better to die as a tiger than as a dog.'"[100] Whether as dogs or "human-viral hybrids," as Ahuja puts it, Haitians were horrifically dehumanized on Guantánamo Bay.[101] But their freedom dreams continued. Reunited with his fiancée, Derosier hoped, "I would like to be somebody, to be a light for society." Herard Jean-Bernard, thirty-five, shared that sentiment: "More than anything else, I want to make something of myself. . . . I want to learn something and take it back to my brothers and sisters there [in Haiti] and my children. I don't want my kids to go through what I went through."[102] Even Success continued chasing her freedom dreams: "Even though I lost my mother, father and baby I think of what Aristide said: 'Together we are strong.'" Consequently, she added, "I still feel that I cannot be discouraged because together as Haitians we are strong."[103]

This chapter has considered how AIDS activist media contested the impacts of alienizing logic on Haitians during the early years of the AIDS pandemic. Showing the long-standing links between the way that the gay media like the *New York Native* reported on the Haitian connection to AIDS and how AIDS Community TV documented ACT UP and allies' advocacy on behalf of imprisoned Haitian migrants reveals some of the complexities of coalition building and the importance of alternative media to creating and promoting alternative perspectives to the mainstream. Despite the devastating impacts of the CDC's designation of Haitians as at high risk for AIDS and the severity of the Guantánamo Bay HIV prison camp, relatively little scholarship has documented how US communities resisted and challenged such treatment. Although both Haitians and homosexuals were alienized from the beginning of the AIDS pandemic, virtually no scholarship has considered connections that existed between them, not to mention homosexual Haitians. I do not mean to overstate the connections or give them more space than is warranted. Obviously, the attention that these media paid to Haitian issues is tiny compared to their emphasis on many other issues, and, for many, that was how it should be. For instance, in response to a question about the demise of ACT UP, Williams explained that she agreed that issues like housing, Haitians, and immigration led to ACT UP's crumbling. Similarly, former ACT UP member and *Native* journalist d'Adesky noted in her ACT UP Oral History Project interview that, generally speaking, and in her memory, ACT UP did not reach out to or actively coalesce with Haitian communities.[104] In a conversation I had with her in March 2013, she noted there were certainly coalitional moments because of a few members' dedication. She also explained that, in general, immigration issues caused tension within ACT UP because migrants involved in ACT UP wanted a broader focus, whereas the loudest voices in ACT UP—US citizen, white, middle-class gay men—focused on medication and US policy.[105]

Thus, this chapter does not argue that the mostly white AIDS activist media makers considered in this chapter are heroic or beyond reproach. In addition to the commentary in the previous paragraph, it is well documented that confrontational AIDS activist groups like ACT UP struggled with their own constituencies or other organizations who were Black or of color. Cathy J. Cohen explains that "in contrast to the more aggressive political tactics of civil disobedience, the political strategies of African American communities were much less confrontational, with compromise and education being key."[106] For example, BAM!, which was featured in some of the AIDS Community TV episodes on Haiti, clearly engaged with civil disobedience against the detention, but the group also focused on educational outreach to Black communities in the city.[107] These different approaches emerged from groups' relationships to white supremacist capitalism in the United States and the fact that for many Black, Indigenous, and other activists of color, racial identifications are, for very material reasons, primary.

Moreover, no matter the advocacy for groups like detained Haitians whom activists rarely if ever had to face directly, racism proliferated in largely queer AIDS activist groups like ACT UP. Brett C. Stockdill writes that one of the Black gay participants in his study of AIDS activism, Steven, struggled with Black organizations' refusal to do direct action but was also critical of groups like ACT UP Los Angeles, which he described as possessing "'the mentality of a white boy's club.' He asked: 'Why can't I keep these Latino and black people involved in ACT UP? And it was because ACT UP was very stubborn in its ways and it didn't make black people feel any more at home than it would have been going to a Republican meeting.'"[108] Such critique is damning and not surprising at the same time. It speaks to the reality that organizing and agitating within white supremacist contexts, which are virtually all contexts in the United States, are perpetually vexed. This also means that solidarity and coalitional work will be full of contradictions too.

Despite the failures and flaws of AIDS activists—media makers and others—understanding how AIDS activist media responded to and challenged how ban and quarantine severely impacted Haitians is an important part of the public memory of HIV/AIDS. The revitalization of this memory is crucial for learning to build coalitions that address such complexities in the present and future. As Juhasz writes of the importance of what she calls "queer archive activism," it is necessary to "relodge those frozen memories in contemporary contexts so that they, and perhaps we, can be reanimated."[109]

CONCLUSION

Against the Alienizing Nation.

> The mass immigration so thoughtlessly triggered in 1965 risks
> making America an *alien nation*—not merely in the sense that the
> numbers of aliens in the nation are rising to levels last seen in the
> nineteenth century; not merely in the sense that America will
> become a freak among the world's nations because of the unprece-
> dented demographic mutation it is inflicting on itself; not merely in
> the sense that Americans themselves will become alien to each other,
> requiring an increasingly strained government to arbitrate between
> them; but, ultimately, in the sense that Americans will no longer share
> in common what Abraham Lincoln called in his First Inaugural
> Address *"the mystic chords of memory, stretching from every battle field*
> *and patriot grave, to every living heart and hearth stone, all over this*
> *broad land . . ."*
>
> And that when the time comes to strike those chords, no sweet
> sound will result.
>
> —PETER BRIMELOW, *Alien Nation*

I BEGIN THIS CONCLUSION WITH AN EPIGRAPH FROM THE 1995
national best-selling, xenophobic screed *Alien Nation* because my identification and discussion of the "alienizing nation" in this book directly intervenes in the persistent and pernicious logic *Alien Nation* inhabits and
promotes. This logic remains just as powerful at the time I am writing and,
I would wager, at the time you, dear reader, are reading this book, as it has
always been since the first settlers arrived on the continent. Brimelow's
book is nothing special; it is part of a genre of books, authored mostly by
white men, that sound various alarms about subjects like affirmative
action, immigration, or family values from a racist, nativist point of view.
They are usually trash to read—arrogantly written, completely unreflexive,
and with an unsurprisingly skewed use of facts. But books like Brimelow's

do highlight characteristics of the nation that are no longer polite to discuss in public but that are absolutely foundational to and constitutive of the project of the United States of America.[1] When Brimelow says, for example, that "the American nation has always had a specific ethnic core. And that core has been white," he is not wrong.[2] In fact, he identifies precisely what the so-called founding fathers had in mind in 1789 when they extended voting rights only to white, property-owning men or in 1790 when Congress bounded the right to naturalize as a US citizen to "any alien, being a free white person."[3] As Brimelow puts it is how the founders of the United States saw it. Of course, the manner in which people who belong to the US nation enact alienizing logic differs, but opportunities abound. This book has shown how HIV/AIDS became one such opportunity for diverse actors in the United States to enact alienizing logic on groups of people—many who were largely already alienized for other reasons—through quarantine and ban.

In significant ways, coalition politics is a framework that undergirds this book's methodological approach and argument. This framework, however, has several shortcomings. For example, Tiffany Lethabo King wonders if coalition "has been weighted down in political speak." More precisely, King notes, "Scholars and activists often attend to and trouble coalition politics while neglecting to scrutinize interracial erotic, sexual, and in turn, political alliances and affinities, particularly their own."[4] A refusal to think about coalition politics in relation to our most intimate attachments can keep discussions of coalition in the realm of the abstract and disembodied. King writes about a context different from my own, but the tendency she identifies is relevant here and beyond this book. After all, for a book about HIV/AIDS and queer politics, it has a surprisingly small amount of erotic content! Moreover, King mentions how the coalition called "people of color" can erase Blackness and Indigeneity, flattening particularities.[5] These critiques are crucial to bear in mind when writing about race.

Nevertheless, I believe that this book offers a strong rationale for the significance of what I have called "coalitional gestures," in which seemingly separate groups reach out to one another in solidarity.[6] I also believe this book points to the necessity of what Aimee Carrillo Rowe calls "coalitional subjectivity," wherein we understand not only our own struggles but also ourselves as integral to the struggles and subjectivities of others.[7] The work of AIDS media makers and queer AIDS activists more broadly evidence the power of coalitional gestures. At the same time, coalitional gestures are impure because even in extending them, they, too, can alienize. One of my hopes is that by thinking through alienizing processes, we will begin to grasp the "alien" as a coalitional position that incorporates seemingly disparate groups within its purview. There are certainly limitations to this framework, and it may end up functioning in a similar manner to "people of color" by flattening differences in ways that reproduce alienizing logic. Yet continuing to consider coalition is worthwhile. As an already-antagonistic position to the nation-state and national citizenship, alien may serve as an analytic to help us challenge the pernicious logic and practices of alienizing. This is what Mae Ngai's notion of "alien citizenship" makes so transparent.[8]

One contribution of this book is to highlight the significant police power of public health that politicians, governmental officials, and members of the populace employ to alienize people. It is unsurprising that just after the time period tracked by this book ends, in 1994, residents in California deliberated on Proposition 187, the so-called Save Our State initiative that, in part, sought to prevent undocumented migrants from using non-emergency health care. Unlike the Lyndon LaRouche and William Dannemeyer propositions in the 1980s, Californians approved Proposition 187, catalyzing a long legal battle. National commonsense arguments related to the economic and cultural impacts migrants had on the state, similar to the rationales for approving the ban on HIV-positive migrants, featured centrally in proponents' rhetoric.[9] We must connect these policies to national-level laws such as the 1996 Illegal Immigrant Responsibility and Reform Act, signed by President Bill Clinton, which similarly minimized access to public benefits for even legal migrants. These pieces of legislation are akin to anti-welfare laws based on the frightful and fictive figure of the "welfare queen." Alienizing logic animates such laws and their associated rhetoric whether voted on by citizens, approved by elected officials, or used as a mechanism for right-wing fundraising. Such laws rely in part on the threat of disease to justify penalizing and criminalizing alienized persons and populations. Their targets are predictable.

Another contribution of this book is to join the other works evidencing the need to read the official rhetoric of politicians and public health officials and the people who influence them, like religious leaders and journalists, alongside the rhetoric of activists, advocates, and others directly impacted by what officials do. Different voices matter differently, but reading them alongside one another helps to depict more fully the stakes and situations of a specific historical moment. It is an imperative to feature the voices of those most impacted alongside the people trying to defend them and the people doing the damage, even when we have the most access to the latter's claims and actions. Attending to the multivocality and diverse strategies of all stakeholders is a political and an archival challenge. This book is imperfect in this regard, but the imperative of centering people who normally do not make it into archives, let alone into news reports, must be attempted if we want scholarship to have any role in liberatory and radical movements.

The voices of HIV-positive people of color, especially Black people like Haitians, have not played a central role in the majority of scholarship written about HIV/AIDS. In my own research, they often appeared ephemerally in primary sources. As the late José Esteban Muñoz writes, "Work that attempts to index the anecdotal, the performative, or what I call the ephemeral as proof is often undermined by the academy's officiating structures."[10] Charles E. Morris III reiterates this point: "As queer rhetorical scholars, hobbled on the one hand by such silences, and on the other by benevolent colleagues who, smelling blood, ratchet up the professional standards that constitute our distinctive burden of proof, we must keenly recognize that to succeed we must become the deftest of archivist-rhetors, or archival queers."[11] Emphasizing the ephemeral refuses this norm; this book reflects a queer politics that others can use to animate their own scholarly projects.

At its heart, this book performs a critique of citizenship and the entire project of the United States. I am not the first to make such a critique. Fundamentally, any such critique is indebted to Chicano/a/x and Latino/a/x studies, Asian American studies, Indigenous studies, gender studies, Black studies, and immigration studies. I am most indebted to the latter two in this undertaking. The biggest takeaway of this book, which I began as a study of AIDS and immigration, is that Blackness, both as an area of study and as it manifests in citizenship and immigration, must be central because Blackness resides at the center of the alienizing nation and resistances to it. In the remainder of this conclusion, I elaborate on this point, using Brimelow's fears about the alien nation to generate some additional insights about the alienizing nation.

Brimelow, though an "alien" himself, laments a particular character of the United States' becoming and potential being as a result of the 1965 Immigration Act. The act is generally remembered for eliminating race-based quotas, thereby opening up new possibilities for people from countries, particularly in Asia, to migrate to the United States. The act did increase migration, but it did not completely liberalize immigration law as Brimelow suggests. Eithne Luibhéid argues that because the act also ensured that nearly three-fourths of legal migrants to the United States would come through so-called family reunification, most migration channels remained closed for anyone without desirable skills, high income, or heteronormative family already in the United States.[12] Still, it remains true that this act ended the era of formal racial quotas and opened up possibility for the United States to fulfill its promise as "a nation of immigrants." Brimelow understands this potential as a becoming that not only fundamentally threatens to alter the white nation, but if becoming results in being, the United States will be a "freak" among its peers.

The use of the word "freak" is especially revealing of Brimelow's anxieties about the modern US nation. A freak is a monster, or at least monstrous, a word extending from the Latin *monstrum*—a bad omen, that which evokes fear. Rosemarie Garland Thomson suggests that "freak discourse is both imbricated in and reflective of our cultural transformation into modernity." She explains that freak discourse actually maps the trajectory of modernity's narrative: "What was once sought after as revelation becomes pursued as entertainment; what aroused awe now inspires horror; what was taken as a portent shifts to a site of progress. In brief, wonder becomes error."[13] Garland Thomson and other scholars of race, gender, sexuality, and disability have discussed this mapping in relation to exceptional human bodies—in particular racialized, queer, and disabled bodies. In modern times, freakish bodies are bodies in error.

Although human bodies are typically the subject of freak discourse, we can also make an analogy to the exceptional national body, made transparent in the classic idea of "American exceptionalism." What has made the "grand experiment" of these united states exceptional is its melting pot, its founding in revolution, its form of representative democracy, and its brand of freedom that is supposedly foreign to the European countries that US colonizers fled. But the grand experiment has always provoked anxiety, particularly around the purity and fitness of the national body with so many different types of people mixed in. This exceptional national body was once a wonder, but would it also become an error? Would the experiment, like Frankenstein, be taken too far? Brimelow's concern about being a "freak" is a concern about the health of the national body. Health for Brimelow, like so many of the architects of this nation, refers primarily to race and culture, but those fears have always been simultaneously about migrant sexuality, gender ideologies, and overall mental and physical fitness for the nation. Some cultures and races and their practices and "inferior stock" create dis-ease for the nation. To become an alien nation is to become a freak nation—a nation full of freaks, a dis-eased nation, and a nation freakish to other modern, white nations. Although this concern seems to be about reputation, it is only that inasmuch as the internal quality of the US nation would make it inferior to whiter, "purer" nations.

Brimelow's reliance on the racist, ableist, normative term "freak" further reveals this fact as we move into Brimelow's next concern: for the nation itself, particularly (white) US Americans' standing among one another in the present. If the nation is full of freaks, not only will it be inferior to other nations, but how will citizens recognize one another if they live in an alien/freak nation? How will they peacefully coexist? The answer, of course, is that they will not, at least not without significant government intervention. If citizens are too strange to one another, the argument goes, the nation simply cannot survive. The mortal threat that is the inability to recognize one's self in their fellow citizens is of course a strong rationale to find ways to enact the alienizing logic.

This fear of survival led Brimelow to his most significant concern, which is that if US citizens are alien to one another, they will no longer share "the mystic chords of memory," words he pulled from President Abraham Lincoln's first inaugural address, delivered in March 1861 on the precipice of civil war with seven southern states having already seceded.[14] This address is not Lincoln's most famous, but his final words have been widely praised for their literary and epideictic quality.[15] David Zarefsky notes that this speech is fundamentally about the question of secession, with Lincoln intending to frame the situation in such a way that if a war broke out, the southern states would be regarded as the aggressors.[16] For Lincoln, "the mystic chords of memory" are aspirational, what he hopes for and envisions for the union, and that hope is a sentimental appeal to remain in the union in order to continue to perfect it, to reach the melodic harmony. For Brimelow, the "mystic chords" are that which exist or, in his mind, once existed and are in grave danger of never being recoverable. The longing for harmony that Lincoln and Brimelow share result in what some will be surprised to see is a shared worldview. For both, alienizing logic animates their positions.

Although Lincoln personally disagreed with the institution of slavery, his treatment of slavery in the speech reveals his grounding in white supremacy, which will help to illuminate why Brimelow turns to this speech, the depth of alienizing logic in the United States, and what is at stake in preserving it. Lincoln began his address by assuring southerners that, as he has said many times before, he had no intention of intervening in the institution of slavery. His opening anticipates the president-who-freed-the-enslaved's ultimate objective: to preserve the imperfect union and implore those who would divide it to engage by other means. Just prior to what Brimelow quotes, Lincoln pleads, "We are not enemies, but friends. We must not be enemies. Though passion may have strained it must not break our bonds of affection." Lincoln's shift from "are" to "must" is instructive. Lincoln insists that "we," the citizens of the United States, whether in the North or the South, are not enemies, but he simultaneously commands "us" not to be. He demands friendship despite, or perhaps because of, his support of slavery and genocide. No matter that slavery should contradict the values upon which the United States was ostensibly built, for Lincoln and for Brimelow, the alternative to holding tight to these bonds of white supremacist, nationalist affection is civil war. Thus, Brimelow implies that if the alien nation comes to be, it can, in effect, expect a civil war. This thesis insists that white racial, ethnic, and cultural harmony must be preserved to prevent extreme forms of state violence.

It is important to remember that Lincoln spent a significant portion of his first inaugural address not only expressing his tacit support for slavery's right to exist but also affirming the right of southern property owners to reclaim their human property when they became fugitives. He affirmed states' rights, saying it did not matter whether that property was reclaimed by national or state authorities, but the law of the land must be upheld. Enslavement and capture, two of the most extreme forms of state violence, cannot feature as such in Lincoln's worldview; when he implores his audience that "we must not be enemies," he affirms that the assurance of this alienizing right is that which will keep "us" in union. Slavery may be a scourge on the United States and a contradiction of its avowed principles of life, liberty, and the pursuit of happiness, but these contradictions are not sufficient reason for "us" to be unfriendly to one another, to start a war. According to Lincoln, "we" can—we must—hold that contradiction and still be whole. In fact, even when we disagree with the actions of this imperfect union, we must do the duty of alienizing. The rhetoric of this union will be stronger than what we do to other human beings among us. What can and must keep the union together is a belief in the claims the union makes about itself in its Constitution and Declaration of Independence. Thus, what keeps us together, how we prevent ourselves from becoming alien to one another, is to uphold the right to alienize: to enslave, to capture, to displace, and to kill. To remain whole, we must keep alive the potential to alienize. Put simply, slavery is constitutive of us. We become a people in our inalienable right to alienize. And if we take away this right, *that* is the undoing of this union. We would have to become something else. To alienize, whether by genocide, lynching, the plantation, the reservation, the ghetto, the internment camp, the prison, the hospital, quarantine, ban, or deportation, is our engine—not just economically, but culturally—and for Lincoln, within an alienizing nation, we must still be friends. To untie the binds of slavery would be to undo the union of friendship, and Lincoln would do all he could to keep the white, alienizing nation.

The alienizing potential—toward the enslaved, the Indigenous, the poor, the alien citizen of color, the migrant—is the bond required for the sovereignty of the nation, these united states, and the masters. Keeping this bond is the possibility to govern. Lincoln extends the branch of friendship on the promise of the ability to alienize—to rule over—even if we don't like it. This is the birth *and the life* of a nation, the homosocial reproductivity of nationhood. Although his premise defies his principles, Lincoln put aside his misgivings, assuring he would not take away the inalienable right to alienize, to rule over, to sovereignty. Lincoln was willing to cede the blood of the enslaved in order to maintain the soil of the nation. It is sacrificial.

Lincoln stakes his claim on the presumption of the vulnerability of the national body. Of course, in one obvious way, his fears made sense on the brink of civil war. But this enduring fear of the national body's vulnerability excuses, enables, and allows violence against the alienized for the sake of the greater project: the white union and all its promises. But the national body is premised on the alienizing logic *and power* of white supremacy, and it was and is actually not vulnerable at all. This national body was and is a vicious, powerful, unrelenting association. In part this is because of the national body's pliability, its dexterity in order to preserve its inalienable right to alienize.

Even a nation that diversifies its citizenry can preserve this right to alienize because, ultimately, it is not dependent on being or becoming but doing. If we move to a twenty-first century example, we can see how being white is not the same as the doing of white supremacy. The doing is invitational: you, no matter whether you are white, can do it too. You can do friendship by targeting, by alienizing the enemy. Zygmunt Bauman argues that the stranger, and we might say alien, is what blurs the friend/enemy binary. The stranger is neither friend nor enemy, but we can have friendship and avoid enemyship by targeting other strangers/aliens. In her revision of this claim, Sara Ahmed claims that the stranger/alien only becomes that by *being recognized* as such.[17] The stranger is always in our midst. Thus, within white supremacy, one does not have to *be* white to recognize another as alien. This ability to recognize another as a stranger/ alien helps to illustrate the distinction between being white and doing white supremacy, a distinction that is central to upholding the alienizing nation. Doing white supremacy can legitimize one who might otherwise be recognized as a stranger/alien. He can still *do* friendship. Even those recognized as strangers can take opportunities to do white supremacy, which means they have use value for the alienizing nation. In this way, to belong or to have friendship is not about identity but identification to an ideology and through a logic of alienizing.

This dynamic and therefore the power of the alienizing nation can be seen in the case of George Zimmerman, the mixed-race Latino and self-appointed neighborhood watchman who killed seventeen-year-old Black youth Trayvon Martin in Florida in 2012. Zimmerman lynched a Black youth and avoided murder charges because of Florida's "stand your ground" law. But Zimmerman did not stand *his* ground, he stood *our* ground, the sovereign ground of the state of Florida and the United States. He did white supremacy by supposedly defending a white neighborhood against the threat of Blackness. Blackness is, and always has been in the United States, an opportunity to enact alienizing logic in the form of cap-ture, incarceration, and murder. Blackness creates the opportunity to do the bidding of white supremacy, even if the murder is not at the hands of a white person. Lincoln licensed the right to alienize because it is required to preserve the home, the proper, property-owning polity. Zimmerman, though not wholly white, made good on that license. Thus, more than a century after Lincoln's affirmation of the right to alienize in order to pre-serve this imperfect union, the nation remains invulnerable because of the power of white supremacy and the power of alienizing logic in constitut-ing it. What Lincoln and Brimelow fear—the breaking of bonds—are within alienizing logic virtually impossible. Opportunities will always arise and be taken in order to preserve the alienizing nation. Quarantine and ban, as manifestations of alienizing logic, are then as American as apple pie. They helped to preserve the bonds of friendship among those so endowed.

This book has offered one instance among many that shows how the threat of the alien nation feared by Lincoln, Brimelow, and so many others is combated by the alienizing nation, the nation that operates by the logic of expulsion, exclusion, and extermination. Thus, where Brimelow is concerned about a potential state of being for the nation, I am concerned about the nation's doing. The alienizing nation may no longer be in the midst of a civil war, but it is premised on exerting extreme forms of state violence against any of those, citizen or migrant, who do not conform to the state's white supremacist, anti-Black, ableist, heteropatriarchal, capitalist norms. The alienizing nation seeks opportunities to enact its logic, and disease repeatedly becomes one such opportunity. *The Borders of AIDS* has documented the ways that HIV/AIDS was—and continues to be—one incredible opportunity for alienizing logic to manifest against the most maligned people in the United States. I have also shown how alienizing logic's manifestations in quarantine and ban come to be justified as rational, commonsense responses to grave threats to the nation. This is not to say that the politicians, public health officials, and others who advocated for quarantine and ban were all ill-intentioned or bad people. It is to say that they expressed the deep logic of the alienizing nation.

But perhaps the most important contribution of this book is that in it, I have documented the ways afflicted communities refused their treatment and fought back. Their imperfect tactics—sometimes also doing the bidding of the alienizing nation by participating in anti-Blackness or reinscribing the divide and conquer logic of worthy and unworthy—are important to interrogate in order to hone our collective abilities to build coalitions to fight alienizing logic. But then, as now, these struggles are always incomplete, can often be categorized as failures in the immediate, and given the way archives and public memory work, are often relegated to a footnote or are forgotten all together. Nevertheless, the stakes for documenting our challenges and continuing to challenge the alienizing nation remain high: this logic is the very material out of which the United States was built and survives. Rather than longing for those mystic chords of memory, we must break the cords that bind them.

EPILOGUE

The statues are falling down. They are not actually falling, of course. Groups of committed, masked activists (not just anarchists or would-be Zapatistas but people concerned about one another's health) have collectively used their strength to topple stone and metal memorials of racist historical figures ranging from Confederate leaders such as Stonewall Jackson and Robert E. Lee to colonial murderer Christopher Columbus to notorious Philadelphia mayor Frank Rizzo. To date, Washington and Lincoln memorials remain unscathed, with the exception of the Emancipation Memorial, designed by Thomas Ball in 1876, in Washington, DC, with a copy erected in Boston a few years later.[1] In this nineteenth-century memorial, Lincoln dons a full suit and stands above a kneeling enslaved Black man dressed only in a loin cloth. Lincoln stares down at the man, with one arm leaning against a platform holding the Emancipation Proclamation and the other outstretched over the man's head as if he is anointing him. The kneeling man is Archer Alexander, who escaped enslavement and helped the Union army only to be returned to slaveholders under the Fugitive Slave Act.[2] Alexander's eyes look upward while the cuffs of the broken chains of slavery dangle at his wrists and ankles. After both Harvard University students and a petition with over twelve thousand signatures called for the statue's removal, the Boston Arts Commission voted unanimously to remove the statue.[3] Activists have also turned attention to the original Emancipation Memorial in Washington, DC, funded largely by formerly enslaved people.

The statue has always been controversial. At the statue's unveiling in Washington, DC, on April 14, 1876—on the eleventh anniversary of Lincoln's assassination—Frederick Douglass gave an impassioned speech. Scholars have widely considered this speech as they have the relationship between Lincoln and Douglass, and so I do not intend to rehearse those arguments here.[4] What I want to draw attention to is the oft-cited section that comes early in the speech, when Douglass, who had a complicated personal relationship with whiteness,[5] proclaimed that Lincoln "was pre-eminently the white man's President, entirely devoted to the welfare of white men. He was ready and willing at any time during the first years of his administration to deny, postpone, and sacrifice the rights of humanity in the colored people to promote the welfare of the white people of this country."[6] This claim makes sense as Douglass clearly had as his delicate task complicating Lincoln's legacy by honoring that he oversaw the fall of slavery and insisting that he was no great liberator. Douglass's statement echoes Lincoln from the first inaugural address: preserving the imperfect union was always his priority. This priority remains true of every president and most white Americans ever since, no matter the cost to Black, Indigenous, and other people of color. Confederate statues become an acceptable target in this regard, even as they are fiercely defended by Republicans and white nationalists, because they reflect the severing of the nation. Overt racists or Indigenous murderers like Columbus are also acceptable targets to a majority for similar reasons. US American "heroes" such as Lincoln and founding fathers such as Jefferson and Washington who held slaves generally remain untouchable. If not for the demeaning depiction of Blackness in the Emancipation Memorial, it too would be beyond reproach.

Contemporary Black liberationists rebelling in response to yet more police and vigilante murders of unarmed Black people hammer cracks in the foundations of the pedestals not just of these statues but the very structures that enable honoring and upholding white supremacy. In the moment I write, they are closer than ever before to pushing society up against what was previously beyond reproach—not just supposedly heroic American monuments but the abolition of police and Immigration and Customs Enforcement, the release of the imprisoned, and more. The very structures that have built the alienizing nation are, I believe and hope, under duress. And all this while COVID-19 ravishes Black, Indigenous, and other communities of color. And while police and vigilante murder of Black people and others in the United States happens with astonishing frequency, perhaps disease became an opportunity in another way. Stay-at-home orders creating weeks of quarantine and isolation perhaps gave space for the anger to build and for people to realize that no matter the risk, the possible rewards for freedom were bigger.

I don't know. Historians and others will interpret this moment with the privilege of greater distance than I have. Furthermore, due to my own underlying condition, against my political sensibilities, I have sat these protests out, quarantining for months now in my comfortable east Austin home with my partner and my animal companions. What I do know, and as I stated in the introduction to this book, is that AIDS has, and will always have, lessons for moments when the alienizing nation violently and subtly enacts its logic. We will be well served by learning them and, more importantly, drawing on them to confront whatever we face.

NOTES

PROLOGUE

1. Lauren Berlant, *Cruel Optimism* (Durham, NC: Duke University Press, 2011), 4.
2. Laura LeMoon, "What the Early AIDS Epidemic Can Teach Us about COVID-19," *HIV Plus Magazine*, March 12, 2020, www.hivplusmag.com /opinion/2020/3/12/what-early-aids-epidemic-can-teach-us-about-covid-19.
3. Mathew Rodriguez, "COVID-19 and HIV Are Not the Same. But They're Similar in Many Ways That Matter," *The Body*, April 9, 2020, www.thebody .com/article/covid-19-aids-not-same-but-similar-in-many-ways.
4. "COVID-19 in Racial and Ethnic Minority Groups," Centers for Disease Control and Prevention, accessed June 25, 2020, www.cdc.gov/coronavirus /2019-ncov/need-extra-precautions/racial-ethnic-minorities.html.
5. Graeme Wood, "What's Behind the COVID-19 Racial Disparity?" *The Atlantic*, May 27, 2020.
6. While I don't want to give this much oxygen here, it is important to note that many, mostly white US Americans were taking to the streets to demand their right to work, get their hair cut, go to bars, and congregate as they pleased without the inconvenience of masks.
7. Hal Dardick, "No Apparent COVID-19 Spread from George Floyd Protests," *Chicago Tribune*, July 2, 2020; and Akshay Syal, "Black Lives Matter Protests Haven't Led to COVID-19 Spikes," *NBC News*, June 24, 2020.
8. Ali Rogin and Amna Nawaz, "'We Have Been through This Before,' Why Anti-Asian Hate Crimes Are Rising amid Coronavirus," *PBS News Hour*, June 25, 2020.
9. Jessica Schaldebeck, "Coronavirus Cases at Immigrant Detention Centers Could Be 15 Times Higher Than ICE Reports, Study Says," *New York Daily News*, July 2, 2020.
10. Thomas H. Maugh II and Davan Maharaj, "AIDS No. 1 Cause of Death of Young Men in California," *Los Angeles Times*, June 16, 1993.
11. Johns Hopkins University of Medicine Coronavirus Resource Center, "Mortality Analyses," accessed August 11, 2020, https://coronavirus.jhu.edu/data/mortality.

TERMINOLOGY

1. Eithne Luibhéid, "Introduction: Queer Migration and Citizenship," in *Queer Migrations: Sexuality, U.S. Citizenship, and Border Crossings*, ed. Eithne

Luibhéid and Lionel Cantú Jr. (Minneapolis: University of Minnesota Press, 2005).

2. Eithne Luibhéid, "Sexuality, Migration, and the Shifting Line between Legal and Illegal Status," *GLQ* 14, no. 2–3 (2008): 289–316.

INTRODUCTION: THE ALIENIZING NATION

1. David Kaufman, "How the Pride March Made History," *New York Times*, June 16, 2020.

2. Trevor Hoppe, *Punishing Disease: HIV and the Criminalization of Sickness* (Berkeley: University of California Press, 2017); and Asha Persson and Christy Newman, "Making Monsters: Heterosexuality, Crime and Race in Recent Western Media Coverage of HIV," *Sociology of Health and Illness* 30, no. 4 (2008): 632–46.

3. Annie Hill, "SlutWalk as Perifeminist Response to Rape Logic: The Politics of Reclaiming a Name," *Communication and Critical/Cultural Studies* 13, no. 1 (2016): 23–39.

4. Sara Ahmed, *Strange Encounters: Embodied Others in Post-Coloniality* (London: Routledge, 2000).

5. *OED Online*, s.v. "alien, adj. and n," accessed December 26, 2019, www.oed .com.

6. Keith Cunningham-Parmeter, "Alien Language: Immigration Metaphors and the Jurisprudence of Otherness," *Fordham Law Review* 79 (2011): 613–66.

7. Edwin F. Ackerman, "The 'Illegal Alien' as a Category of Analysis: A Methodological Intervention," *Journal of Language and Politics* 13, no. 3 (2014): 563–79.

8. Zygmunt Bauman, "Making and Unmaking of Strangers," *Thesis Eleven* 43, no. 1 (1995): 1.

9. Bauman, 2.

10. On the stranger as foundational to building state order, see Bonnie Honig, *Democracy and the Foreigner* (Princeton, NJ: Princeton University Press, 2001).

11. Ahmed, *Strange Encounters*.

12. Katarzyna Marciniak, *Alienhood: Citizenship, Exile, and the Logic of Difference* (Minneapolis: University of Minnesota Press, 2006), xiii.

13. Ayelet Shachar, Rainer Bauböck, Irene Bloemraad, and Maarten Vink, eds., *The Oxford Handbook of Citizenship* (Oxford: Oxford University Press, 2017); and Amy L. Brandzel, *Against Citizenship: The Violence of the Normative* (Urbana: University of Illinois Press, 2016).

14. Linda Bosniak, *The Citizen and the Alien: Dilemmas of Contemporary Membership* (Princeton, NJ: Princeton University Press, 2006), 13.

15. Joseph Nevins, *Operation Gatekeeper: The Rise of the "Illegal Alien" and the Making of the U.S.-Mexico Boundary* (New York: Routledge, 2002); Eithne Luibhéid, "Sexuality, Migration, and the Shifting Line between Legal and Illegal Status," *GLQ* 14, no. 2–3 (2008): 289–315; and Jenna M. Loyd, Matt

Mitchelson, and Andrew Burridge, eds., *Beyond Walls and Cages: Prisons, Borders, and Global Crisis* (Athens: University of Georgia Press, 2012).

16. Adelaida R. Del Castillo, "Illegal Status and Social Citizenship: Thoughts on Mexican Immigrants in a Postnational World," *Aztlan* 27, no. 2 (2002): 9–32; Renato Rosaldo, "Cultural Citizenship and Educational Democracy," *Cultural Anthropology* 9, no. 3 (1994): 402–11; and Aihwa Ong, "Cultural Citizenship as Subject-Making: Immigrants Negotiate Racial and Cultural Boundaries in the United States," *Current Anthropology* 37, no. 5 (1996): 737–62.

17. Aihwa Ong, *Buddha Is Hiding: Refugees, Citizenship, the New America* (Berkeley: University of California Press, 2003), 217.

18. Avigail Eisenberg and Patti Tamara Lenard, "The Theory and Politics of the Second-Class Citizenship," *Politics, Groups, and Identities* 8, no. 2 (2020): 213–15.

19. Bosniak, *Citizen and the Alien.*

20. Mae M. Ngai, *Impossible Subjects: Illegal Aliens and the Making of Modern America* (Princeton, NJ: Princeton University Press, 2004), 8. An expansive body of social scientific and humanities literature explores various iterations of the production of formations akin to what Ngai calls "alien citizens." See, e.g., David Bacon, *Illegal People: How Globalization Creates Migration and Criminalizes Immigrants* (Boston: Beacon Press, 2008); David Cole, *Enemy Aliens: Double Standards and Constitutional Freedoms in the War on Terrorism* (New York: New Press, 2003); Lisa A. Flores, *Deportable and Disposable: Public Rhetoric and the Making of the "Illegal" Immigrant* (State College: Pennsylvania State University Press, 2020); Erika Lee, *America for Americans: A History of Xenophobia in the United States* (New York: Basic Books, 2019); Erika Lee, *At America's Gates: Chinese Immigration during the Exclusion Era, 1882–1943* (Chapel Hill: University of North Carolina Press, 2004); Lisa Lowe, *Immigrant Acts: On Asian American Cultural Politics* (Durham, NC: Duke University Press, 1996); Patrisia Macías-Rojas, *From Deportation to Prison: The Politics of Immigration Enforcement in Post-Civil Rights America* (New York: New York University Press, 2016); Kunal M. Parker, *Making Foreigners: Immigration and Citizenship Law in America, 1600–2000* (New York: Cambridge University Press, 2015); Jasbir K. Puar, *Terrorist Assemblages: Homonationalism in Queer Times* (Durham, NC: Duke University Press, 2007); Saskia Sassen, *Guests and Aliens* (New York: New Press, 1999); and Elliott Young, *Alien Nation: Chinese Migration in the Americas from the Coolie Era through World War II* (Chapel Hill: University of North Carolina Press, 2014).

21. Brett C. Stockdill, *Activism against AIDS: At the Intersection of Sexuality, Race, Gender, and Class* (Boulder, CO: Lynne Rienner Publishers, 2003), 2. Others that share this concern include Sabrina Marie Chase, *Surviving HIV/AIDS in the Inner City: How Resourceful Latinas Beat the Odds* (New Brunswick, NJ: Rutgers University Press, 2011); Cathy J. Cohen, *The Boundaries of Blackness: AIDS and the Breakdown of Black Politics* (Chicago: University of Chicago Press, 1999); and ACT UP/NY and Women and AIDS Book Group, eds., *Women, AIDS & Activism* (Boston: South End Press, 1990).

22. There is a long history in the United States of the relationship between disease and alienizing logic. See, e.g., Amy L. Fairchild, *Science at the Borders: Immigrant Medical Inspection and the Shaping of the Modern Industrial Labor Force* (Baltimore: Johns Hopkins University Press, 2003); Alan M. Kraut, *Silent Travelers: Germs, Genes, and the "Immigrant Menace"* (Baltimore: Johns Hopkins University Press, 1994); Howard Markel and Alexandra Minna Stern, "The Foreignness of Germs: The Persistent Association of Immigrants and Disease in American Society," *Milbank Quarterly* 80, no. 4 (2002): 757–88; John Mckiernan-González, *Fevered Measures: Public Health and Race at the Texas-Mexico Border, 1848–1942* (Durham, NC: Duke University Press, 2012); and Natalia Molina, "Borders, Laborers, and Racialized Medicalization: Mexican Immigration and US Public Health Practices in the 20th Century," *American Journal of Public Health* 101, no. 6 (2011): 1024–31.

23. There is an expansive body of work that explores racism and colonialism in the history of public health and medical practice. Some important studies in this regard include Neel Ahuja, *Bioinsecurities: Disease Interventions, Empire, and the Government of Species* (Durham, NC: Duke University Press, 2016); Warwick Anderson, *Colonial Pathologies: American Tropical Medicine, Race, and Hygiene in the Philippines* (Durham, NC: Duke University Press, 2006); Warwick Anderson, *The Cultivation of Whiteness Science, Health, and Racial Destiny in Australia* (Durham, NC: Duke University Press, 2006); Michelle T. Moran, *Colonizing Leprosy: Imperialism and the Politics of Public Health in the United States* (Chapel Hill: University of North Carolina Press, 2007); and Samuel Kelton Roberts Jr., *Infectious Fear: Politics, Disease, and the Health Effects of Segregation* (Chapel Hill: University of North Carolina Press, 2009).

24. Susan L. Smith, *Sick and Tired of Being Sick and Tired: Black Women's Health Activism in America, 1890–1950* (Philadelphia: University of Pennsylvania Press, 1995), 5.

25. As Smith also argues, consistent public health and medical maltreatment of Black people in the United States has also led Black folks, perhaps especially women, to organize on behalf of their communities. See also Alondra Nelson, *Body and Soul: The Black Panther Party and the Fight against Medical Discrimination* (Minneapolis: University of Minnesota Press, 2011).

26. Nayan Shah, *Contagious Divides: Epidemics and Race in San Francisco's Chinatown* (Berkeley: University of California Press, 2001), 4. See also Natalia Molina, *Fit to Be Citizens? Public Health and Race in Los Angeles, 1879–1939* (Berkeley: University of California Press, 2006).

27. Markel and Stern, "Foreignness of Germs," 757.

28. Mckiernan-González, *Fevered Measures*; Erica Rand, *The Ellis Island Snow Globe* (Durham, NC: Duke University Press, 2005); and Alexandra Minna Stern, "Buildings, Boundaries, and Blood: Medicalization and Nation-Building on the U.S.-Mexico Border, 1910–1930," *Hispanic American Historical Review* 79, no. 1 (1999): 41–81.

29. Annie Hill, "Breast Cancer's Rhetoricity: Bodily Border Crisis and Bridge to Corporeal Solidarity," *Review of Communication* 16, no. 4 (2016): 281–98.

30. Susan Sontag, *Illness as Metaphor and AIDS and Its Metaphors* (New York: Doubleday, 1990), 100.

31. Paula A. Treichler, *How to Have Theory in an Epidemic: Cultural Chronicles of AIDS* (Durham, NC: Duke University Press, 1999), 329.

32. E.g., Dennis Altman, *AIDS in the Mind of America: The Social, Political, and Psychological Impact of a New Epidemic* (New York: Anchor Press, 1986); Michael Callen, *Surviving AIDS* (New York: HarperPerennial, 1990); Peter F. Cohen, *Love and Anger: Essays on AIDS, Activism, and Politics* (Binghamton, NY: Harrington Press, 1998); Douglas Crimp, *Melancholia and Moralism: Essays on AIDS and Queer Politics* (Cambridge, MA: MIT Press, 2002); Martin Duberman, *Hold Tight Gently: Michael Callen, Essex Hemphill, and the Battlefield of AIDS* (New York: New Press, 2014); Steven Epstein, *Impure Science: AIDS, Activism, and the Politics of Knowledge* (Berkeley: University of California Press, 1996); Deborah B. Gould, *Moving Politics: Emotion and ACT UP's Fight against AIDS* (Chicago: University of Chicago Press, 2009); Richard A. McKay, *Patient Zero and the Making of the AIDS Epidemic* (Chicago: University of Chicago Press, 2017); David Román, *Acts of Intervention: Performance, Gay Culture, and AIDS* (Bloomington: Indiana University Press, 1998); and Randy Shilts, *And the Band Played On: Politics, People, and the AIDS Epidemic* (New York: St. Martin's Press, 1987).

33. E.g., Ronald Bayer and Gerald M. Oppenheimer, *AIDS Doctors: Voices from the Epidemic: An Oral History* (Oxford: Oxford University Press, 2000); Victoria A. Harden, *AIDS at 30: A History* (Washington, DC: Potomac Books, 2012); and Perry N. Halkitis, *The AIDS Generation: Stories of Survival and Resistance* (Oxford: Oxford University Press, 2014).

34. Margot Canaday, *The Straight State: Sexuality and Citizenship in Twentieth-Century America* (Princeton, NJ: Princeton University Press, 2009); David K. Johnson, *The Lavender Scare: The Cold War Persecution of Gays and Lesbians in the Federal Government* (Chicago: University of Chicago Press, 2006); Joey Mogul, Andrea Ritchie, and Kay Whitlock, *Queer (in)Justice: The Criminalization of LGBT People in the United States* (Boston: Beacon Press, 2011); Eric A. Stanley and Nat Smith, eds., *Captive Genders: Trans Embodiment and the Prison Industrial Complex* (Oakland, CA: AK Press, 2011); Ryan Conrad, ed., *Against Equality: Queer Revolution Not Mere Inclusion* (Oakland, CA: AK Press, 2014); Kath Weston, *Families We Choose: Lesbians, Gays, Kinship* (New York: Columbia University Press, 1991); Sarah Schulman, *Ties That Bind: Familial Homophobia and Its Consequences* (New York: New Press, 2009); and Eithne Luibhéid, *Entry Denied: Controlling Sexuality at the Border* (Minneapolis: University of Minnesota Press, 2002).

35. Michele Tracy Berger, *Workable Sisterhood: The Political Journey of Stigmatized Women with HIV/AIDS* (Princeton, NJ: Princeton University Press, 2004); see also Darius Bost, *Evidence of Being: The Black Gay Cultural Renaissance and the Politics of Violence* (Chicago: University of Chicago Press, 2018); Héctor Carrillo, *The Night Is Young: Sexuality in Mexico in the Time of AIDS* (Chicago: University of Chicago Press, 2002); Chase, *Surviving*

HIV/AIDS; Gena Corea, *The Invisible Epidemic: The Story of Women and AIDS* (New York: HarperCollins, 1992); Alyson O'Daniel, *Holding On: African American Women Surviving AIDS* (Lincoln: University of Nebraska Press, 2016); and Celeste Watkins-Hayes, *Remaking a Life: How Women Living with HIV/AIDS Confront Inequality* (Berkeley: University of California Press, 2019).

36. Jennifer Brier has been the notable exception in this regard. See Jennifer Brier, *Infectious Ideas: U.S. Political Responses to the AIDS Crisis* (Chapel Hill: University of North Carolina Press, 2009); and Jennifer Brier, "The Immigrant Infection: Images of Race, Nation, and Contagion in the Public Debates on AIDS and Immigration," in *Modern American Queer History*, ed. Allida M. Black (Philadelphia: Temple University Press, 2001).

37. Jih-Fei Cheng, Alexandra Juhasz, and Nishant Shahani, *AIDS and the Distribution of Crises* (Durham, NC: Duke University Press, 2020).

38. It is important to note that just as medications became more available in 1996, "the epidemic became disproportionately a disease of African Americans." See Linda Villarosa in Marlon M. Bailey, Darius Bost, Jennifer Brier, Angelique Harris, Johnnie Ray Kornegay III, Linda Villarosa, Dagmawi Woubshet, Marissa Miller, and Dana D. Hines, "Souls Forum: The Black AIDS Epidemic," *Souls* 21, no. 2–3 (2019): 217.

39. Ted Kerr, "A History of Erasing Black Artists and Bodies from the AIDS Conversation," *Hyperallergic*, December 31, 2015, https://hyperallergic.com/264934/a-history-of-erasing-black-artists-and-bodies-from-the-aids-conversation.

40. Bost, *Evidence of Being*, 16.

41. Bost; Katherine McKittrick, *Demonic Grounds: Black Women and the Cartographies of Struggle* (Minneapolis: University of Minnesota Press, 2006); and Tiffany Lethabo King, *The Black Shoals: Offshore Formations of Black and Native Studies* (Durham, NC: Duke University Press, 2019).

42. King, 30.

43. Cheng, Juhasz, and Shahani, *AIDS and the Distribution of Crises*, 2.

CHAPTER ONE: A BRIEF RHETORICAL HISTORY OF QUARANTINE

1. Felicia R. Lee, "Bench of Memory at Slavery's Gateway," *New York Times*, July 28, 2008.

2. Popular history in South Carolina views the history in this way. A marker on the island notes "tens of thousands" of Black people arriving at this port. See, e.g., Bob Janiskee, "Sullivan's Island Was the African American Ellis Island," *National Parks Traveler*, March 3, 2009, www.nationalparkstraveler.org/2009/03/sullivan-s-island-african-american-ellis-island. More recently, some historians have questioned this taken-for-granted narrative, suggesting that only as many as 5 percent to 20 percent of arriving Africans came through Sullivan's Island. See Robert Behre, "Historian Sheds New Light on How Many Slaves Might Have Been Quarantined on Sullivan's Island, but No One Knows

for Sure," *Post and Courier* (Charleston, NC), August 25, 2017. Historian Peter H. Wood first made the problematic comparison to Ellis Island. Peter H. Wood, *Black Majority: Negroes in Colonial South Carolina from 1670 through the Stono Rebellion* (New York: Knopf, 1975).

3. Suzannah Smith Miles, *Writings of the Islands: Sullivan's Island and Isle of Palms* (Columbia, SC: History Press, 2004).

4. See, e.g., Joe Feagin and Zinobia Bennefield, "Systemic Racism and U.S. Health Care," *Social Science and Medicine* 103 (2014): 7–14; Betsy Hartmann, *Reproductive Rights and Wrongs: The Global Politics of Population Control* (Boston: South End Press, 1995); John M. Hoberman, *Black and Blue: The Origins and Consequences of Medical Racism* (Berkeley: University of California Press, 2012); James H. Jones, *Bad Blood: The Tuskegee Syphilis Experiment* (New York: Free Press, 1981); Rebecca Skloot, *The Immortal Life of Henrietta Lacks* (New York: Crown, 2010); and Harriet A. Washington, *Medical Apartheid: The Dark History of Medical Experimentation on Black Americans from Colonial Times to the Present* (New York: Harlem Moon, 2006).

5. Rhetorical history is not a singular thing. It can refer to several methodological approaches that bring together rhetoric and history. See David Zarefsky, "Four Senses of Rhetorical History," in *Doing Rhetorical History: Concepts and Cases*, ed. Kathleen Turner (Tuscaloosa: University of Alabama Press, 2003), 19–32. My approach in this chapter is perhaps most akin to Celeste Michelle Condit and John Louis Lucaites's rhetorical history of the concept of "equality" in public discourse in the United States. See Celeste Michelle Condit and John Louis Lucaites, *Crafting Equality: America's Anglo-African Word* (Chicago: University of Chicago Press, 1993).

6. Richard A. McKay, *Patient Zero and the Making of the AIDS Epidemic* (Chicago: University of Chicago Press, 2017), 44.

7. McKay, 44.

8. Scott W. Stern, *The Trials of Nina McCall: Sex, Surveillance, and the Decades-Long Government Plan to Imprison "Promiscuous" Women* (Boston: Beacon Press, 2018).

9. Brock C. Hampton, "Development of the National Maritime Quarantine System of the United States," *Public Health Reports* 55, no. 28 (July 12, 1940): 1241–93.

10. George Rosen, *A History of Public Health*, expanded ed. (Baltimore: Johns Hopkins University Press, 1993).

11. Mark Harrison, *Contagion: How Commerce Has Spread Disease* (New Haven, CT: Yale University Press, 2012), 8. Ragussa was located in what is now Croatia.

12. *OED Online*, s.v. "quarantine, n.," accessed February 5, 2019, www.oed.com.

13. Rosen, *History of Public Health*, 45.

14. Alison Bashford, "Maritime Quarantine: Linking Old World and New World Histories," in *Quarantine: Local and Global Histories*, ed. Alison Bashford (London: Palgrave Macmillan, 2016), 5. Of course, isolation existed at

locations other than ports too. There are records of isolating people with
plague, for example.

15. Harrison, *Contagion*, 13–14.

16. Bashford, "Maritime Quarantine," 5.

17. Alan M. Kraut, *Silent Travelers: Germs, Genes, and the "Immigrant Menace"* (Baltimore: Johns Hopkins University Press, 1994), 3.

18. Priscilla Wald, *Contagious: Cultures, Carriers, and the Outbreak Narrative* (Durham, NC: Duke University Press, 2008), 8.

19. Bashford, "Maritime Quarantine," 9.

20. Howard Markel, *Quarantine! East European Jewish Immigrants and the New York City Epidemics of 1892* (Baltimore: Johns Hopkins University Press, 1997); Howard Markel, *When Germs Travel: Six Major Epidemics That Have Invaded America and the Fears They Have Unleashed* (New York: Pantheon Books, 2004); and Howard Markel and Alexandra Minna Stern, "The Foreignness of Germs: The Persistent Association of Immigrants and Disease in American Society," *Milbank Quarterly* 80, no. 4 (2002): 757–88.

21. G. Thomas Goodnight, "The Personal, Technical, and Public Spheres of Argument: A Speculative Inquiry into the Art of Public Deliberation," *Journal of the American Forensic Association* 18, no. 4 (1982): 214–27.

22. This was how Dr. John H. Griscom, the new president of the third Quarantine and Sanitary Convention, put it in his welcome speech at the convention. See *Proceedings and Debates of the Third National Quarantine and Sanitary Convention* (New York: Edmund Jones, 1859), 16.

23. Hampton, "National Maritime Quarantine System."

24. Joseph Jones, *Outline of the History, Theory and Practice of Quarantine: Relation of Quarantine to Constitutional and International Law and to Commerce* (New Orleans, LA: E.A. Brandao, 1883).

25. "78. A Bill for Compelling Vessels and Persons Coming, and Goods Brought from Infected Places, to Perform Quarantine, 18 June 1779," *Founders Online*, National Archives, accessed August 9, 2019, https://founders.archives .gov/documents/Jefferson/01-02-02-0132-0004-0078. Original source is *The Papers of Thomas Jefferson*, vol. 2, *1777–18 June 1779*, ed. Julian P. Boyd (Princeton, NJ: Princeton University Press, 1950), 524–26.

26. Hampton, "National Maritime Quarantine System."

27. *Laws of Maryland*, 1793, Session, Ch. LVI, accessed August 9, 2019, https://msa .maryland.gov/megafile/msa/speccol/sc2900/sc2908/000001/000645/pdf /am645--54.pdf.

28. Kenneth R. Foster, Mary F. Jenkins, and Anna Coxe Toogood, "The Philadelphia Yellow Fever Epidemic of 1793," *Scientific American* 279, no. 2 (1998): 88–93.

29. "To Thomas Jefferson from Henry Remsen, 1 October 1793," *Founders Online*, National Archives, accessed August 9, 2019, https://founders.archives.gov /documents/Jefferson/01-27-02-0175. Original source is *The Papers of Thomas Jefferson*, vol. 27, *1 September–31 December 1793*, ed. John Catanzariti (Princeton, NJ: Princeton University Press, 1997), 173–75.

30. For more on competing theories of disease, see Cindy Patton, *Globalizing AIDS* (Minneapolis: University of Minnesota Press, 2002).

31. Foster, Jenkins, and Toogood, "Philadelphia Yellow Fever Epidemic," 90.

32. Simon Finger, *Contagious City: The Politics of Public Health in Early Philadelphia* (Ithaca, NY: Cornell University Press, 2012), 138.

33. Jones, *Outline of the History*.

34. Jones, 10.

35. "A Schooner with Yellow Fever on Board Runs Away from Quarantine at Fortress Monroe," *New York Times*, June 27, 1868, 5.

36. "Quarantine Abuses: Still Further Charges against the Quarantine Officials," *New York Times*, August 16, 1871, 5; and "Frauds on Commerce: Shameful Outrages on the Part of Health Officer Carnochan," *New York Times*, February 23, 1872, 2.

37. Letter from Wilson Jewell to John H. Griscom, which served as the introduction to *Proceedings and Debates*, 5.

38. Harold M. Cavins, "The National Quarantine and Sanitary Conventions of 1857 to 1860 and the Beginnings of the American Public Health Association," *Bulletin of the History of Medicine* 13 (1943): 404–26.

39. *Proceedings and Debates*, 23; and "Quarantine and Sanitary Convention: Third Annual Meeting—Second Day's Proceedings," *New York Times*, April 29, 1959, 4.

40. Cavins, "National Quarantine and Sanitary Conventions."

41. *Proceedings and Debates*, 287.

42. *Proceedings and Debates*, 320.

43. *Proceedings and Debates*, 325.

44. Jerrold M. Michael, "The National Board of Health: 1879–1883," *Public Health Reports* 126, no. 1 (2011): 123–29.

45. An Act to Prevent the Introduction of Contagious or Infectious Disease into the United States, 45th Cong., Sess. II, 20 Stat. L. 37 (April 29, 1878); and Hampton, "National Maritime Quarantine System," 1250.

46. Mariola Espinosa, "The Threat from Havana: Southern Public Health, Yellow Fever, and the US Intervention in the Cuban Struggle for Independence, 1878–1898," *Journal of Southern History* 72, no. 3 (2006): 548.

47. W. G. Smillie, "The National Board of Health, 1879–1883," *American Journal of Public Health* 33, no. 8 (1943): 926.

48. Smillie, 930.

49. Nayan Shah, *Contagious Divides: Epidemics and Race in San Francisco's Chinatown* (Berkeley: University of California Press, 2001).

50. John Mckiernan-González, *Fevered Measures: Public Health and Race at the Texas-Mexico Border, 1848–1942* (Durham, NC: Duke University Press, 2012).

51. Eithne Luibhéid, *Entry Denied: Controlling Sexuality at the Border* (Minneapolis: University of Minnesota Press, 2002).

52. Jas. Simpson, M.D., H. Gibbons Jr., M.D., and W. A. Douglass, M.D., "Quarantine Affairs," *Daily Evening Bulletin*, August 5, 1882.

53. It is important to note that in the late twentieth and early twenty-first centuries, states again began to test whether immigration was solely a federal matter. Proposition 187 (1994) in California, Proposition 200 (2004) and SB 1070 (2010) in Arizona, and HB 56 (2011) in Alabama are challenges to who has the right to regulate immigration.

54. Benjamin Harrison, "Accepting First Nomination, September 11, 1888," in *The Papers and Public Addresses of Benjamin Harrison, Twenty-Third President of the United States, March 4, 1889 to March 4, 1893* (Washington, DC: Government Printing Office, 1893), 4.

55. Kraut, *Silent Travelers*, 51; and William F. Lewis, "Telling America's Story: Narrative Form and the Reagan Presidency," *Quarterly Journal of Speech* 73 (1987): 292.

56. An act in amendment to the various acts relative to immigration and the importation of aliens under contract or agreement to perform labor, 51st Cong., Sess. II Chap. 551, 26 Stat. 1084 (March 3, 1891).

57. Kraut, *Silent Travelers*, 66.

58. "Address, December 9, 1891," in *The Papers and Public Addresses of Benjamin Harrison, Twenty-Third President of the United States, March 4, 1889 to March 4, 1893* (Washington, DC: Government Printing Office, 1893), 100.

59. Markel, *Quarantine!*

60. Markel.

61. "Will It Spread to Us," *Morning Oregonian* (Portland), August 24, 1892.

62. "To Keep Out Cholera," *Boston Daily Advertiser*, August 25, 1892.

63. "Cholera's Onward March: Incapacity and Filth in Russia Help Its Progress," *New York Times*, July 5, 1892, 5.

64. "Dangerous Immigration," editorial, *New York Times*, July 25, 1892, 4.

65. "Progress of the Cholera: The Epidemic Spreading Rapidly in Hamburg," *New York Times*, August 29, 1892, 5.

66. "Progress of the Cholera," 5.

67. "The Only Safe Course," *New York Times*, September 1, 1892, 4.

68. Walter Wyman, Charles Foster, and Benjamin Harrison, "President's Proclamation," *Atchison (KS) Daily Globe*, September 2, 1982.

69. "Will Stop Immigration: What Steamship Men Say of the Twenty Day Quarantine," *New York Times*, September 2, 1892, 2.

70. "Two Suspicious Cases: Otherwise the City Is Free from the Asiatic Scourge," *New York Times*, September 30, 1892, 5. Interestingly, even as the fear of cholera subsided on the East Coast of the United States, fears continued further west. For example, on October 1, 1892, the Kingdom of Hawaii passed an act to prevent cholera from entering the kingdom, closing all ports but the one in Honolulu and requiring health inspection of all vessels arriving there. See "Special Quarantine Regulations against Cholera: An Act to Prevent the Infection of Cholera in the Hawaiian Islands," Hawaiian Kingdom, October 1, 1892.

71. An Act Granting Additional Quarantine Powers and Imposing Additional Duties upon the Marine-Hospital Service, 27 Stat. L. 449 (February 15, 1893).

72. William H. Allen, "The Rise of the National Board of Health," *Annals of the American Academy of Political and Social Science* 15 (1900).

73. Susan Sontag, *Illness as Metaphor* (New York: Farrar, Straus and Giroux, 1978).

74. Marcia G. Gaudet, *Carville: Remembering Leprosy in America* (Jackson: University Press of Mississippi, 2004), 7.

75. Peter Hartlaub, "How San Francisco's Chinatown Rose from Ashes, after Decades of Struggle," *San Francisco Chronicle*, October 3, 2015, www.sfchronicle.com/oursf/article/Our-SF-Chinatown-rises-from-ashes-after-decades-6546489.php.

76. "Anti-Coolie Meeting," *Daily Evening Bulletin* (San Francisco), November 13, 1861.

77. "Leprosy among the Chinese," *Idaho Signal* (Lewiston), May 31, 1873.

78. "Leprosy," *St. Louis Globe-Democrat* (reprinted from *New York Sun*), May 8, 1879.

79. See, e.g., James C. White, "The Question of Contagion and Leprosy," *American Journal of the Medical Sciences* no. 168 (October 1982).

80. Julia Rivera Elwood, *Known Simply to the Rest of the World as Carville—100 Years: 1894–1994* (Carville, LA: United States Public Health Service, Gillis W. Long Hansen's Disease Center, 1994), 46.

81. Gaudet, *Carville*, 17.

82. "Detained in Quarantine," *Idaho Daily Statesman* (Boise), June 26, 1899, 1.

83. "Plague Spreads in China," *New Haven (CT) Evening Register*, November 28, 1899, 11.

84. "Bubonic Plague in Honolulu," *Evening News* (San José), January 4, 1900, 1; and "Shotgun Quarantine," *Morning World-Herald* (Omaha, NE), January 9, 1900, 8.

85. "San Francisco in Fear of the Plague," *Evening News* (San José), March 7, 1900, 1.

86. "Plague Cordon Is Maintained," *Evening News* (San José), March 8, 1900, 1.

87. "The Bubonic Plague," *Santa Fe New Mexican*, March 12, 1900, 1.

88. "Bubonic Plague," *Morning Olympian* (Olympia, WA), May 19, 1900, 1.

89. "Chinese Resist," *Idaho Daily Statesman* (Boise), May 22, 1990, 1. As Nayan Shah notes, Chinese newspapers reported on several incidents of Chinese getting gravely ill after taking the vaccination, so the worries were not merely conspiratorial. See Shah, *Contagious Divides*, 138.

90. "Greatly Exaggerated," *Age Herald* (Birmingham, AL), May 23, 1900, 3.

91. "Health Board Made Mistake," *Evening News* (San José), May 28, 1900, 1.

92. T. V. Powderly, "Immigration's Menace to the National Health," *North American Review* 175, no. 548 (1902): 53–60.

93. Craig Phelan, *Grand Master Workman: Terence Powderly and the Knights of Labor* (Westport, CT: Greenwood Press, 2000).

94. T. V. Powderly, "A Menacing Irruption," *North American Review* 147, no. 381 (1888): 165. On the prevalence of digestion metaphors with regard to immigration, see KC Councilor, "Feeding the Body Politic: Metaphors of Digestion in

Progessive Era US Immigration Discourse," *Communication and Critical/Cultural Studies* 14, no. 2 (2017): 139–57.

95. Powderly, "Menacing Irruption," 166.

96. Powderly, "Immigration's Menace," 60.

97. For more on turn of the century eugenics, see Nancy Ordover, *American Eugenics: Race, Queer Anatomy, and the Science of Nationalism* (Minneapolis: University of Minnesota Press, 2003).

98. Alfred C. Reed, "The Medical Side of Immigration," *Popular Science Monthly* 80 (April 1912): 390.

99. Alfred C. Reed, "Immigration and the Public Health," *Popular Science Monthly* 83 (October 1913): 320–38.

100. Throughout the twentieth century, a bodily inspection for venereal disease was a mandated part of the medical examination as dictated by the Public Health Service. See United States Public Health Service, *Guidelines for Medical Examination of Aliens*, 1984. As of the time of this writing in 2020, the Centers for Disease Control and Prevention (CDC) still looks for syphilis and gonorrhea in the medical examination. They are grounds for exclusion based on their designation (along with tuberculosis and leprosy) as "communicable diseases of public health significance." See Centers for Disease Control and Prevention, "Medical Examination: Frequently Asked Questions," updated February 22, 2017, www.cdc.gov/immigrantrefugeehealth/exams/medical-examination-faqs.html#4.

101. Natalia Molina, *Fit to Be Citizens? Public Health and Race in Los Angeles, 1879–1939* (Berkeley: University of California Press, 2006), 8.

102. Alexandra Minna Stern, *Eugenic Nation: Faults and Frontiers of Better Breeding in Modern America* (Berkeley: University of California Press, 2016).

103. Frederic J. Haskin, "The Real Border Raids," *Lexington (KY) Herald*, July 22, 1916, 4.

104. "Mexican Women Cause a Riot at the Border," *Columbus (OH) Daily Enquirer*, January 29, 1917, 1.

105. Stern, *Eugenic Nation*, 67.

106. Markel and Stern, "Foreignness of Germs," 776.

107. Markel and Stern, 774.

108. Cong. Rec. 5089 (May 13, 1952).

109. Phillipa Levine, *Prostitution, Race and Politics: Policing Venereal Disease in the British Empire* (New York: Routledge, 2003), 2.

110. Allan M. Brandt, *No Magic Bullet: A Social History of Venereal Disease in the United States since 1880* (New York: Oxford University Press, 1985), 85.

111. Brandt, *No Magic Bullet*; and John Parascandola, *Sex, Sin, and Science: A History of Syphilis in America* (Westport, CT: Praeger, 2008).

112. Chamberlain-Kahn Act of 1918, Pub. L. No. 65-193, 40 Stat. 845 (1918).

113. Brandt, *No Magic Bullet*, 53; and Wendy E. Parmet, "AIDS and Quarantine: The Revival of an Archaic Doctrine," *Hofstra Law Review* 14, no. 1 (1985): 66.

114. Stern, *Trials of Nina McCall*, 5. See also David J. Pivar, *Purity and Hygiene: Women, Prostitution, and the "American Plan," 1900–1930* (Westport, CT: Greenwood Press, 2002).

115. Stern, *Trials of Nina McCall*, 97.

116. On this point but in a different context, see Laura Briggs, *Reproducing Empire: Race, Sex, Science, and U.S. Imperialism in Puerto Rico* (Berkeley: University of California Press, 2002).

117. Elmer Scott, "Makes Interpretation of Social Disease Law," *Dallas Morning News*, October 6, 1918, 11.

118. Stern, *Trials of Nina McCall*.

119. Stern, 240. It is important to also recognize that during this time, laws targeting "wayward" Black women functioned as effective quarantines, placing them in jails or work camps for extensive periods. See Saidiya Hartman, *Wayward Lives, Beautiful Experiments: Intimate Histories of Social Upheaval* (New York: W. W. Norton, 2019).

120. Peter Baldwin, *Disease and Democracy: The Industrialized World Faces AIDS* (Berkeley: University of California Press, 2005), 4.

CHAPTER TWO: AIDS AND THE RHETORIC OF QUARANTINE

1. Andrea Peterson and Annie-Rose Strasser, "Kansas Bill Seeks to Quarantine HIV-Positive People," *Think Progress*, March 28, 2013, https://thinkprogress .org/kansas-bill-seeks-to-quarantine-hiv-positive-people-ce1c6f4ce936/; John Celock, "Kansas Ban on AIDS Quarantines May Be Repealed in Public Health Reform," *HuffPost*, March 19, 2013, www.huffpost.com/entry/kansas-aids -quarantine_n_2908815; and Dan Avery, "Kansas 'Infectious Diseases' Bill Could Quarantine People with HIV and AIDS," *Queerty*, March 27, 2013, www.queerty.com/kansas-infectious-diseases-bill-could-quarantine-people -with-hiv-and-aids-20130327.

2. Kansas Department of Health and Environment, "State Health Department Addresses Concerns with Substitute for House Bill 2183," press release, March 29, 2013, accessed December 1, 2019, www.kdheks.gov/news/web _archives/2013/03292013a.htm.

3. Centers for Disease Control, "Epidemiologic Notes and Reports Possible Transfusion-Associated Acquired Immune Deficiency Syndrome (AIDS)— California," *Morbidity and Mortality Weekly Report* 31, no. 48 (December 10, 1982).

4. Centers for Disease Control, "Current Trends Prevention of Acquired Immune Deficiency Syndrome (AIDS): Report of Inter-Agency Recommendations," *Morbidity and Mortality Weekly Report* 32, no. 8 (March 4, 1983).

5. American Association of Physicians for Human Rights, "CDC Preparing for Quarantine," *Update*, March 26, 1986, 8.

6. Randy Shilts, *And the Band Played On: Politics, People, and the AIDS Epidemic* (New York: St. Martin's Press, 1987).

7. Michael Worobey, Thomas D. Watts, Richard A. McKay, Marc A. Suchard, Timothy Granade, Dirk E. Teuwen, Beryl A. Koblin, Walid Heneine, Philippe Lemey, and Harold W. Jaffe, "1970s and 'Patient o' HIV-1 Genomes Illuminate Early HIV/AIDS History in North America," *Nature: International Journal of Science* 539 (2016): 98–101. See also Richard A. McKay, *Patient Zero and the Making of the AIDS Epidemic* (Chicago: University of Chicago Press, 2017). Priscilla Wald maintains that like AIDS, Dugas was "rapidly Africanized," further signaling how racialized xenophobic discourses constituted understanding of the origins of AIDS. See Priscilla Wald, *Contagious: Cultures, Carriers, and the Outbreak Narrative* (Durham, NC: Duke University Press, 2008), 216.

8. "The AIDS-ASFV Hypothesis, 1983–1987," *New York Native*, February 22, 1993, 5.

9. Cindy Patton, "From Nation to Family: Containing African AIDS," in *The Lesbian and Gay Studies Reader*, ed. Henry Abelove, Michele Aina Barale, and David M. Halperin (New York: Routledge, 1993), 127–38.

10. Michael Specter, "Discovery Indicates Link of AIDS, Monkey Virus; Insights Sought on Disease's Lethality," *Washington Post*, April 9, 1987, A20.

11. James Brooke, "In Cradle of AIDS Theory, a Defensive Africa Sees a Disguise for Racism," *New York Times*, November 19, 1987.

12. Mark Vandervelden, "Return of the Pink Triangle," *Mom . . . Guess What?* 45 (August 1982): 1.

13. Jeffrey A. Bennett, *Banning Queer Blood: Rhetorics of Citizenship, Contagion, and Resistance* (Tuscaloosa: University of Alabama Press, 2009).

14. Susan Goldfarb, "Homosexuals Complain about Blood Banks' Anti-AIDS Policy," *United Press International*, May 16, 1983.

15. Jan Ziegler, "Falwell Urges Action on AIDS," *United Press International*, July 12, 1983.

16. While calling for mandatory testing and quarantine, Falwell also reportedly offered to contribute money for AIDS research. See Gary W. Spokes, "AIDS Update," *New York City News*, August 24, 1983, 10.

17. Joseph McQuay, "Group Favors Closing All Gay Businesses," *Gaze*, January 1984, 8.

18. These polls came from media companies such as New York Daily News-Eyewitness News (1985), Washington Post-ABC News (1985), New York Times-CBS News (1985), Los Angeles Times (1985, 1986), NBC News-Wall Street Journal (1986), Harris-The Observer (1986), Gallup (1986, twice in 1987), and MD Magazine (1987).

19. See, e.g., Rick Hampson, "AIDS Leaves 2 City Jail Inmates Dead, Seven Hospitalized," *Associated Press*, June 1, 1983; Steve Geissinger, "Special Prison Unit Houses State's AIDS-Plagued Inmates," *Associated Press*, February 9, 1986; Associated Press, "Judge Delays School Admission of Girl with AIDS," *New York Times*, August 25, 1988, B13; and Laurie Garrett, "The Army's 'HIV Hotel'; Fort Hood First in Military to Segregate Soldiers with AIDS Virus," *Newsday*, February 26, 1989, 5.

20. Jennifer Brier, *Infectious Ideas: U.S. Political Responses to the AIDS Crisis* (Chapel Hill: University of North Carolina Press, 2009), 3.

21. Peter Baldwin, *Disease and Democracy: The Industrialized World Faces AIDS* (Berkeley: University of California Press, 2005), 3.

22. C. Everett Koop, *Surgeon General's Report on Acquired Immune Deficiency Syndrome* (Washington, DC: US Department of Health and Human Services, 1986).

23. National Academy of Sciences, *Confronting AIDS: Directions for Public Health, Health Care, and Research* (Washington, DC: National Academies Press, 1986), 16, https://doi.org/10.17226/938.

24. It is probably worth noting that the term "hooker," as applied to prostitutes, likely extends from its earlier slang usage to describe a thief.

25. See, e.g., COYOTE (Call Off Your Old Tired Ethics) Rhode Island, http://coyoteri.org/wp/.

26. Paula A. Treichler, *How to Have Theory in an Epidemic: Cultural Chronicles of AIDS* (Durham, NC: Duke University Press, 1999); and Gena Corea, *The Invisible Epidemic: The Story of Women and AIDS* (New York: Harper Collins, 1992).

27. The CDC reports, "There is a lack of population-based studies on persons who exchange sex." See Centers for Disease Control and Prevention, "HIV Risk among Persons Who Exchange Sex for Money or Nonmonetary Items," September 21, 2018, www.cdc.gov/hiv/group/sexworkers.html. See also Scott W. Stern, *The Trials of Nina McCall: Sex, Surveillance, and the Decades-Long Government Plan to Imprison "Promiscuous" Women* (Boston: Beacon Press, 2018).

28. See, e.g., Phillipa Levine, *Prostitution, Race and Politics: Policing Venereal Disease in the British Empire* (New York: Routledge, 2003); and Stern, *Trials of Nina McCall*.

29. Stern, 261.

30. René Esparza, "Black Bodies on Lockdown: AIDS Moral Panic and the Criminalization of HIV in Times of White Injury," *Journal of African American History* 104, no. 2 (2019): 252. Esparza's work is helpful in outlining some of the relationships between HIV criminalization and quarantine; however, some of his analysis is problematic as he identifies Carlotta Locklear—a Black woman—as white, and he builds some of his analysis around her having a white racial identity.

31. Douglas Crimp, "Portraits of People with AIDS," in *Cultural Studies*, ed. Lawrence Grossberg, Cary Nelson, and Paula Treichler (New York: Routledge, 1991), 118.

32. Crimp, 118.

33. Evelynn Hammonds, "Race, Sex, and AIDS: The Construction of 'Other,'" *Radical America* 20, no. 6 (1987): 29.

34. Darius Bost, *Evidence of Being: The Black Gay Cultural Renaissance and the Politics of Violence* (Chicago: University of Chicago Press, 2018), 17.

35. Tiffany Lethabo King, *The Black Shoals: Offshore Formations of Black and Native Studies* (Durham, NC: Duke University Press, 2019), 23.

36. King, *Black Shoals*, 25; and C. Riley Snorton, *Black on Both Sides: A Racial History of Trans Identity* (Minneapolis: University of Minnesota Press, 2017).

37. Stephen H. Marshall, "The Political Life of Fungibility," *Theory and Event* 15, no. 3 (2012), www.muse.jhu.edu/article/484457.

38. Saidiya Hartman, *Scenes of Subjection: Terror, Slavery, and Self-Making in Nineteenth-Century America* (New York: Oxford University Press, 1997), 20.

39. King, *Black Shoals*, 30.

40. Judd Everhart, "Lawmaker Considering Quarantine of AIDS Victims," *Associated Press*, January 25, 1984. A report appeared in a Yale student publication, the *New Journal*, in December 1983. See Scott W. Stern, "Rethinking Complicity in the Surveillance of Sex Workers: Policing and Prostitution in America's Model City," *Yale Journal of Law and Feminism* 31, no. 2 (2020): 435.

41. Steven Hamm, "AIDS Symptoms Unconfirmed: Prostitute Fears for Safety," *New Haven Register*, February, 15, 1984, as quoted in Stern, "Rethinking Complicity," 436.

42. Christine Guilfoy, "Quarantine Law Introduced: Media Indicts Woman Rumored to Have AIDS," *Gay Community News*, March 24, 1984, as quoted in Stern, "Rethinking Complicity," 436.

43. "Prostitute Who Possibly Has AIDs Missing in Alleged Bail Jump," *Associated Press*, February 22, 1984.

44. "Police Search for Runaway AIDS Victim," *United Press International*, February 22, 1984, www.upi.com/Archives/1984/02/22/Police-search-for-runaway-AIDS-victim/5046446274000. For more on how media promote "moral panics" during pandemics, see Marina Levina, *Pandemics and the Media* (New York: Peter Lang, 2012).

45. Associated Press, "Escapee Gives Up," *New York Times*, February 28, 1984, 4. Other sources claim she was held on $27,500 bail. See "Police Searching for Prostitute and Suspected AIDS Victim," *Associated Press*, February 22, 1984.

46. Michael S. Gerber, "Arresting Ebola Carriers Will Not Curb Virus," op-ed, *Hartford (CT) Courant*, October 20, 2014, www.courant.com/opinion/op-ed/hc-op-gerber-do-not-criminalize-ebola-carriers-102-20141020-story.html.

47. "Suspected AIDS Carrier Freed," *Associated Press*, May 4, 1984.

48. Stern, "Rethinking Complicity."

49. Connecticut amended its quarantine laws so that they could apply to people with AIDS. See P.A. 84-336, § 1, 1984 Conn. Acts - (Reg. Sess.) (amending CONN. GEN. STAT. 19a-221: An Act Concerning Quarantine Measures).

50. Everhart, "Lawmaker Considering Quarantine."

51. "Prostitute Thinks She Has AIDS; Will Work Anyway," *Associated Press*, January 5, 1985.

52. Alyson O'Daniel, *Holding On: African American Women Surviving HIV/AIDS* (Lincoln: University of Nebraska Press, 2016), 18.

53. "Controversial Possible AIDS Victim Dies," *Associated Press*, January 15, 1985; and Christine Guilfoy, "Quarantine Bill Passes in Connecticut," *Gay Community News*, June 2, 1984, 3.

54. "ACLU in First Legal Challenge to AIDS-Related Quarantine," *Front Page* 9 (May 17, 1988): 10. It is challenging to find a comprehensive summary of this case, and some small details that do exist differ among existing sources. For example, William B. Rubenstein claims the woman was known as "Robin," her apparent first name, not Jane Doe. See William B. Rubenstein, "Law and Empowerment: The Idea of Order in the Time of AIDS," *Yale Law Journal* 98 (1989): 975–97. See also Carol Leigh, "No Mandatory Testing! A Feminist Prostitute Speaks Out," *On the Issues* 10 (1988), www.ontheissuesmagazine.com/1988vol10/vol10_1988_3.php; DiAna DiAna, "Talking That Talk," in *Women, AIDS & Activism*, ed. ACT UP/NY and Women and AIDS Book Group (Boston: South End Press, 1990), 219–222; and Kenneth Vogel, "Discrimination on the Basis of HIV Infection: An Economic Analysis," *Ohio State Law Journal* 49 (1989): 965–98.

55. Zoe Leonard and Polly Thistlethwaite, "Prostitution and HIV Infection," in *Women, AIDS & Activism*, ed. ACT UP/NY and Women and AIDS Book Group (Boston: South End Press, 1990), 177–85.

56. DiAna, "Talking That Talk," 220.

57. This case coincided with the ACLU's publishing of a position paper on the law and quarantine to address the problems with public health officials having virtually unchecked powers to quarantine and to dissuade passing any new quarantine legislation targeting people with HIV/AIDS, especially because prostitutes and intravenous drug users would be the most obvious targets. See American Civil Liberties Union AIDS and Civil Liberties Project, "Isolation or Quarantine of HIV-Infected Persons," 1988, Series II, Field Files: AIDS Project: Alphabetical Files: Quarantine (Excludes Publications), 1985–1988, and The National Gay and Lesbian Taskforce Records, 1973–2000: Series II: Field Files box 126, folder 50; both at Cornell University Libraries, retrieved from Archives of Sexuality and Gender, accessed July 9, 2020.

58. Patrick E. Gauen, "AIDS Privacy vs. Prevention," *St. Louis Post-Dispatch*, May 5, 1991, 1B.

59. Gauen, 1B. Some sources also maintain that Horton suggested she would infect as many people as she could and that she knowingly shared needles and even one time slashed her wrist and tried to get her blood on two people. See "HIV-Positive Woman Ordered Quarantined," *United Press International*, April 25, 1991; and Daniel R. Browning, "Alton Woman Is Accused of Spreading AIDS Risk," *St. Louis Post-Dispatch*, April 24, 1991, 1A. Her attorney maintained that she "had been unfairly portrayed and was no threat at all." See Patrick E. Gauen and Charles Bosworth Jr., "Woman with AIDS Defended," *St. Louis Post-Dispatch*, May 24, 1991, 8A.

60. Terry Hughes Column, "An Outsider, Even at Place She Calls Home," *St. Louis Post-Dispatch*, April 25, 1991, 3A.

61. Marlon A. Walker and Denise Hollinshed, "Woman Held Tight by Grip of Streets," *St. Louis Post-Dispatch*, July 31, 2011, B1.

62. Column, "An Outsider," 3A. Horton was also referred to as a fugitive (see, e.g., Patrick Gauen, "Fugitive Called Less of a Threat," *St. Louis Post-Dispatch*,

June 4, 1991, 4B; and Patrick Gauen, "Madison County Fugitive Who Has AIDS May Give Herself Up," *St. Louis Post-Dispatch*, July 11, 1991, 5A) and a menace (see, e.g., Daniel R. Browning, "Alton Woman Given Month of Freedom," *St. Louis Post-Dispatch*, October 9, 1991, 4C; and Column, "An Outsider").

63. Saidiya Hartman, *Wayward Lives, Beautiful Experiments: Intimate Histories of Social Upheaval* (New York: W. W. Norton, 2019), xv.

64. Charles Bosworth Jr., "Alton Woman with AIDS Virus Has Baby," *St. Louis Post-Dispatch*, October 3, 1991, 7A.

65. Gauen, "AIDS Privacy."

66. Gauen.

67. Terry Hillig, "Prostitution Sweep Nets Familiar Face," *St. Louis Post-Dispatch*, June 19, 2003, B1; and Walker and Hollinshed, "Woman Held Tight," B1.

68. Celeste Watkins-Hayes, *Remaking a Life: How Women Living with HIV/AIDS Confront Inequality* (Berkeley: University of California Press, 2019), 113. The concerns of predominantly white gay AIDS organizations and activists differed from those of Black communities. Often this meant that Black communities were left out of the work these better-funded organizations did. As Black gay writer Joseph Beam wrote in 1986, "The State (a euphemism for white people) has never been concerned with the welfare of Black people. So it comes as no surprise to me that the Philadelphia AIDS Task Force (PATF) has trouble getting AIDS information to North Philadelphia, that the New York City Gay Men's Health Crisis (GMHC) outreach doesn't quite make it to Harlem, or that the efforts of Washington, D.C.'s Whitman-Walker Clinic (WWC) fail to extend east of the Anacostia River. It is not a matter of whether their racism is intentional or unintentional. We die 'by accident' daily and the state is a witness who documents that demise." See Joseph Beam, "Caring for Each Other," *Black/Out: The Magazine of the National Coalition of Black Lesbians and Gays* 1, no. 1 (Summer 1986): 9. Black AIDS activists built on a long tradition of Black health activism in major cities to address the particular needs of Black communities. For example, Blacks Educating Blacks About Sexual Health Issues (BEBASHI) in Philadelphia took a harm reduction approach. As J.T. Roane writes, "In a context in which public health advocates sought to examine the proliferation of the disease through narrow accounts of sexual behavior or drug usage, resulting in limited interventions, BEBASHI sought to explode behavioral models incapable of accounting for racism, patriarchy, economic segregation, and history." See J.T. Roane, "Black Harm Reduction Politics in the Early Philadelphia Epidemic," *Souls* 21, no. 2–3 (2019): 146.

69. The risk doesn't mean that prostitutes did not organize against their treatment. During these years, prostitutes testified before government panels and challenged provisions such as mandatory testing in court. See Scott W. Stern, "The Venereal Doctrine: Compulsory Examinations, Sexually Transmitted Infections, and the Rape/Prostitution Divide," *Berkeley Journal of Gender, Law and Justice* 34 (2019): 149–214; and Stern, *Trials of Nina McCall*, 259.

70. Richard Luna, "Psychologist Urges Quarantine of Gays," *United Press International*, January 4, 1985.

71. Leon Daniel, "The Sideshow at a Conservatives' Convention," *United Press International*, March 1, 1985.

72. Evelyn Schlatter and Robert Steinback, "10 Anti-Gay Myths Debunked," *Intelligence Report*, February 27, 2011, www.splcenter.org/fighting-hate /intelligence-report/2011/10-anti-gay-myths-debunked.

73. Joy Buchanan, "County Public Health Official Leaves Job at 78," *Los Angeles Times*, April 1, 2004; and Richard Luna, "Psychologist Urges Quarantine of Gays," *United Press International*, January 4, 1985.

74. Chuck Patrick, "Newstalk: Post Referendum Analysis," *TWT*, January 25–31, 1985, 25.

75. Ken Herman, "Texas AIDS Victims Could Face Quarantine," *Associated Press*, October 22, 1985.

76. "Haughton Wants State to Give Him Quarantine Rights," *Montrose Voice*, no. 258 (October 4, 1985): 1.

77. Buchanan, "County Public Health Official."

78. It was widely reported that Bridges was a prostitute, but in one report, gay activist Ray Hill insisted that Bridges was not nor had ever been a prostitute. See "Fabian Bridges Leaves Hospital, Finds Refuge with Friends," *Montrose Voice*, no. 259 (October 11, 1985): 3.

79. See, e.g., Hector Amaya, *Citizenship Excess: Latina/os, Media, and the Nation* (New York: New York University Press, 2013); Rodger Streitmatter, *Unspeakable: The Rise of the Gay and Lesbian Press in America* (Boston: Faber and Faber, 1995); and Todd Vogel, ed. *The Black Press: New Literary and Historical Essays* (New Brunswick, NJ: Rutgers University Press, 2001).

80. Linda Wyche, "Gay Community Protests at Minneapolis TV Station," *Montrose Voice*, no. 265 (November 22, 1985): 1, 4.

81. PBS, "AIDS: A National Inquiry," *Frontline*, aired March 25, 1986.

82. Pete Diamond, "Fabian Bridges: 'Let Me Be Somebody,'" *Montrose Voice*, no. 282 (March 21, 1986): 5.

83. "Fabian Bridges Leaves Hospital."

84. E. R. Shipp, "Concern over Spread of AIDS Generates a Spate of New Laws Nationwide," *New York Times*, October 26, 1985, 30.

85. "Proposed Confinement Would Apply Only in Rare Cases, Texas Official Says," *Associated Press*, October 23, 1985; and Wyche, "Gay Community Protests."

86. "Defiant AIDS Victim Checks into Hospital," *Los Angeles Times*, October 3, 1985, 2.

87. "Bridges Re-Hospitalized, Doctors Defend Past Action," *Montrose Voice*, no. 260 (October 18, 1985): 5.

88. PBS, "AIDS: A National Inquiry."

89. Diamond, "Fabian Bridges."

90. Wyche, "Gay Community Protests."

91. Schipp, "Concern over Spread."

92. Herman, "Texas AIDS Victims."

93. Ken Herman, "Health Panel Gives Tentative Approval to AIDS Quarantine," *Associated Press*, December 15, 1985.

94. Ken Herman, "Texas Health Commissioner Kills Proposal for AIDS Quarantine," *Associated Press*, January 16, 1986.

95. Howard Rosenberg, "'FRONTLINE' AIDS CONTROVERSY Documentary Makers' Relentless Focus on the Lethal Life Style of a Dying Fabian Bridges Puts Minneapolis Station and PBS in the Spotlight," *Los Angeles Times*, March 27, 1986, Entertainment sec., 1.

96. G. Robert Lowry, "Texas Health Officials Withdraw Quarantine Plan," *United Press International*, January 16, 1986.

97. We get no real indication of McIntyre's gender identity. An article in *The Advocate* describes McIntyre as a "transvestite," whereas others make mention of cross-dressing but do not assign an identity. McIntyre said only the following about wearing skirts, heels, and wigs: "I never thought about it. I just always did it. It was just something that came natural to me to do." See Dudley Clendinen, "Dilemma for Southern Prosecutors: Streets or Prison for AIDS Carrier?" *New York Times*, January 2, 1987, A12.

98. Clendinen, A12.

99. Dave Walter, "Transvestite Quarantined in Jackson," *The Advocate*, March 31, 1987, 13.

100. David Beard, "AIDS Carrier Swears Off Prostitution; Says He's Moving to California," *Associated Press*, February 13, 1987.

101. Clendinen, "Dilemma for Southern Prosecutors," A12.

102. In July 2019, I asked Tommy Mayfield if he had any additional information about McIntyre or what happened to him. He emailed back, "I had tried to forget Mr. McIntyre and was reasonably successful in doing so until I got your e-mail. Going strictly from memory, I recall the following about the case:

    1. Mr. McIntyre had been the subject of a quarantine order pursuant to one of our Public Health statutes.
    2. Despite the quarantine order, he persisted in practicing his profession openly in the Battlefield Park area of Jackson where he was arrested.
    3. Nobody, myself included, knew what to do with him. While the matter was pending, as I recall, he simply dropped off the radar and I had not heard of him until your e-mail. I assume he relocated since I have no knowledge of his being arrested again in this jurisdiction.
    4. Mr. McIntyre is of the Black race.
    5. He was not transgender. He was simply a skillful cross-dresser."

103. Beard, "AIDS Carrier Swears Off."

104. David Beard, "Authorities Issue Quarantine against Prostitute with AIDS," *Associated Press*, February 12, 1987.

105. Associated Press, "Male Prostitute in Mississippi Put under Quarantine Order," *New York Times*, February 12, 1987, B7.

106. Beard, "AIDS Carrier Swears Off."

107. Walter, "Transvestite Quarantined," 127.

108. See, e.g., Elizabeth Crisp, "Wife Faces Jail Time for Secret HIV Status," *HIV Justice Network*, May 2008, http://criminalhivtransmission.blogspot.com/2008/05.

109. Tamar Lewin, "Rights of Citizens and Society Raise Legal Muddle on AIDS," *New York Times*, October 14, 1987, A1.

110. Cristine Russell, "AIDS Rights vs. Safety; Plans to Restrict Carriers Gain Momentum," *Washington Post*, December 16, 1985, A1.

111. Steven W. Thrasher, "'Tiger Mandingo,' a Tardily Regretful Prosecutor, and the 'Viral Underclass,'" *Souls* 21, no. 2–3 (2019). See also Joseph F. Lawless, "The Deceptive Fermata of HIV-Criminalization Law: Rereading the Case of 'Tiger Mandingo' through the Juridico-Affective," *Columbia Journal of Gender and Law* 35, no. 1 (2017): 117–59; and Jesús Gregorio Smith, "The Crime of Black Male Sexuality: Tiger Mandingo and Black Male Vulnerability," in *Home and Community for Queer Men of Color: The Intersection of Race and Sexuality*, ed. Jesús Gregorio Smith and C. Winter Han, 149–71 (Lanham, MD: Lexington Books, 2020).

112. Trevor Hoppe, *Punishing Disease: HIV and the Criminalization of Sickness* (Berkeley: University of California Press, 2017), 5.

113. Robin Toner, "LaRouche Savors Fame That May Ruin Him," *New York Times*, April 4, 1986, A1.

114. "Initiative to Allow Quarantine Makes Ballot," *Associated Press*, June 25, 1986.

115. "Initiative to Allow Quarantine."

116. Doug Willis, "California AIDS Ballot Measure Alarms Medical Community," *Associated Press*, June 30, 1986.

117. Willis.

118. Richard Labonte, "'No on 64' Running Scared," *Update*, October 15, 1986, A-1, 11.

119. "California Catholic Bishops Attack LaRouche AIDS Initiative," *Associated Press*, September 16, 1986.

120. "Prop. 64 Would Cost SF $69 Million," *Update*, July 23, 1986, A-5.

121. Labonte, "'No on 64.'"

122. Jay Matthews, "LaRouche's Call to Quarantine AIDS Victims Trails in California," *Washington Post*, October 26, 1986, A9.

123. "LaRouche Goes Down in CA," *Rag Times*, December 1986, 1, 3.

124. Tom Patterson, "Prop 64 Dies, but Threat Lives," *Bi-line*, December 1986, 15.

125. "Contra Costa Leaders Say No to P.A.N.I.C.," *East Bay Alternative* 1, no. 3 (1987): 10.

126. "New LaRouche Initiative Makes June '88 Ballot," *Bravo! Newsmagazine*, December 3–9, 1987, 10.

127. "Facts on Proposition 69," *East Bay Alternative* 2, no. 1 (June–July 1988): 3.

128. Linda Deutsch, "LaRouche Undaunted by Defeat of AIDS Initiative," *Associated Press*, June 8, 1988.

129. Darrell Morgan, "Dannemeyer's Devastating AIDS Initiative," *Bravo! Newsmagazine*, June 30–July 6, 1988, 3, 6, 14.

130. Associated Press, "Florida Considering Locking Up Some Carriers of the AIDS Virus," *New York Times*, January 27, 1988, A15.

131. Robin Epstein, "Florida Tries to Deal with AIDS," *St. Petersburg Times*, July 12, 1988, 1D.

132. Brent Kallestad, "Governor's Plan Seeks Quarantine of Non-Compliant AIDS Carriers," *Associated Press*, April 6, 1988.

133. Kallestad.

134. Diane Hirth and John Grogan, "AIDS Quarantine Is Endorsed," *Sun Sentinel* (Fort Lauderdale, FL), April 8, 1988, www.sun-sentinel.com/news/fl-xpm-1988 -04-08-8801220655-story.html.

135. Jackie Hallifax, "Martinez Signs Anti-Discrimination, Detention Package," *Associated Press*, July 7, 1988; and Donna O'Neal, "$18 Million AIDS Plan Becomes Law," *Orlando (FL) Sentinel*, July 7, 1988, www.orlandosentinel.com /news/os-xpm-1988-07-07-0050220163-story.html.

136. See, e.g., Deanna Cann, Sayward E. Harrison, and Shan Qiao, "Historical and Current Trends in HIV Criminalization in South Carolina: Implications for the Southern HIV Epidemic," *AIDS and Behavior* 23 (2019): 233–41; Scott Burris and Edwin Cameron, "The Case against Criminalization of HIV Transmission," *Journal of the American Medical Association* 300, no. 5 (2008): 578–81; and Hoppe, *Punishing Disease.*

137. Margot Canaday, *The Straight State: Sexuality and Citizenship in Twentieth-Century America* (Princeton, NJ: Princeton University Press, 2009); and David K. Johnson, *The Lavender Scare: The Cold War Persecution of Gays and Lesbians in the Federal Government* (Chicago: University of Chicago Press, 2006).

138. William Dannemeyer, *Shadow in the Land: Homosexuality in America* (San Francisco: Ignatius Press, 1989).

139. United Press, "Anti-Gay Adviser Stirs Controversy," *San Francisco Chronicle*, August 19, 1985, 7; and Tara Stevens, "Congressman's New AIDS Adviser," *Washington Post*, August 19, 1985, D3.

140. Robin Goldstein and Jean O. Pasco, "Dannemeyer to Represent Bush at AIDS Event," *Orange County (CA) Register*, September 10, 1988.

141. Michael Whitney, "Helms Calls for Quarantine of AIDS Carriers," *United Press International*, June 14, 1987.

CHAPTER THREE: NATIONAL COMMON SENSE AND
THE BAN ON HIV-POSITIVE MIGRANTS

1. Jorge Cortiñas, "Immigrant Bashing and HIV/AIDS," *The Slant*, September 1994, 20.

2. A key exception to this absence is Jennifer Brier, *Infectious Ideas: U.S. Political Responses to the AIDS Crisis* (Chapel Hill: University of North Carolina Press, 2009).

3. In the papers of Lowell P. Weicker Jr., Weicker is described in this manner. See http://dev1.shanti.virginia.edu/lowellweicker/people/gov-lowell-palmer-weicker-jr.

4. See, e.g., Rona Morrow, "AIDS and Immigration: The United States Attempts to Deport a Disease," *University of Miami Inter-American Law Review* 20, no. 1 (1988–1989): 131–73.

5. Nancy E. Allin, "The AIDS Pandemic: International Travel and Immigration Restrictions and the World Health Organization's Response," *Virginia Journal of International Law* 28 (1987–1988): 1043–64; and Alan M. Kraut, *Silent Travelers: Germs, Genes, and the "Immigrant Menace"* (Baltimore: Johns Hopkins University Press, 1994), 51.

6. Sean M. Baker, "Prevention at Our Borders? Testing Immigrants for AIDS," *Suffolk Transnational Law Journal* 12 (1988–89): 331–61; Ronald Bayer, *Private Acts, Social Consequences: AIDS and the Politics of Public Health* (New York: Free Press, 1989); Nancy J. Eckhardt, "The Impact of AIDS on Immigration Law: Unresolved Issues," *Brooklyn Journal of International Law* 14 (1988): 223–48; W. R. Lange and E. M. Dax, "HIV Infection and International Travel," *American Family Physician* 36, no. 3 (1987): 197–204; Lynn Acker Starr, "The Ineffectiveness and Impact of the Human Immunodeficiency Virus (HIV) Exclusion in U.S. Immigration Law," *Georgetown Immigration Law Journal* 3 (1989): 87–111; and Morrow, "AIDS and Immigration."

7. At this time, the HHS secretary was Margaret Heckler, who, though appointed by Reagan, was viewed as ineffective by other members of the Reagan administration and was pushed out on December 13, 1985, just under a month after Mason as acting assistant secretary for health put forth his recommendation. One report from the *Executive Intelligence Review*, a Lyndon LaRouche publication, notes that he essentially acted as secretary through much of 1985 because of the controversy around Heckler. See James O. Mason, "AIDS No Threat, Says CDC's Mason," *Executive Intelligence Review* 13, no. 41 (1986): 27, https://larouchepub.com/eiw/public/1986/eirv13n41-19861017/eirv13n41-19861017.pdf. The controversy surrounding Heckler had to do with a messy divorce in early 1985. She reportedly had denied her husband sex since 1963. The couple reached a settlement in February in order to avoid what would have likely been embarrassing testimony for Heckler and the Reagan administration (United Press International, "Hecklers Reach Divorce Accord," *New York Times*, February 14, 1985, A18). Heckler produced what was known as the Heckler Report, with the full title "Report of the Secretary's Task Force on Black and Minority Health," which detailed racial disparities impacting Blacks and Latinos (1985; full text at https://minorityhealth.hhs.gov/assets/pdf/checked/1/ANDERSON.pdf). It is unclear whether things would have gone differently under her full leadership. She made false assurances about the safety of the nation's blood supply, and she also reportedly never talked to Reagan about AIDS (PBS, "Interview, Margaret Heckler," *Frontline*,

January 11, 2006, www.pbs.org/wgbh/pages/frontline/aids/interviews/heckler
.html).

8. Importantly, this regulation did not impact non-immigrants, who continued to only undergo medical examinations at the discretion of a consular official in the country of origin or immigration officer at a port of entry.

9. Department of Health and Human Services, 51 Fed. Reg. 15,354-5 (Apr. 23, 1986).

10. Department of Health and Human Services, 52 Fed. Reg. 21,352 (June 8, 1987). See also 52 Fed. Reg. 32,540-44 (Aug. 28, 1987).

11. As a side note, it is clear that the IRCA was on the minds of senators in the debates over Helms's amendment. As one example, Senator Alan Simpson brought up this point in the May 21, 1987, debates, noting, "If you are going to add the AIDS test—and I must say I think we should do that—if you are going to add the AIDS test to the tests of legal immigrants, you surely ought to add it to those who are being admitted under the aegis of illegal immigrants" (133 Cong. Rec. 13,464 [1987]). Despite advocating this position, he was also aware of the dicey ethical implications of his position, stating, "I think if then we are to test for AIDS, then we have to remember that these people will not then be legalized and yet what do we do? Deport them then to their country? And knowing and respecting their right of privacy—and I think we have to do that—then are you going to send a person back to their country with confidential information that he is positive on the exposure to AIDS or leave him here, he or she here, on the basis that they can stay in the United States but they are deportable if they are found?" (133 Cong. Rec. 13,464 [1987]). In the June 2 debate, it is clear IRCA will be included, and these ethical concerns that Simpson raises are nowhere in the record.

12. Bernard Weinraub, "Health Officials Seek AIDS Test for Immigrants," *New York Times*, May 16, 1987; and Allin, "AIDS Pandemic."

13. *Interpreter Releases: An Information Service on Immigration, Naturalization and Related Matters* 64 (1987): 873–74.

14. Court E. Golumbic, "Closing the Open Door: The Impact of the Human Immunodeficiency Virus Exclusion on the Legalization Program of the Immigration Reform and Control Act of 1986," *Yale Journal of International Law* 5, no. 1 (1990): 162–89.

15. Bettina M. Fernandez, "HIV Exclusion of Immigrants under the Immigration Reform & Control Act of 1986," *La Raza Law Journal* 5 (1992): 65–107; Eckhardt, "Impact of AIDS"; Lange and Dax, "HIV Infection"; and Bayer, *Private Acts, Social Consequences.*

16. Jorge Cortiñas, "Case Examples of Persons Assisted by the Coalition for Immigrant and Refugee Rights/HIV Task Force that Demonstrate Nature and Consequences of Counseling by the INS Designated Civil Surgeons," August 10, 1989, San Francisco LGBT General Subjects Ephemera Collection (hereafter SUB EPH)—AIDS box (hereafter B) 2 (Cons-M), folder (hereafter F) "Discrimination Immigration," GLBT Historical Society (hereafter GLBT HS). See also CIRRS Position Paper dated April 2, 1990, which would have been

testimony delivered to a congressional hearing in February but was canceled; National Gay and Lesbian Task Force Series II, 1989–1991 (hereafter NGLTF S II, 1989–1991), Field Files (hereafter FF): AIDS Project (hereafter AP): Immigration: Reports-Positions (hereafter R-P), B119, F6, Archives of Sexuality and Gender (ASG).

17. Marvin Howe, "Aliens Testing Positive for AIDS Are Said to Be Giving Up on Legalization," *New York Times*, August 18, 1989, B1.

18. Supplemental Appropriations Act of 1987, Pub. L. No. 100-71, 101 Stat. 391 (July 11, 1987).

19. Brier, *Infectious Ideas*, 93–94. Brier also notes that even though the commission included many social conservatives, its recommendations included calls for significantly more government funding (98).

20. 133 Cong. Rec. 13,451 (1987).

21. 133 Cong. Rec. 11,270 (1987).

22. See, e.g., C. Everett Koop, *Surgeon General's Report on Acquired Immune Deficiency Syndrome* (Washington, DC: US Department of Health and Human Services, 1986). In his report, Koop advocated information and education as the best way to prevent the spread of the AIDS virus.

23. Leslie Maitland Werner, "Education Chief Presses AIDS Tests," *New York Times*, May 1, 1987; and Weinraub, "Health Officials."

24. I use "AIDS" here as opposed to HIV because that is Helms's language.

25. Department of Health and Human Services, 51 Fed. Reg. 15,355 (Apr. 23, 1986).

26. Robert L. Ivie, "Speaking 'Common Sense' about the Soviet Threat: Reagan's Rhetorical Stance," *Western Journal of Speech Communication* 48 (1984): 44.

27. 133 Cong. Rec. 13,451 (1987).

28. 133 Cong. Rec. 13,452 (1987).

29. Jennifer Brier, "The Immigrant Infection: Images of Race, Nation, and Contagion in the Public Debates on AIDS and Immigration," in *Modern American Queer History*, ed. Allida M. Black (Philadelphia: Temple University Press, 2001), 257.

30. Simon Watney, "Missionary Positions: AIDS, 'Africa,' and Race," *Critical Quarterly* 31, no. 3 (1989): 45–62.

31. 133 Cong. Rec. 13,451 (1987).

32. 133 Cong. Rec. 13,452 (1987).

33. Reportedly, the AMA eventually supported mandatory testing for migrants and prisoners. See Werner, "Education Chief." "A.M.A. Backs AIDS Testing of Two Groups," *New York Times*, June 24, 1987. The CDC did not recommend mandatory testing, preferring voluntary testing. The PHS was also on record at this time against mandatory testing, despite what it proposed for adding HIV infection to the exclusion list.

34. 133 Cong. Rec. 13,452 (1987).

35. 133 Cong. Rec. 13,452–3 (1987).

36. 133 Cong. Rec. 13,453 (1987).

37. The *Congressional Record* shows that several senators and representatives gave speeches on the floor between 1981 and 1987 and that a handful of committees

held hearings to address AIDS. But prior to this instance, no serious and sustained debate about how to address the AIDS crisis had occurred in the full Senate.

38. It is important to mention that several senators worried about the costs associated with the proposal in the original section of the appropriations bill that called for $30 million to help provide medications to poor people who have AIDS. This concern differed from that about the costs of mandatory testing, although sometimes the same senator had both concerns.

39. Brier, "Immigrant Infection," 259.

40. Another interesting exception only briefly mentioned in the debate were those who were hired to protect the nation's interests and were already exempt from civilian rules, such as members of the US military and foreign service agents.

41. William F. Lewis, "Telling America's Story: Narrative Form and the Reagan Presidency," *Quarterly Journal of Speech* 73 (1987): 292; Ivie, "Speaking 'Common Sense,'" 44.

42. John Lyne, "Science Controversy, Common Sense, and the Third Culture," *Argumentation and Advocacy* 42 (2005): 38–42.

43. 133 Cong. Rec. 13,453 (1987).

44. 133 Cong. Rec. 13,453 (1987).

45. 133 Cong. Rec. 13,453 (1987).

46. 133 Cong. Rec. 13,454 (1987).

47. 133 Cong. Rec. 13,454 (1987).

48. 133 Cong. Rec. 13,454 (1987).

49. *AIDS Research: Hearings before Senate Committee on Labor and Human Resources*, 100th Cong. 266 (May 15, 1987) (testimony of James O. Mason, Director, Centers for Disease Control), 58.

50. 133 Cong. Rec. 13,457 (1987).

51. 133 Cong. Rec. 13,473 (1987).

52. Danforth essentially confirmed this point later in the debate, though not because he was being "a nervous Nelly" as Helms suggested or because he wanted to tiptoe around the issue. As he put it, these amendments come out of panic and in a panic situation: "Nobody wants to say, 'oh, I voted for or against testing' or 'I voted for or against $30 million'" (133 Cong. Rec. 13,479 [1987]). This unwillingness to act is even more sobering because, once again, this is the first time the full Senate debated the issue of HIV/AIDS.

53. 133 Cong. Rec. 13,477 (1987).

54. 133 Cong. Rec. 13,477 (1987).

55. 133 Cong. Rec. 14,119 (1987).

56. Reagan publicly mentioned AIDS and touted his administration's response to it for the first time on April 1, 1987, at remarks he gave to members of the College of Physicians in Philadelphia. However, Reagan spoke about AIDS for just over three minutes of the twenty-seven-minute speech. He described his administration's response as like "an emergency room operation." "We've thrown everything we have into it. We've declared AIDS public health enemy number one," Reagan said. This was a gross overstatement. See Ronald Reagan

Presidential Library, "President Reagan's Remarks to the Members of the College of Physicians," April 1, 1987, YouTube video, 27:07, posted December 22, 2016, www.youtube.com/watch?v=v5UuYDqPq8o.

57. "Conference Opening Greets Bush with Boos," *Journal of AID Atlanta*, June 1987, 6.

58. "Vigil Remembers Deceased, Protests Reagan," *Journal of AID Atlanta*, June 1987, 6.

59. "Vigil Remembers Deceased," 6.

60. Charles Perrow and Mauro F. Guillén, *The AIDS Disaster: The Failure of Organizations in New York and the Nation* (New Haven, CT: Yale University Press, 1990), 18.

61. "President Reagan's amfAR Speech," May 31, 1987, www.pbs.org/wgbh/pages /frontline/aids/docs/amfar.html.

62. Mark Gabrish Conlan, "Reagan Calls for Testing, Draws Fire," *Bravo! Newsmagazine*, June 4–10, 1987, 6.

63. 133 Cong. Rec. 14,284 (1987).

64. 133 Cong. Rec. 14,285 (1987).

65. 133 Cong. Rec. 14,286 (1987).

66. 133 Cong. Rec. 14,288–9 (1987).

67. Antonio Gramsci, *Selections from the Prison Notebooks* (New York: International Publishers, 1971).

68. Kristen Hoerl, "Cinematic Jujitsu: Resisting White Hegemony through the American Dream in Spike Lee's *Malcolm X*," *Communication Studies* 59, no. 4 (2008): 355–70; John Lyne, "Science Controversy, Common Sense, and the Third Culture," *Argumentation and Advocacy* 42 (2005): 38–42; and Joshua Welsh, "Common Sense and the Rhetoric of Technology," *POROI: An Interdisciplinary Journal of Rhetorical Analysis and Invention* 10, no. 1 (2014): Article 3.

69. 133 Cong. Rec. 18,331 (1987).

70. N. Ordover, "Defying *Realpolitik*: Human Rights and the HIV Entry Bar," *Scholar and Feminist Online* 10, no. 1–2 (2011/2012), http://sfonline.barnard .edu/a-new-queer-agenda/defying-realpolitik-human-rights-and-the-hiv -entry-bar.

71. One of the few examples is a report in *Chicago Outlines*: Johanna Stoyva, "US Senate Backs AIDS Virus Antibody Testing of Immigrants," *Chicago Outlines*, June 18, 1987, 9.

72. Susan Okie, "Public Health Experts Raise Doubts on Plan to Test Immigrants for AIDS," *Washington Post*, July 15, 1987, A14; and Sandra G. Boodman, "AIDS Policy: A Question of Behavior Modification," *Washington Post*, June 11, 1987, A15.

73. Health Ominbus Extension of 1988, Pub. L. No. 100-607 (November 4, 1988).

74. Ignatius Bau, Pat Dunn, Monica Hernandez, and Jorge Cortiñas of CIRRS, Letter to "Immigrant/AIDS/Gay and Lesbian Organizations," January 24, 1990, Jorge Cortiñas Papers (hereafter JC Papers), collection number 1998-42 (hereafter 1998-42), B2, F17—Correspondence, Out, GLBT HS.

75. Allen White, "ACT UP, CDC Target INS Policy," *Bay Area Reporter*, March 1, 1990.

76. Philip J. Hilts, "Agency Says AIDS Should Not Bar Entry to US," *New York Times*, February 27, 1990, A18.

77. Bruce Lambert, "Now, No Haitians Can Donate Blood," *New York Times*, March 14, 1990, A20.

78. George Bush, "Remarks to the National Leadership Coalition on AIDS," Arlington, VA, March 29, 1990, www.presidency.ucsb.edu/documents/remarks -the-national-leadership-coalition-aids.

79. Brier, "Immigrant Infection," 255.

80. Associated Press, "Bush Says Nation Is on 'Wartime Footing' against AIDS, Assails Bias," *Los Angeles Times*, March 29, 1990.

81. Malcolm Gladwell, "President Calls for End to AIDS Discrimination," *Washington Post*, March 30, 1990, A4.

82. Michael Specter, "Major Groups Plan to Boycott San Francisco AIDS Meeting," *Washington Post*, December 13, 1989, A2.

83. Philip J. Hilts, "US to Ease Passport Curbs on Visitors Infected with AIDS Virus," *New York Times*, January 17, 1990, B6.

84. Warren E. Leary, "Visa Rules Eased for Foreigners with AIDS," *New York Times*, April 14, 1990, Sec. 1, 7.

85. Cliff O'Neill, "Activists Lock Up INS HQ," *Bay Area Reporter*, April 12, 1990, 24.

86. Peter Altman, "INS Office Occupied," *Bay Area Reporter*, May 3, 1990, 1.

87. Malcolm Gladwell, "US Creating Special Visas amid Dispute on AIDS Policy," *Washington Post*, April 14, 1990, A2; and Philip J. Hilts, "Disease Control Center Says AIDS Shouldn't Bar US Entry," *New York Times*, February 28, 1990, A24.

88. Malcolm Gladwell, "HHS Can Lift AIDS-Virus Immigration Barrier, Opinion Says," *Washington Post*, May 23, 1990, A9.

89. Immigration Act of 1990, Pub. L. No. 101-649, 104 Stat. 4978 (November 29, 1990).

90. The only time I can find reference to HIV/AIDS in the immigration debates is in the House Conference Report on the act. Representative Hamilton Fish (R-NY) mentioned "important changes" the law would make, including getting rid of the homosexual exclusion and "the opportunity for the administration to change its policy on the exclusion of HIV-positive aliens." Representative Theodore Weiss (D-NY) similarly noted that the law would give HHS "the power to remove AIDS from the list of diseases for which a visitor maybe excluded." He went on, "The Bush administration now must act expeditiously on this newly granted power" (136 Cong. Rec. 36,846 [1990]).

91. Philip J. Hilts, "In Shift, Health Chief Lifts Ban on Visitors with the AIDS Virus," *New York Times*, January 4, 1991, A1.

92. Hilts.

93. Department of Health and Human Services, 56 Fed. Reg. 2,484 (Jan. 23, 1991).

94. See, e.g., Ignatius Bau and Pat Dunn, "Request for Comments on Proposed HHS Regulation Removing HIV Infection from INS Exclusion List," letter to CIRRS members and others, February 6, 1991, in National Lawyers Guild AIDS Network Records, 1985–1993 (hereafter NLGAN Records, 1985–1993), collection number MSS 94-25 (hereafter MSS-94-25), carton (hereafter C) 1, F "Removal of Ban," University of California, San Francisco Library (hereafter UCSFL).

95. John S. James, "HIV Travel/Immigration Ban: Background, Documentation," *AIDS Treatment News*, 1991, www.aids.org/2010/10/hiv-travelimmigration -ban.

96. Malcolm Gladwell, "Reversal of AIDS Exclusion Is Said to Be Shelved," *Washington Post*, May 25, 1991, A6; and letter from AMA Executive Vice President James S. Todd to Senator Edward Kennedy, May 23, 1991, NGLTF S II, 1989–1991, FF: AP: I: Legislation/Regulation (hereafter L-R), B119, F4, ASG.

97. James, "HIV Travel/Immigration Ban."

98. Karen De Witt, "US, in Switch, Plans to Keep Out People Infected with AIDS Virus," *New York Times*, May 26, 1991, Sec. 1, Part 1, 1; and Department of Health and Human Services, 56 Fed. Reg. 25,000 (May 31, 1991). De Witt reports forty thousand letters, whereas James reports only thirty-five thousand.

99. De Witt, "US, in Switch."

100. About the Christian Action Network, see www.christianaction.org/about.

101. Martin Mawyer Letter, Christian Action Network, March 1991, NGLTF S II, 1989–1991, FF: AP: I: L-R, B119, F4, ASG.

102. For example, in 1983, Falwell infamously referred to AIDS as the "gay plague," a moniker that circled widely among evangelicals (Sue Cross, "Falwell Wants Attack on 'Gay Plague,'" *Associated Press*, July 5, 1983). Dannemeyer notoriously linked HIV/AIDS with homosexuality in the most grotesque of ways, including in a 1985 speech in Congress advocating that gay men be banned from giving blood, in part premised on his belief that angry homosexuals with AIDS would pollute the blood supply out of spite and that hospitals run by male homosexuals were discriminating against health providers by telling them not to wear gowns, masks, and gloves when treating AIDS patients (131 Cong. Rec. 25,491 [1985]). In June 1989, Dannemeyer entered into the *Congressional Record* a screed title "What Homosexuals Do," in which he makes numerous wild links between gay sex and AIDS (135 Cong. Rec. 13950-53 [1989]), and in a November 1989 speech advocating for the expulsion of Representative Barney Frank (D-MA), he describes AIDS as the "alter ego" of homosexuality (135 Cong. Rec. 27078 [1989]). These views are concretized in his 1989 book, *A Shadow in the Land*, about the influence of the homosexual movement in the United States.

103. Robert Pear, "Health Dept. Loses in AIDS Rule Dispute," *New York Times*, May 28, 1991, A18.

104. Robert Pear, "Ban on Aliens with AIDS to Continue for Now," *New York Times*, May 30, 1991, A23.

105. Press release, ACT UP Golden Gate, May 30, 1991, JC Papers, 1998-42, B1, F20—Press Conference May 30, 1991, GLBT HS.

106. "Help Fight HIV Immigrant Exclusion, AIDS Action Council, June 12, 1991, NLGAN Records, 1985–1993, MSS-94-25, C1, F "Removal of Ban," UCSFL.

107. "ACT UP Protests Immigration Restrictions," ACT UP Golden Gate Media Advisory, June 19, 1991, JC Papers, 1998-42, B1, F20—Press Conference May 30, 1991, GLBT HS.

108. Philip J. Hilts, "US Policy on Infected Visitors Keeps AIDS Meeting out of Country," *New York Times*, August 17, 1991, 6.

109. Howard W. French, "HIV Could Cut Haitian Entry to US," *New York Times*, December 14, 1991, 3.

110. Sam Fulwood III, "Status of HIV-Positive Haitians Debated," *Los Angeles Times*, February 21, 1992, A4.

111. George Gedda, "HIV-Infected Haitians Pose Dilemma," *Associated Press*, February 20, 1992.

112. James Rowley, "Haitian Refugees with AIDS Virus to Remain at Guantanamo Bay Base," *Associated Press*, March 9, 1992.

113. Jorge Cortiñas' Rap at the Resistance Haiti Demo, March 23, 1992, Tomás Fábregas Papers (hereafter TF Papers), collection 1996-44 (hereafter 1996-44), B1, F1, GLBT HS.

114. David Lauter and Marlene Cimons, "Clinton to Drop Travel Ban on HIV Patients," *Los Angeles Times*, February 5, 1993.

115. Lynne Duke, "Haitians Hope Strike Will Open Safe Haven," *Washington Post*, February 11, 1993, A4.

116. John Pacenti, "Jackson Vows to Join Haitian Refugees' Hunger Strike," *Associated Press*, February 14, 1993. In some sources, Elma Verdieu's names are in opposite order. I am not sure which is correct.

117. "AIDS and Immigration," op-ed, *Washington Post*, February 12, 1993, A26.

118. Richard Cole, "Haitian Hunger Strikers Not Impressed by Clinton's Promises," *Associated Press*, February 10, 1993. Like Elma Verdieu, in some sources, Michel Vilsaint's names are in opposite order. I am not sure which is correct, but I have chosen this order after seeing a May 12, 1993, letter signed by him (TF Papers, 1996-44, B2, F3, GLBT HS).

119. Helen Dewar, "Senate, 76–23, Votes to Bar HIV-Infected Immigrants," *Washington Post*, February 19, 1993, A2.

120. Adam Clymer, "House, Like Senate, Votes to Ban HIV Immigrants, *New York Times*, March 12, 1993, A11.

121. Cited in A. Naomi Paik, *Rightlessness: Testimony and Redress in US Prison Camps since World War II* (Chapel Hill: University of North Carolina Press, 2016), 136.

122. Clymer, "House, Like Senate."

123. ACT UP New York Records, Reel 27, B37, F3-4, New York Public Library.

124. Elizabeth Kurylo, "Jackson Goal: Admit HIV-Infected Haitian Refugees 'Trapped' at US Base, He Says," *Atlanta Journal and Constitution*, February 17, 1993, A9.

125. "AIDS Control Act of 1993," S. 59, January 21, 1993. Importantly, the language "dangerous contagious disease" was no longer the language of the HHS or the Immigration and Nationality Act, as the language was updated in 1990 to "communicable disease of public health significance."

126. 139 Cong. Rec. 2,702 (1993).

127. Grace Kyungwon Hong, "Existentially Surplus: Women of Color Feminism and the New Crises of Capitalism," *GLQ* 18, no. 1 (2012): 87–106.

128. 139 Cong. Rec. 2,849 (1993).

129. 139 Cong. Rec. 2,852–3 (1993).

130. 139 Cong. Rec. 2,849 (1993).

131. 139 Cong. Rec. 2,870 (1993).

132. 139 Cong. Rec. 3,015 (1993).

133. 139 Cong. Rec. 2,852 (1993).

134. 139 Cong. Rec. 2,853 (1993).

135. Cedric J. Robinson, *Black Marxism: The Making of the Black Radical Tradition*, 2nd ed. (Chapel Hill: University of North Carolina Press, 2000).

136. Adam M. Geary, *Antiblack Racism and the AIDS Epidemic: State Intimacies* (New York: Palgrave Macmillan, 2014), 129.

137. 139 Cong. Rec. 2,861 (1993).

138. 139 Cong. Rec. 2,860 (1993).

139. 139 Cong. Rec. 2,860 (1993).

140. 139 Cong. Rec. 2,863 (1993).

141. 139 Cong. Rec. 3,015 (1993).

142. 139 Cong. Rec. 2,870–1 (1993).

143. Paul Farmer, *Pathologies of Power: Health, Human Rights, and the New War on the Poor* (Berkeley: University of California Press, 2003); and Paik, *Rightlessness*.

144. 139 Cong. Rec. 3,012 (1993).

145. 139 Cong. Rec. 2,864 (1993).

146. 139 Cong. Rec. 2,860 (1993).

147. 139 Cong. Rec. 2,851 (1993).

148. 139 Cong. Rec. 2,851 (1993).

149. 139 Cong. Rec. 2,860 (1993).

150. 139 Cong. Rec. 2,862 (1993).

CHAPTER FOUR: BOYCOTTS AND PROTESTS OF THE INTERNATIONAL AIDS CONFERENCES

1. "INS Recommends Freeing Dutch Visitor with AIDS," *Associated Press*, April 7, 1989.

2. Sandra G. Boodman, "US Ban on Tourists with HIV Surprises Some Lawmakers," *Washington Post*, April 19, 1989, A2.

3. "Detained AIDS Expert to Fight for Change in Law," *United Press International*, April 8, 1989.

4. Associated Press, "Alien with AIDS Ordered Freed," *New York Times*, April 8, 1989, 9.

5. Boodman, "US Ban on Tourists."

6. Boodman.

7. "Foreigners with AIDS to Be Permitted Limited Entry to U.S.," *Washington Post*, May 19, 1989, A20.

8. ACT NOW was a coalition of AIDS activist groups from the United States, Canada, Mexico, Europe, and Australia formed at the 1987 March on Washington for Lesbian and Gay Rights. See ACT UP Golden Gate Records 1988–1993 (hereafter AUGG Records, 1988–1993), collection number MSS 98-47 (hereafter MSS 98-47), box (hereafter B) 1, folder (hereafter F) 6, University of California, San Francisco Library (hereafter UCSF L).

9. Phaedra C. Pezzullo, "Contextualizing Boycotts and Buycotts: The Impure Politics of Consumer-Based Advocacy in an Age of Global Ecological Crises," *Communication and Critical/Cultural Studies* 8, no. 2 (2011): 124–45.

10. James C. Scott, *Domination and the Arts of Resistance: Hidden Transcripts* (New Haven, CT: Yale University Press, 1992).

11. Monroe Friedman, *Consumer Boycotts: Effecting Change through the Marketplace and the Media* (New York: Routledge, 1999), 3.

12. Pezzullo, "Contextualizing Boycotts and Buycotts," 125.

13. On tensions between boycotts as economic tactics and their rhetorical dimensions, see also Franklyn S. Haiman, "Nonverbal Communication and the First Amendment: The Rhetoric of the Streets Revisited," *Quarterly Journal of Speech* 68, no. 4 (1982): 371–83; Kirt H. Wilson, "Interpreting the Discursive Field of the Montgomery Bus Boycott: Martin Luther King Jr.'s Holt Street Address," *Rhetoric and Public Affairs* 8, no. 2 (2005): 299–326; and Anna M. Young, Adria Battaglia, and Dana L. Cloud, "(Un)Disciplining the Scholar Activist: Policing the Boundaries of Political Engagement," *Quarterly Journal of Speech* 96, no. 4 (2010): 427–35.

14. Emily Beaulieu and Susan D. Hyde, "In the Shadow of Democracy Promotion: Strategic Manipulation, International Observers, and Election Boycotts," *Comparative Political Studies* 42, no. 3 (2009): 392–415.

15. Ayodele Samuel Jegede, "What Led to the Nigerian Boycott of the Polio Vaccination Campaign?," *PLoS Medicine* 4, no. 3 (2007): 417–22.

16. Colin Blakemore, Richard Dawkins, Denis Noble, and Michael Yudkin, "Is a Scientific Boycott Ever Justified? Practical Guidance Is Needed to Uphold the Universality of Science," *Nature* 421 (January 23, 2003): 314.

17. Ronald E. Kennedy, "Political Boycotts, the Sherman Act, and the First Amendment: An Accommodation of Competing Interests," *Southern California Law Review* 55 (1981–1982): 983–1030.

18. Gordon M. Orloff, "The Political Boycott: An Unprivileged Form of Expression," *Duke Law Journal* (1983): 1076.

19. Orloff, 1077.

20. Claudia Mills, "Should We Boycott Boycotts?," *Journal of Social Philosophy* 27, no. 3 (1996): 136.

21. Mills, 148.

22. American Association of University Professors, "On Academic Boycott," September–October 2006, www.aaup.org/report/academic-boycotts.

23. Ernst Benjamin, "Reflections on Academic Boycotts," *Academe* 92, no. 5 (2006): 80–83.

24. Nick Riemer, "A Question of Academic Freedom," *Jacobin*, July 31, 2017, www .jacobinmag.com/2017/07/bds-boycott-divest-sanctions-palestine-israel -academic-universities.

25. Therese J. Lee, "Democratizing the Economic Sphere: A Case for the Political Boycott," *Lecturer and Other Affiliate Scholarship Series* 3 (2012): 1, http:// digitalcommons.law.yale.edu/ylas/3.

26. Steven Salaita, "Speaking of Palestine and Academic Freedom," *Mondoweiss*, April 24, 2017, http://mondoweiss.net/2017/04/speaking-palestine-academic.

27. Salaita.

28. "History of the IAS—Episode 1," www.iasociety.org/Who-we-are/About-the -IAS/25th-anniversary-of-the-IAS/Episode-1.

29. "Scientists to Be Confronted with Social Challenge of AIDS," *United Press International*, June 3, 1989.

30. Daniel Q. Haney, "12,000 Gather for Biggest AIDS Conference Ever," *Associated Press*, June 3, 1989.

31. "Scientists to Be Confronted."

32. Philip J. Hilts, "Federal Inquiry Finds Misconduct by a Discoverer of the AIDS Virus," *New York Times*, December 31, 1992. The federal inquiry discovered that in a 1984 scientific paper, he "'falsely reported' a critical fact" and thereby "intentionally misled colleagues to gain credit for himself and diminish credit due his French competitors."

33. Cheryl Clark, "Scientists Vow Boycott over AIDS Uproar," *San Diego Union Tribune*, June 11, 1989, A2.

34. Stevie Cameron, "The Growing Movement to Restrict AIDS Victims' Freedom to Travel," *Globe and Mail* (Canada), May 11, 1989.

35. Daniel Q. Haney, "Protest Delays Conference," *Associated Press*, June 4, 1989; and Rebecca Kolberg, "Scientific, Social Forces Clash at AIDS Gathering," *United Press International*, June 10, 1989.

36. Michelle Lalonde and Andre Picard, "AIDS Activists Disrupt Opening of Conference," *Globe and Mail* (Canada), June 5, 1989.

37. Robert Manor, "AIDS Antics: Joke Protesters Nearly Steal Show at Conference," *St. Louis Post-Dispatch*, June 11, 1989.

38. Andre Picard, "AIDS Montreal Conference: Activists Voice Anger at TB Comparison, Testing Hints," *Globe and Mail* (Canada), June 6, 1989.

39. Andre Picard, "AIDS Montreal Conference: Put End to Discrimination over AIDS, Student Pleads," *Globe and Mail* (Canada), June 7, 1989.

40. Rebecca Kolberg, "Scientific, Social Forces Clash at AIDS Gathering," *United Press International*, June 10, 1989.

41. Clark, "Scientists Vow Boycott," A2.

42. Robert M. Wachter, *The Fragile Coalition: Scientists, Activists, and AIDS* (New York: Palgrave Macmillan, 1991).

43. Deborah B. Gould, *Moving Politics: Emotion and ACT UP's Fight against AIDS* (Chicago: University of Chicago Press, 2009).

44. From the finding aid for Sixth International Conference on AIDS records, 1988–1990 (UCSF Library and Center for Knowledge Management, Archives and Special Collections), http://socialarchive.iath.virginia.edu/xtf/view?docId =international-conference-on-aids-6th-1990--san-francisco-cr.xml.

45. Tomás Fábregas, Memo to ACT UP Golden Gate, "US Policy on HIV Infected Foreigners," August 6, 1991. See Jorge Cortiñas Papers (hereafter JC Papers), collection number 1998-42 (hereafter 1998-42), B1, F8, GLBT Historical Society (hereafter GLBT HS).

46. Peter McIntyre, "Aids Meeting Faces Boycott over Rules on Entry to US," *Independent* (UK), November 20, 1989.

47. "International AIDS Conference May Move from SF," *United Press International*, April 27, 1989.

48. Kelly Toughill, "US Eases Visa Rules for AIDS Conference," *Toronto Star*, April 17, 1990. It is difficult to say who first called for the boycott as stories conflict. Some sources say the UK consortium was the first. See McIntyre, "Aids Meeting Faces Boycott," 3.

49. "Third World Charities Set to Boycott Aids Forum," *Guardian* (UK), November 20, 1989; and McIntyre, "Aids Meeting Faces Boycott."

50. Michael Specter, "Major Groups Plan to Boycott San Francisco AIDS Meeting; US Restrictions on Immigration Criticized," *Washington Post*, December 13, 1989, A2.

51. Quoted in McIntyre, "Aids Meeting Faces Boycott."

52. "National Association of People With AIDS Withdraws Participation in Sixth International Conference," *PR Newswire*, December 1, 1989.

53. Jane Coutts, "AIDS Groups Urge Boycott of Conference, Cite US Law," *Globe and Mail* (Canada), January 31, 1990.

54. Philip J. Hilts, "U.S. Urged to End Screening on AIDS," *New York Times*, December 13, 1989, B4.

55. Malcolm Gladwell, "U.S. Creating Special Visas amid Dispute on AIDS Policy," *Washington Post*, April 14, 1990, A2.

56. Andrew Orkin, "Boycott Casts Shadow over San Francisco AIDS Conference," *Canadian Medical Association Journal* 142, no. 12 (1990): 1411.

57. "Visa Requirements for HIV-Infected Individuals," Advanced Conference Program, Sixth International Conference on AIDS Records, collection AR 91-19, B1, F3, UCSFL.

58. Eric Sawyer, "Absolutely Fabregas," *Poz* (June 1997), www.poz.com/articles /241_12368.shtml.

59. Orkin, "Boycott Casts Shadow," 1412; and Andrew Orkin, "Policy Protests, Scientific Spats Take Centre Stage at Sixth International AIDS Conference," *Canadian Medical Association Journal* 143, no. 4 (1990): 312.

60. "Restrictions Set Off AIDS Session Boycott," *St. Louis Post-Dispatch*, June 15, 1990.

61. Christie McLaren, "Canada Joins Boycott of Major AIDS Conference; Health Minister Cites Restrictive US Immigration Law," *Globe and Mail* (Canada), June 16, 1990.

62. This appeared to be one of the first protests against INS, but on June 23, 1989, ACT UP SF organized a protest at the "Immigration and Naturalization 'Service'" office, which may be the first. Unfortunately, the English- and Spanish-language flyers from the ACT UP Golden Gate records announcing the protest are the only materials I could find related to actions in 1989 in any of the archival materials consulted for this chapter. See AU GG Records, 1988–1993, MSS 98-47, B1, F1, UCSFL.

63. ACT UP, press release, February 23, 1990, JC Papers, 1998-42, B1, F12, GLBT HS.

64. Allen White, "ACT UP, CDC Target INS Policy," *Bay Area Reporter*, March 1, 1990, 1.

65. Jesus Reyes, rally speech, February 27, 1990, JC Papers, 1998-42, B1, F12, GLBT HS.

66. "Shut Down the INS—National Phone Zap," press release, March 28, 1990, JC Papers, 1998-42, B1, F13, GLBT HS.

67. ACT UP SF, letter to other organizations, May 7, 1990 (May 10, 1990 in Spanish), JC Papers, 1998-42, B1, F16, GLBT HS.

68. NAMES Project, "Statement for VIth International Conference on AIDS in San Francisco," May 10, 1990, AU GG Records, 1988–1993, MSS 98-47, B1, F6, UCSFL.

69. ACT UP, "Calendar of Events during the Sixth International Conference on AIDS," June 4, 1990, AU GG Records, 1988–1993, MSS 98-47, B1, F1, UCSFL.

70. ACT UP and ACT Now, "Speaking across Borders Program," June 17, 1990, JC Papers, 1998-42, B1, F14, GLBT HS.

71. ACT UP, press release, June 18, 1990, JC Papers, 1998-42, B1, F15, GLBT HS.

72. ACT UP SF, "An Open Letter to President Bush," June 18, 1990, JC Papers, 1998-42, B1, F15, GLBT HS.

73. Paul Taylor, "Activists Push for AIDS Funds; Gay Groups Threatening to Disrupt US Conference in Fight to Speed Research," *Globe and Mail* (Canada), June 20, 1990.

74. "AIDS Protest Gets Rough," *Toronto Star*, June 20, 1990, A19.

75. Jefferson Morley, "Louis Sullivan: Can Health Policy Be Set without Confrontation?" *Los Angeles Times*, August 12, 1990, M3.

76. Actions and Events 1987–1997, Conference on AIDS, Sixth International (San Francisco) AA90.0620 1990, 7, MS ACT UP Los Angeles Records: Actions and Events 1987–1997 B6, F43, ONE National Gay & Lesbian Archives, retrieved from Archives of Sexuality and Gender.

77. Dennis Conkin, "Sullivan Slams ACT UP Protestors," *Bay Area Reporter*, June 28, 1990, 4.

78. Sixth International AIDS Conference, *C-SPAN*, June 24, 1990, www.c-span .org/video/?12863-1/sixth-international-aids-conference.

79. Paul Taylor, "Protest Disrupts Close of AIDS Conference; Activists, Scientists Decry US Policy," *Globe and Mail* (Canada), June 25, 1990. See also AU GG Records, 1988–1993, MSS 98-47, B1, F6, UCSFL.

80. Gould, *Moving Politics*, 287.

81. As cited in Gould, 288.

82. Although not a point I can elaborate on here, it is worth noting that Gould argues that the traction of disparagement of the confrontational tactics of ACT UP was determined not by whether the critiques were right or wrong but by "queers' perceptions about their standing vis-à-vis mainstream society" (326).

83. Kramer said, "Now we must make history again. WE MUST SCREAM AND FIGHT LIKE FURIOUS FUCKING GODDAMN TIGERS FOR OUR DRUGS AND OUR RESEARCH AND OUR CURE. WE MUST RIOT IN SAN FRANCISCO." See Larry Kramer, "A Call to Riot," *Outweek*, March 18, 1990, 38, AU GG Records, 1988–1993, MSS 98-47, B1, F16, UCSFL.

84. "New York's ACT UP to Attend San Francisco AIDS Conference," press release from ACT UP NY, June 8, 1990, AU GG Records, 1988–1993, MSS 98-47, B1, F6, UCSFL.

85. Orkin, "Policy Protests, Scientific Spats."

86. Taylor, "Protest Disrupts."

87. C-SPAN, "Sixth International AIDS Conference."

88. Diane Bernard, "Three Decades before Coronavirus, Anthony Fauci Took Heat from AIDS Protestors," *Washington Post*, May 20, 2020.

89. C-SPAN, "Sixth International AIDS Conference."

90. In an open letter to the Florence conference penned by someone only going by the initial "N," N explains why they could not be at the conference as a result of being an HIV-positive immigrant living in the United States. N calls on conference goers to denounce US policies. N., "An Open Letter to the VII International AIDS Conference," June 12, 1991, JC Papers, 1998-42, B2, F7, GLBT HS.

91. The 1991 conference in Florence, Italy, was also subject to some protests, and there was some controversy surrounding it. Conservative US Congress members charged that the IAC "serves as a junket for federal employees." Dannemeyer sent a letter to HHS secretary Sullivan just before the conference, and shortly thereafter, the government reduced the number of scientists it covered "from nearly 1000 to about 200." See Steve Stenberg, "Controversy Reigns as AIDS Talks Open," *Atlanta Journal and Constitution*, June 17, 1991, A10. Many worried about what this meant for advancement toward a vaccine.

92. "Future AIDS Confab in Jeopardy," *Outweek*, July 18, 1990, 20.

93. Letter from Jorge Cortiñas of the ACT UP GG Immigrant Working Group, May 24, 1991, JC Papers, 1998-42, B1, F19, GLBT HS.

94. "An Open Letter to President Bush," May 30, 1991, JC Papers, 1998-42, B1, F20, GLBT HS.

95. Jorge Cortiñas speech, May 30, 1991, JC Papers, 1998-42, B1, F20, GLBT HS.
96. Malcolm Gladwell, "Reversal of AIDS Exclusion Is Said to Be Shelved; 4-Year Bar to Immigration Criticized as Discriminatory and Medically Unjustified," *Washington Post*, May 25, 1991, A6.
97. ACT UP press release, June 17, 1991, Tomás Fábregas Papers (hereafter TF Papers), collection 1996-44 (hereafter 1996-44), B1, F2, GLBT HS.
98. "Revised Speech for Dr. Max Essex at the Closing Ceremony," part of a press package dated June 25, 1991, JC Papers, 1998-42, B2, F1, GLBT HS.
99. "ACT UP Protests Immigration Restrictions," media advisory, June 19, 1991, JC Papers, 1998-42, B1, F23, GLBT HS.
100. Letter from ACT UP GG, June 14, 1991, JC Papers, 1998-42, B1, F23, GLBT HS.
101. "Remarks of Bob Nelson," Interreligious Coalition on AIDS, June 26, 1991, JC Papers, 1998-42, B1, F23, GLBT HS.
102. Julie Rioux, Dana Van Gorder, and John Willoughby, "AIDS Hysteria at Our Borders," summer 1991, National Lawyers Guild AIDS Network Records, 1985–1993, collection number MSS 94-25, carton 1, F "Removal of Ban," UCSFL. Rioux was with the institute's International AIDS Center. Van Gorder was the community relations officer for the IAC. Willoughby's specific role is unclear.
103. "Rally Targets Immigration Restrictions," press advisory, July 20, 1991, JC Papers, 1998-42, B1, F25, GLBT HS.
104. It is worth again noting that not all AIDS activists were on the same page. Even before Bush's announcement that he would essentially keep the ban in place, Project Inform, perhaps more accurately described as an advocacy group for HIV-positive people than an activist group, backtracked on its earlier position. Having been persuaded by Essex's speech at the Florence conference in which he stated that canceling the conference may have been precisely what the Bush administration wanted, Project Inform supported a conference in Boston regardless of the immigration or travel issue. See Jay Lipner, Jesse Dobson, and Martin Delaney, the Project Inform Advocacy Committee, "Save the VIIIth International AIDS Conference," sent July 30, 1991, JC Papers, 1998 42, B2, F11, GLBT HS.
105. Philip J. Hilts, "U.S. To Admit Some Immigrants with AIDS under New Health Policy," *New York Times*, August 3, 1991, 7.
106. "U.S. Immigration Policy Restrictions and the Eighth International Conference on AIDS," August 1991, JC Papers, 1998-42, B2, F8, GLBT HS.
107. "Prisoner of an Obsolete HIV Policy," *Independent* (UK), August 9, 1991.
108. ACT UP Immigration Working Group letter to ACT UP Members, 1992, TF Papers, 1996–44, B1, F2, GLBT HS.
109. Immigration Working Group, letter to Dr. Jonathan Mann, May 25, 1992, TF Papers, 1996-44, B1, F5, GLBT HS.
110. Sarah Boseley, "Drive to End US Curb on HIV Visitors," *The Guardian* (UK), March 5, 2002, https://actupny.org/actions/Immigration.html.
111. Tomás Fábregas, letter to Fernard Deauval, March 25, 1992, TF Papers, 1996-44, B1, F4, GLBT HS.

112. Steven Epstein, *Impure Science: AIDS, Activism and the Politics of Knowledge* (Berkeley: University of California Press, 1996), 221–22.

113. Elizabeth Taylor, "Remarks," news conference on worldwide travel and immigration restrictions, July 23, 1992, Amsterdam, TF Papers, 1996-44, B2, F5, GLBT HS.

114. "Statement of Tomás Fábregas," amfAR press conference, July 23, 1992, TF Papers, 1996-44, B2, F5, GLBT HS.

115. "Statement of Tomás Fábregas," July 25, 1992, TF Papers, 1996-44, B2, F5, GLBT HS.

116. See, e.g., Urvashi Vaid, *Virtual Equality: The Mainstreaming of Lesbian and Gay Liberation* (New York: Anchor Books/Doubleday, 1995).

117. Gould, *Moving Politics*, 178.

118. Marke B., "The Week ACT UP Shut SF Down," *48hills.org*, June 16, 2015, www.48hills.org/2015/06/16/the-week-act-up-shut-sf-down.

119. N. Ordover, "Defying *Realpolitik*: Human Rights and the HIV Entry Bar," *Scholar and Feminist Online* 10, no. 1–2 (2011/2012), http://sfonline.barnard .edu/a-new-queer-agenda/defying-realpolitik-human-rights-and-the-hiv -entry-bar.

CHAPTER FIVE: AIDS ACTIVIST MEDIA AND THE "HAITIAN CONNECTION"

Epigraph: Ron Howell, "Held HIV Haitians Feel Deserted," *Newsday*, February 15, 1993, 13.

1. Anna Quindlen, "Public and Private; Set Her Free," opinion, *New York Times*, November 18, 1992, A27.

2. "Lucha contra" is Spanish for "fight against," and "koupab" is Haitian Creole for "guilty."

3. DIVA TV/AIDS Community Television, October 30, 1992, Video 01230-A, AIDS Activist Videotape Collection, 1985–2000 (hereafter AAVC, 1985–2000), New York Public Library, Manuscripts and Archives Division (hereafter NYPL). See also DIVA TV/AIDS Community Television, October 16, 1992, Video 00876.

4. DIVA TV and the role of media activism in facilitating the goals of AIDS activists has been widely addressed. See, e.g., Ann Cvetkovich, "Video, AIDS, and Activism," in *Art, Activism, & Oppositionality: Essays from* Afterimage, ed. Grant H. Kester (Durham, NC: Duke University Press, 1991), 182–98; Roger Hallas, *Reframing Bodies: AIDS, Bearing Witness, and the Queer Moving Image* (Durham, NC: Duke University Press, 2009); Lucas Hildebrand, "Retroactivism," *GLQ* 12, no. 2 (2006): 303–17; and Alexandra Juhasz, "WAVE in the Media Environment: Camcorder Activism and the Making of *HIV TV*," *Camera Obscura: Feminism, Culture, and Media Studies* 10, no. 1 28 (1992): 134–51.

5. Martha M. Solomon, ed., *A Voice of Their Own: The Woman Suffrage Press, 1840–1910* (Tuscaloosa: University of Alabama Press, 1991); Rodger Streitmatter, *Unspeakable: The Rise of the Gay and Lesbian Press in America* (Boston:

Faber and Faber, 1995); and Bernell Tripp, *Origins of the Black Press: New York, 1827–1847* (Northport, AL: Vision, 1992).

6. Roger Hallas, "The Witness in the Archive," *Scholar and Feminist Online* 2, no. 1 (2003): para. 17.

7. "Queer" was not yet a reclaimed term when the *Native* began, and so using the term to describe their activism is anachronistic. However, the *Native* was undoubtedly a proto-queer organization that pushed ideas and theories that were anti-establishment, unpopular, and in-your-face. For these reasons and for the sake of ease, I categorize the *Native* and other media in this chapter as "queer."

8. Darius Bost, *Evidence of Being: The Black Gay Cultural Renaissance and the Politics of Violence* (Chicago: University of Chicago Press, 2018), 2.

9. Emily M. Drew, "'Coming to Terms with Our Own Racism': Journalists Grapple with the Racialization of Their News," *Critical Studies in Media Communication* 28, no. 4 (2011): 353–73.

10. I bring up this point to acknowledge that there are likely sources that I have missed, particularly those produced by Haitians in either French or Haitian Creole that center Haitian voices in ways that the media makers I consider here never could. Viviane Namaste has suggested as much in a critique of an earlier version of my work. Her own work on Haitians in Montreal, published in French and English, evidences her point. This point is well taken and speaks to my own limitations as a researcher. See Viviane Namaste, "Five AIDS Histories Otherwise: The Case of Haitians in Montreal," in *AIDS and the Distribution of Crises*, ed. Jih-Fei Cheng, Alexandra Juhasz, and Nishant Shahani (Durham, NC: Duke University Press, 2020); and Viviane Namaste, *Savoirs Créoles: Leçons du Sida pour L'histoire de Montréal* (Montréal: Mémoire d'encrier, 2019).

11. Philip J. Hilts, "Haitian Doctors Uncover Clue to Mystery of Deadly AIDS," *Washington Post*, October 23, 1983, A12.

12. Paul Farmer, *AIDS & Accusation: Haiti and the Geography of Blame*, 2nd ed. (Berkeley: University of California Press, 2006). See also Paul Farmer, *The Uses of Haiti*, 2nd ed. (Monroe, ME: Common Courage Press, 2003); and Cindy Patton, *Inventing AIDS* (New York: Routledge, 1990). Several reports in the mainstream press and medical journals linked Haiti and HIV/AIDS, often in problematic ways. See, e.g., Lawrence K. Altman, "The Doctor's World; the Confusing Haitian Connection to AIDS," *New York Times*, August 16, 1983, C2; Robin Marantz Henig, "AIDS a Disease's Deadly Odyssey," *New York Times*, February 6, 1983, 28; Hilts, "Haitian Doctors," A12; Jean-Robert Leonidas and Nicole Hyppolite, "Haiti and the Acquired Immunodeficiency Syndrome," *Annals of Internal Medicine* 98, no. 6 (1983): 1020–21; Peter Moses and John Moses, "Haiti and the Acquired Immunodeficiency Syndrome," *Annals of Internal Medicine* 99, no. 4 (1983): 565; and Jane Teas, "Could AIDS Agent Be a New Variant of African Swine Fever Virus?," *The Lancet* 321, no. 8330 (1983): 923. More recently, the Haitian connection has been reintroduced by an evolutionary biologist from the University of Arizona.

See "HIV First Came to the U.S. in 1969," *Gay People's Chronicle*, November 2, 2007, 5.

13. Altman, "Doctor's World."

14. Joe Dolce, "The Politics of Fear," *New York Native*, no. 69 (1983): 16.

15. Marlise Simons, "For Haiti's Tourism, the Stigma of AIDS Is Fatal," *New York Times*, November 29, 1983, A2.

16. It is also worth noting that while the *New York Times* first published a story on a "rare cancer" afflicting homosexuals on July 3, 1981, Dr. Lawrence Mass, a regular writer for the *Native*, first published about an "exotic disease" apparently victimizing gay men two months earlier. This was the first report in the United States. See Lawrence Mass, "Disease Rumors Largely Unfounded," *New York Native*, May 18, 1981, 7.

17. Douglas Crimp, "How to Have Promiscuity in an Epidemic," *October* 43 (1987): 238.

18. Steven Epstein, *Impure Science: AIDS, Activism, and the Politics of Knowledge* (Berkeley: University of California Press, 1996), 101.

19. The boycott impacted the circulation of the *Native* so much that it finally folded in 1997. See Robin Pogrebin, "Controversial Gay Magazine Shuts Down," *New York Times*, January 9, 1997; and "Death of a Watchdog," *Spin*, April, 1997, 145.

20. Scholars generally distinguish between advocacy and activist journalism, but in both cases, this kind of journalism is clear about its point of view and functions in the service of a movement or particular political objective. See Sue Careless, "Advocacy Journalism," *The Interim*, May 2000, https://web.archive.org/web/20050429050614/http://www.theinterim.com/2000/may/10advocacy.html.

21. See Mass's comment about Larry Kramer's praise here: Lawrence D. Mass, "Larry Mass Looks Back on 25 Years of AIDS Reporting, Activism," *Gay City News* 5, no. 19 (2006).

22. Robert Lawless, *Haiti's Bad Press* (Rochester, VT: Schenkman Books, 1992), xiii.

23. Lawrence K. Altman, "Five States Report Disorders in Haitians' Immune Systems," *New York Times*, July 9, 1982.

24. Lawrence Mass, "Haitians Linked to Aid Epidemic," *New York Native*, July 19–August 1, 1982, 14.

25. "Time for Prevention: Devising Ways of Evading Aid," *New York Native*, August 16–29, 1982.

26. "Health in a Society of 'Significant Others': New York's Health Commissioner on the Epidemic," *New York Native*, January 31–February 13, 1983, 23.

27. "Time for Prevention," 31.

28. E.g., Anne-christine d'Adesky, "AIDS in Haiti," *New York Native*, December 23–29, 1985; Anne-christine d'Adesky, "Haiti: The Great AIDS Cover-Up: Part Two," *New York Native*, April 21, 1986; Anne-christine d'Adesky, "New Haitan AIDS/ASFV Link," *New York Native*, June 9, 1986, 8; Anne-christine d'Adesky, "Kidneys, Pigs, and Plasma," *New York Native*, June 16, 1986;

Charles L. Ortleb, "Pigs in Belle Glade Test Positive for Antibodies to HTLV-III," *New York Native*, May 26, 1986, 8; Charles L. Ortleb, "The News from Haiti," *New York Native*, August 18, 1986; and Charles L. Ortleb, "Belle Glade Mystery Deepens," *New York Native*, June 9, 1986.

29. Dolce, "Politics of Fear," 18. See also James E. D'Eramo, "Is African Swine Fever Virus the Cause?," *New York Native*, May 23, 1983, 1; and Teas, "Could AIDS Agent."

30. Lawrence K. Altman, "Concern over AIDS Grows Internationally," *New York Times*, May 24, 1983, C1.

31. Ronald K. St. John, "AIDS and African Swine Fever," *The Lancet* 321, no. 8337 (1983): 1335.

32. Emmanuel Arnoux, Jean Michel Guerin, Rodolphe Malebranche, Robert Elie, A. Claude Caroche, Gerard Pierre, Max Millien, and Farouk M. Hamdy, "AIDS and African Swine Fever," *The Lancet* 322, no. 8341 (1983): 110.

33. E.g., d'Adesky, "Cover-Up: Part Two."

34. Ortleb, "Belle Glade Mystery Deepens."

35. Thomas Steele, "CDC Director Says Announcement of AIDS Cause Is Forthcoming," *New York Native*, April 9–22, 1984.

36. The *Native* continued to write about the AIDS-ASFV connection, including revisiting the major moments in the debate in an entire issue: *New York Native*, issue 514, February 22, 1993.

37. See, e.g., Anna Christensen, "AIDS May Be Linked to Haitian Religious Practices," *United Press International*, January 20, 1983; Matt Clark, "AIDS: A Lethal Mystery Story," *Newsweek*, December 27, 1982; Daniel Q. Haney, "Study Calls Immunity Disorder Serious Health Problem for Everyone," *Associated Press*, January 19, 1983; Daniel Q. Haney, "Doctors Question Charge That AIDS Began in Haiti," *Associated Press*, October 19, 1983; and Henig, "AIDS." These causes were also reported in medical journals like the *New England Journal of Medicine*.

38. Dolce, "Politics of Fear," 18.

39. Dolce, 18.

40. Stuart Schear, "Haitians Protest Classification," *New York Native*, October 10–23, 1983, 57.

41. Dolce, "Politics of Fear," 18.

42. Brett Averill, "Roundup of Gays Reported in Haiti," *New York Native*, August 15, 1983, 13.

43. Anne-christine d'Adesky, "Haitian Community Fights AIDS," *New York Native*, December 16–22, 1985, 9.

44. Anne-christine d'Adesky, "Haiti: The Great AIDS Cover-Up," *New York Native*, April 14, 1986.

45. Anne-christine d'Adesky, 16.

46. Anne-christine d'Adesky, 16.

47. In September 1981, President Reagan signed Executive Order 12324, on the "Interdiction of Illegal Aliens," and entered into a "cooperative agreement" with Haitian President Duvalier that allowed the US Coast Guard to intercept

Haitians leaving Haiti by sea, and Duvalier promised he would not punish them upon their return. See the order at www.presidency.ucsb.edu/documents /executive-order-12324-interdiction-illegal-aliens. For more on the interdiction program, see Paul Farmer, *Pathologies of Power: Health, Human Rights, and the New War on the Poor* (Berkeley: University of California Press, 2003); and William G. O'Neill, "The Roots of Human Rights Violations in Haiti," *Georgetown Immigration Law Journal* 7, no. 1 (1993).

48. Brunson McKinley, "US Policy on Haitian Refugees," *U.S. Department of State Dispatch*, June 15, 1992, 472–74.

49. Several of those detained insisted that they were not HIV positive. For example, "'I don't have the HIV,' said Jean-Louis Dallard, 29 . . . 'I don't believe them, why should I?' Dallard said he thought US military doctors would lie to him 'because I am black and because I am Haitian.'" See William Booth, "17 Haitians Freed from 'HIV Prison,'" *Washington Post*, June 15, 1993, A1. They had good reason to be suspicious. *Los Angeles Times* reporters found that "because of problems in identifying and handling blood samples, AIDS [*sic*] testing of Haitian immigrants at the U.S. Navy base at Guantanamo Bay has had an error rate more than 80 times that of other large U.S. screening programs, according to Public Health Service documents." See Marlene Cimons and Melissa Healy, "Haitian Refugee AIDS Tests Render Large Rate of Error," *Los Angeles Times*, April 25, 1992, 14.

50. Michael Ratner, "How We Closed the Guantanamo HIV Camp: The Intersection of Politics and Litigation," *Harvard Human Rights Journal* 11 (1998): 196, see note 41.

51. Thomas L. Friedman, "U.S. To Release 158 Haitian Detainees," *New York Times*, June 10, 1993, 12; and Larry Rohter, "Long Exodus Nears End for HIV-Infected Refugees from Haiti," *New York Times*, June 13, 1993, 24. Activists who visited Guantánamo also reported these conditions in various venues featured on the AIDS Community TV episodes.

52. "Haitian Refugees Ready to Begin New Life," *Stonewall News*, June 28, 1993, 22.

53. Ron Howell, "'A Living Hell,'" *Newsday*, February 11, 1993, 17.

54. Marlene Cimons and Melissa Healy, "Public Health Threat Cited in Isolation of Ill Haitians," *Los Angeles Times*, April 25, 1992, A1.

55. "Haitian, Gay Groups Call for Release of Haitian Refugees," *New York Native*, May 3, 1993, 10.

56. Neel Ahuja, *Bioinsecurities: Disease Interventions, Empire, and the Government of Species* (Durham, NC: Duke University Press, 2016), 182–83.

57. A. Naomi Paik, *Rightlessness: Testimony and Redress in US Prison Camps since World War II* (Chapel Hill: University of North Carolina Press, 2016), 99.

58. Paik, *Rightlessness*, 123.

59. Only a few non-legal scholars have addressed the HIV detention. See Ahuja, *Bioinsecurities*; Farmer, *Pathologies of Power*; Cathy Hannabach, *Blood Cultures: Medicine, Media, and Militarisms* (New York: Palgrave MacMillan, 2015); Jeffrey S. Kahn, *Islands of Sovereignty: Haitian Migration and the Borders of Empire* (Chicago: University of Chicago Press, 2019); Carl

Lindskoog, *Detain and Punish: Haitian Refugees and the Rise of the World's Largest Immigration Detention System* (Gainesville: University of Florida Press, 2018); Jenna M. Loyd and Alison Mountz, *Boats, Borders, and Bases: Race, the Cold War, and the Rise of Migration Detention in the United States* (Oakland: University of California Press, 2018); and Paik, *Rightlessness*. Legal scholars have more fully addressed the detention and its legal implications. See, e.g., Rebecca Kidder, "Administrative Discretion Gone Awry: The Reintroduction of the Public Charge Exclusion for HIV-Positive Refugees and Asylees," *Yale Law Journal* 106, no. 2 (1996): 389–422; Harold Hongju Koh, "The 'Haiti Paradigm' in United States Human Rights Policy," *Yale Law Journal* 103, no. 8 (1994): 2391–435; Harold Hongju Koh and Michael J. Wishnie, "The Story of *Sale v. Haitian Centers Council*: Guantánamo and *Refoulement*," in *Human Rights Advocacy Stories*, ed. Deena R. Hurwitz and Margaret L. Satterthwaite (New York: Thomson Reuters/Foundation Press, 2009), 385–432; and Elizabeth Mary McCormick, "HIV-Infected Haitian Refugees: An Argument against Exclusion," *Georgetown Immigration Law Journal* 7 (1993): 149–72.

60. Brandt Goldstein, *Storming the Court: How a Band of Law Students Fought the President—and Won* (New York: Scribner, 2005).

61. Ratner, "How We Closed." See also Merle English, "Rally Hits Haitian HIV 'Prison Camp,'" *New York Newsday*, September 23, 1992, 28.

62. Some of the same materials available in ACT UP NY's archives are present in the papers of Tomás Fábregas, ACT UP SF, and ACT UP Golden Gate, but as far as I can tell, there was little unique organizing in these chapters. At the time, Crowing Rooster Arts, which produces media related to Haitian struggles for self-determination also produced a video on the Haitian detention, possibly in conjunction with DIVA TV, at least according to ACT UP member Walt Wilder. See Walt Wilder, "Immigration, Guantanamo, and Other Psychosocial Responses at Berlin [for the 9th International AIDS Conference]," ACT UP NY Papers (AUNY Papers), reel (hereafter R) 27, box (hereafter B) 37, folder (hereafter F) 1—Part 2—Emergency Coalition Papers. I have been unable to locate a copy of this video. See http://crowingrooster.org.

63. Assotto Saint, *Spells of a Voodoo Doll: The Poems, Fiction, Essays and Plays of Assotto Saint* (New York: Richard Kasak Books, 1996). In "No More Metaphors (Part Three)," Saint's statement before a court on April 28, 1993, after being arrested for participating in a direct-action protest, Saint explains that in part his actions were on behalf of the detained Haitians (128). Records from Radio Haiti, which was a prominent French and Haitian Creole independent radio station, includes one folder related to AIDS and some mention of Guantánamo. See Radio Haiti Papers, David M. Rubenstein Rare Book and Manuscript Library, Duke University, https://archives.lib.duke.edu/catalog/radiohaitipapers. Other collections concerned with immigration issues more broadly do have records related to the detention. The Caribbean Sea Migration Collection includes some materials related to refugee camps on Guantánamo Bay from 1991–1996. See Caribbean Sea Migration Collection, David M.

Rubenstein Rare Book and Manuscript Library, Duke University, https://
archives.lib.duke.edu/catalog/caribbeansea#contents. The Americans for
Immigrant Justice records, which focus on the non-profit's work in the state of
Florida to support migrants, particularly Haitians, also include project files
and correspondence related to the Haitian detention. See Americans for
Immigrant Justice Records, David M. Rubenstein Rare Book and Manuscript
Library, Duke University, https://archives.lib.duke.edu/catalog
/americansforimmigrantjustice.

64. Götz-Dietrich Opitz, "Transnational Organizing and the Haitian Crisis,
1991–1994," *Journal of Haitian Studies* 8, no. 2 (2002): 122. Writing for the
Guantánamo Memory Project, MA student David Welsh describes an
interview he conducted with Haitian Centers Council attorney Michael
Wishnie that corroborates this view. Welsh further adds that differing views
between Haitians and ACT UP on homosexuality made their collaboration in
support of the detainees challenging. See David Welsh, "Advocacy Groups and
Their Compatibility," Guantánamo Public Memory Project, March 31, 2014,
http://blog.gitmomemory.org/2014/03/31/advocacy-groups-and-their
-compatibility.

65. "United States: Haitians Urge Tough Action against De Facto Regime," *Inter
Press Service*, April 2, 1993.

66. Andres Viglucci, "Mourners' Rage: Haitians Protest AIDS Death, Take Coffin
to INS," *Miami Herald*, May 8, 1993, 1B.

67. Schear, "Haitians Protest Classification," 57. When a leader in the organization
who organized this protest, Coalition Against AIDS Propaganda (KAPAIDS),
was asked whether they would build a coalition with gay activists on AIDS,
spokespeople were reluctant to affirm the possibility, but others quoted in the
article such as Jean-Claude Compas from the Haitian Coalition on AIDS
expressed confidence in their ability to work together.

68. Donatella Lorch, "FDA Policy to Limit Blood Is Protested," *New York Times*,
April 21, 1990; Jonathan M. Katz, "Did the AIDS Panic Make Trump Afraid of
Haitians?" *Politico Magazine*, January 15, 2018; and "April 20th, 1990: 100,000
Haitians Protest against FDA 'Bad Blood' HIV Claims," *L'Union Suite*,
April 20, 2015, www.lunionsuite.com/april-20th1990-100000-haitians-protest
-against-fda-bad-blood-hiv-claims.

69. This point may be confirmed by Tatiana Wah and François Pierre-Louis, who
barely even mention the detention in their discussion of Haitian community
development in New York. See Tatiana Wah and François Pierre-Louis,
"Evolution of Haitian Immigrant Organizations and Community Development in New York City," *Journal of Haitian Studies* 10, no. 1 (2004): 146–64.

70. These groups included the Center for Constitutional Rights, the ACLU
Immigrant Rights Project, the San Francisco Lawyers Committee, and the
Yale Law School's Lowenstein Human Rights Clinic. See Kaplan and Wilder's
November 30, 1992 letter to ACT UP, AUNY Papers, R27, B37, F1, NYPL.

71. James Rowley, "AIDS-Infected Haitians Seeking Asylum Will Be Kept Out of
US," *Associated Press*, March 10, 1992.

72. It is not entirely clear when all of the Haitians were finally let into the United States after the court ordered them released. In *Bioinsecurities*, Ahuja claims that some were detained well into 1994, but he does not cite a source supporting this claim. "Haiti: HIV Positive Refugees Granted US Asylum," *Inter Press Service*, June 15, 1993, said the remaining refugees would be flown out in two weeks. "A Long Wait for a New Life Is Not Quite Over," *New York Times*, July 16, 1993, B1, implied they were all in New York, but thirty-five were still waiting for housing there. The Shut Down Guantánamo Coalition in New York City issued a statement late August 1993 indicating that all of the Haitians in the camp had finally been released (Shut Down Guantánamo Coalition letter, August 27, 1993, AUNY Papers, R67, B89, F5-Miscellaneous Haiti, NYPL).

73. In his 2016–2017 retrospective, Koh not only details the lasting legacy of these legal efforts, but he also provides an expansive reference archive in his notes of the different sites where the efforts have been documented, taken up, and extended. See Harold Hongju Koh, "The Enduring Legacies of the Haitian Refugee Litigation," *New York Law School Law Review* 61 (2016–2017): 31–66.

74. Quoted in Richard Cole, "Haitian Hunger Strikers Not Impressed by Clinton's Promises," *Associated Press*, February 10, 1993.

75. Ratner, "How We Closed," 210.

76. See Richard B. Gregg, "The Ego-Function of the Rhetoric of Protest," *Philosophy and Rhetoric* 4 (1971): 71–91.

77. Ratner, "How We Closed," 219.

78. Minutes from the ACT UP NY Coordinating Committee meeting of March 29, 1992, AUNY Papers, R27, B36, F2, NYPL. I have phrased this in passive voice, because in the minutes, it indicates that ACT UP was asked, but it does not indicate by whom. In her Oral History Project interview, Betty Williams indicates that the CCR made the initial request for ACT UP's help. Michael Ratner of the CCR confirms this in "How We Closed."

79. Betty Williams, interview by Sarah Schulman, August 23, 2008, New York, NY, ACT UP Oral History Project, interview #099, www.actuporalhistory.org /interviews/interviews_17.html#bwilliams.

80. In the archives, there is a flyer indicating a demonstration on Tuesday, September 22, 1992, at the US District Court, Brooklyn Federal Courthouse (AUNY Papers, R27, B37, F6, NYPL). However, there is no additional documentation for this event.

81. Alexandra Juhasz, *AIDS TV* (Durham, NC: Duke University Press, 1995). See also Hildebrand, "Retroactivism."

82. DIVA TV/AIDS Community Television, February 23, 1993, Video 01235, AAVC, 1985–2000, NYPL.

83. DIVA TV clearly worked with very little budget, and so hardly any activists are named in the videos.

84. DIVA TV/AIDS Community Television, Video 00876.

85. DIVA TV/AIDS Community Television, Video 00876.

86. DIVA TV/AIDS Community Television, Video 01235.

87. C. L. R. James, *The Black Jacobins: Toussaint L'ouverture and the San Domingo Revolution*, 2nd ed., revised ed. (New York: Vintage Books, 1989).

88. DIVA TV/AIDS Community Television, Video 00876.

89. DIVA TV/AIDS Community Television, Video 00876.

90. DIVA TV/AIDS Community Television, Video 00876.

91. DIVA TV/AIDS Community Television, Video 01235.

92. Paik, *Rightlessness*; and Lisa Marie Cacho, *Social Death: Racialized Rightlessness and the Criminalization of the Unprotected* (New York: New York University Press, 2012).

93. DIVA TV/AIDS Community Television, Video 01235.

94. DIVA TV/AIDS Community Television, Video 01230-A.

95. DIVA TV/AIDS Community Television, 1993, Video 01234, AAVC, 1985–2000, NYPL.

96. DIVA TV/AIDS Community Television, Video 01234.

97. DIVA TV/AIDS Community Television, Video 01334.

98. Lauren Berlant, "Slow Death (Sovereignty, Obesity, Lateral Agency)," *Critical Inquiry* 33, no. 4 (2007): 754.

99. The deadly effects were long lasting. As of 1998, at least twenty of those detained had died (Garry Pierre-Pierre, "Haitians Bear HIV Alone, Waiting for Word on Asylum," *New York Times*, May 25, 1998, A1). Former ACT UP activist Betty Williams said that by 2003, half of those detained were dead (Lizzy Ratner, "The Legacy of Guantánamo," *The Nation*, July 14, 2003, www.thenation.com/article/archive/legacy-guantanamo).

100. "From New Home in Boston, Haitian Refugee Says Holding Camp Worse Than Prison," *Stonewall News*, July 5, 1993, 14–15.

101. Ahuja, *Bioinsecurities*, 171.

102. Ron Howell, "Finding the 'Promised Land,'" *Newsday*, April 18, 1993, 17.

103. Charles Baillou, "Haitians Detained at US Naval Base Are Activist, Says Forum," *New York Amsterdam News*, February 6, 1993, 4.

104. Anne-christine d'Adesky, interview by Sarah Schulman, April 15, 2003, San Francisco, CA, ACT UP Oral History Project, interview #016, www.actuporalhistory.org/interviews/interviews_03.html#adesky.

105. Phone conversation with Anne-christine d'Adesky, March 27, 2013. d'Adesky did not list their identities, but certainly other sources connected to ACT UP support that it was this constituency that emphasized the United States and treatment.

106. Cathy J. Cohen, *The Boundaries of Blackness: AIDS and the Breakdown of Black Politics* (Chicago: University of Chicago Press, 1999), 341.

107. Brett C. Stockdill, *Activism against AIDS: At the Intersection of Sexuality, Race, Gender, and Class* (Boulder, CO: Lynne Rienner, 2003), 60.

108. Stockdill, *Activism against AIDS*, 75.

109. Alexandra Juhasz, "Video Remains: Nostalgia, Technology, and Queer Archive Activism," *GLQ* 12, no. 2 (2006): 320.

CONCLUSION: AGAINST THE ALIENIZING NATION

Epigraph: Peter Brimelow, *Alien Nation: Common Sense about America's Immigration Disaster* (New York: HarperPerennial, 1995), xxi.

1. The Trump administration has certainly altered this norm.
2. Brimelow, *Alien Nation*, 10.
3. An Act to Establish a Uniform Rule of Naturalization, 1 Stat. 103 (March 26, 1790).
4. Tiffany Lethabo King, *The Black Shoals: Offshore Formations of Black and Native Studies* (Durham, NC: Duke University Press, 2019), 148.
5. See also Jared Sexton, "People-of-Color-Blindness: Notes on the Afterlife of Slavery," *Social Text* 28, no. 2 (2010): 31–56.
6. Karma R. Chávez, *Queer Migration Politics: Activist Rhetoric and Coalitional Possibilities* (Urbana: University of Illinois Press, 2013).
7. Aimee Carrillo Rowe, *Power Lines: On the Subject of Feminist Alliances* (Durham, NC: Duke University Press, 2008).
8. Mae M. Ngai, *Impossible Subjects: Illegal Aliens and the Making of Modern America* (Princeton, NJ: Princeton University Press, 2004).
9. Arizonans approved a similar measure in 2004, Proposition 200, colloquially known as Protect Arizona Now. This, too, faced a lengthy court battle.
10. José Esteban Muñoz, "Ephemera as Evidence: Introductory Notes to Queer Acts," *Women and Performance: A Journal of Feminist Theory* 8, no. 2 (1996): 7.
11. Charles E. Morris III, "Archival Queer," *Rhetoric and Public Affairs* 9, no. 1 (2006): 147.
12. Eithne Luibhéid, "The 1965 Immigration and Nationality Act: An 'End' to Exclusion?," *positions* 5, no. 2 (1997): 501–22.
13. Rosemarie Garland Thomson, "Introduction: From Wonder to Error—a Genealogy of Freak Discourse in Modernity," in *Freakery: Cultural Spectacles of the Extraordinary Body*, ed. Rosemarie Garland Thomson (New York: New York University Press, 1996), 3.
14. Abraham Lincoln, "First Inaugural Address," March 4, 1861, www .abrahamlincolnonline.org/lincoln/speeches/1inaug.htm.
15. Karlyn Kohrs Campbell and Kathleen Hall Jamieson, *Presidents Creating the Presidency: Deeds Done in Words* (Chicago: University of Chicago Press, 2008).
16. David Zarefsky, "Philosophy and Rhetoric in Lincoln's First Inaugural Address," *Philosophy and Rhetoric* 45, no. 3 (2012): 165–88.
17. Sara Ahmed, *Strange Encounters: Embodied Others in Post-Coloniality* (London: Routledge, 2000).

EPILOGUE

1. All Things Considered, "Boston to Remove a Copy of Thomas Ball's 1876 Emancipation Memorial," *NPR*, July 1, 2020.
2. Sean Philip Cotter, "Removal Date to Be Determined for Emancipation Statue in Boston," *Boston Herald*, July 1, 2020.

3. Emily Czachor, "Protesters Clash with D.C. Tour Guide over Removal of Emancipation Memorial," *Newsweek*, June 27, 2020; and Cristela Guerra, "Boston Art Commission Votes Unanimously to Remove Emancipation Memorial," July 2, 2020, www.wbur.org/artery/2020/07/02/boston -emancipation-memorial-park-square-to-be-removed.

4. On the speech, see, e.g., Gregory Stephens, "Arguing with a Monument: Frederick Douglass' Resolution of the 'White Man Problem' in His 'Oration in Memory of Lincoln,'" *Comparative American Studies: An International Journal* 13, no. 3 (2015): 129–45; and Peter C. Myers, "'A Good Work for Our Race To-Day': Interests, Virtues, and the Achievement of Justice in Frederick Douglass's Freedmen's Monument Speech," *American Political Science Review* 104, no. 2 (2010): 209–25. On the relationship between Lincoln and Douglass, see, e.g., James Oakes, *The Radical and the Republican: Frederick Douglass, Abraham Lincoln, and the Triumph of Antislavery Politics* (New York: W. W. Norton, 2008); and John Stauffer, *Giants: The Parallel Lives of Frederick Douglass and Abraham Lincoln* (New York: Twelve, 2008).

5. Gregory Stephens, *On Racial Frontiers: The New Culture of Frederick Douglass, Ralph Ellison, and Bob Marley* (Cambridge: Cambridge University Press, 1999).

6. Frederick Douglass, "Oration by Frederick Douglass, delivered on the occasion of the unveiling of the Freedman's monument in memory of Abraham Lincoln," April 14, 1876, Digital Public Library of America, p. 12, http://dp.la/item/8bc54d540ed276aadd08279bf58136d8.

SELECTED BIBLIOGRAPHY

Ackerman, Edwin F. "The 'Illegal Alien' as a Category of Analysis: A Methodological Intervention." *Journal of Language and Politics* 13, no. 3 (2014): 563–79.

ACT UP/NY and Women and AIDS Book Group, eds. *Women, AIDS, and Activism*. Boston: South End Press, 1990.

Ahmed, Sara. *Strange Encounters: Embodied Others in Post-Coloniality*. London: Routledge, 2000.

Ahuja, Neel. *Bioinsecurities: Disease Interventions, Empire, and the Government of Species*. Durham, NC: Duke University Press, 2016.

Allen, William H. "The Rise of the National Board of Health." *Annals of the American Academy of Political and Social Science* 15 (1900): 51–68.

Allin, Nancy E. "The AIDS Pandemic: International Travel and Immigration Restrictions and the World Health Organization's Response." *Virginia Journal of International Law* 28 (1987–1988): 1043–64.

Altman, Dennis. *AIDS in the Mind of America: The Social, Political, and Psychological Impact of a New Epidemic*. New York: Anchor Press, 1986.

Amaya, Hector. *Citizenship Excess: Latina/os, Media, and the Nation*. New York: New York University Press, 2013.

American Association of University Professors. *On Academic Boycott*. September–October 2006. www.aaup.org/report/academic-boycotts.

Anderson, Warwick. *Colonial Pathologies: American Tropical Medicine, Race, and Hygiene in the Philippines*. Durham, NC: Duke University Press, 2006.

———. *The Cultivation of Whiteness: Science, Health, and Racial Destiny in Australia*. Durham, NC: Duke University Press, 2006.

Bacon, David. *Illegal People: How Globalization Creates Migration and Criminalizes Immigrants*. Boston: Beacon Press, 2008.

Bailey, Marlon M., Darius Bost, Jennifer Brier, Angelique Harris, Johnnie Ray Kornegay III, Linda Villarosa, Dagmawi Woubshet, Marissa Miller, and Dana D. Hines. "Souls Forum: The Black AIDS Epidemic." *Souls* 21, no. 2–3 (2019): 215–26.

Baker, Sean M. "Prevention at Our Borders? Testing Immigrants for AIDS." *Suffolk Transnational Law Journal* 12 (1988–89): 331–61.

Baldwin, Peter. *Disease and Democracy: The Industrialized World Faces AIDS*. Berkeley: University of California Press, 2005.

Bashford, Alison. "Maritime Quarantine: Linking Old World and New World Histories." In *Quarantine: Local and Global Histories*, edited by Alison Bashford, 1–12. London: Palgrave Macmillan, 2016.

Bauman, Zygmunt. "Making and Unmaking of Strangers." *Thesis Eleven* 43, no. 1 (1995): 1–16.

Bayer, Ronald. *Private Acts, Social Consequences: AIDS and the Politics of Public Health*. New York: Free Press, 1989.

Bayer, Ronald, and Gerald M. Oppenheimer. *AIDS Doctors: Voices from the Epidemic: An Oral History*. Oxford: Oxford University Press, 2000.

Beam, Joseph. "Caring for Each Other." *Black/Out: The Magazine of the National Coalition of Black Lesbians and Gays* 1, no. 1 (Summer 1986): 9.

Beaulieu, Emily, and Susan D. Hyde. "In the Shadow of Democracy Promotion: Strategic Manipulation, International Observers, and Election Boycotts." *Comparative Political Studies* 42, no. 3 (2009): 392–415.

Benjamin, Ernst. "Reflections on Academic Boycotts." *Academe* 92, no. 5 (2006): 80–83.

Bennett, Jeffrey A. *Banning Queer Blood: Rhetorics of Citizenship, Contagion, and Resistance*. Tuscaloosa: University of Alabama Press, 2009.

Berger, Michele Tracy. *Workable Sisterhood: The Political Journey of Stigma-tized Women with HIV/AIDS*. Princeton, NJ: Princeton University Press, 2004.

Berlant, Lauren. *Cruel Optimism*. Durham, NC: Duke University Press, 2011.

———. "Slow Death (Sovereignty, Obesity, Lateral Agency)." *Critical Inquiry* 33, no. 4 (2007): 754–80.

Blakemore, Colin, Richard Dawkins, Denis Noble, and Michael Yudkin. "Is a Scientific Boycott Ever Justified? Practical Guidance Is Needed to Uphold the Universality of Science." *Nature* 421 (January 23, 2003): 314.

Bosniak, Linda. *The Citizen and the Alien: Dilemmas of Contemporary Membership*. Princeton, NJ: Princeton University Press, 2006.

Bost, Darius. *Evidence of Being: The Black Gay Cultural Renaissance and the Politics of Violence*. Chicago: University of Chicago Press, 2018.

Brandt, Allan M. *No Magic Bullet: A Social History of Venereal Disease in the United States since 1880*. New York: Oxford University Press, 1985.

Brandzel, Amy L. *Against Citizenship: The Violence of the Normative*. Urbana: University of Illinois Press, 2016.

Brier, Jennifer. "The Immigrant Infection: Images of Race, Nation, and Contagion in the Public Debates on AIDS and Immigration." In *Modern American Queer History*, edited by Allida M. Black, 253–70. Philadelphia: Temple University Press, 2001.

———. *Infectious Ideas: U.S. Political Responses to the AIDS Crisis*. Chapel Hill: University of North Carolina Press, 2009.

Briggs, Laura. *Reproducing Empire: Race, Sex, Science, and U.S. Imperialism in Puerto Rico*. Berkeley: University of California Press, 2002.

Brimelow, Peter. *Alien Nation: Common Sense about America's Immigration Disaster*. New York: HarperPerennial, 1995.

Burris, Scott, and Edwin Cameron. "The Case against Criminalization of HIV Transmission." *Journal of the American Medical Association* 300, no. 5 (2008): 578–81.

Cacho, Lisa Marie. *Social Death: Racialized Rightlessness and the Criminalization of the Unprotected.* New York: New York University Press, 2012.

Callen, Michael. *Surviving AIDS.* New York: HarperPerennial, 1990.

Campbell, Karlyn Kohrs, and Kathleen Hall Jamieson. *Presidents Creating the Presidency: Deeds Done in Words.* Chicago: University of Chicago Press, 2008.

Canaday, Margot. *The Straight State: Sexuality and Citizenship in Twentieth-Century America.* Princeton, NJ: Princeton University Press, 2009.

Cann, Deanna, Sayward E. Harrison, and Shan Qiao. "Historical and Current Trends in HIV Criminalization in South Carolina: Implications for the Southern HIV Epidemic." *AIDS and Behavior* 23 (2019): 233–41.

Carrillo, Héctor. *The Night Is Young: Sexuality in Mexico in the Time of AIDS.* Chicago: University of Chicago Press, 2002.

Carrillo Rowe, Aimee. *Power Lines: On the Subject of Feminist Alliances.* Durham, NC: Duke University Press, 2008.

Cavins, Harold M. "The National Quarantine and Sanitary Conventions of 1857 to 1860 and the Beginnings of the American Public Health Association." *Bulletin of the History of Medicine* 13 (1943): 404–26.

Chase, Sabrina Marie. *Surviving HIV/AIDS in the Inner City: How Resourceful Latinas Beat the Odds.* New Brunswick, NJ: Rutgers University Press, 2011.

Chávez, Karma R. *Queer Migration Politics: Activist Rhetoric and Coalitional Possibilities.* Urbana: University of Illinois Press, 2013.

Cheng, Jih-Fei, Alexandra Juhasz, and Nishant Shahani. *AIDS and the Distribution of Crises.* Durham, NC: Duke University Press, 2020.

Cohen, Cathy J. *The Boundaries of Blackness: AIDS and the Breakdown of Black Politics.* Chicago: University of Chicago Press, 1999.

Cohen, Peter F. *Love and Anger: Essays on AIDS, Activism, and Politics.* Binghamton, NY: Harrington Press, 1998.

Cole, David. *Enemy Aliens: Double Standards and Constitutional Freedoms in the War on Terrorism.* New York: New Press, 2003.

Condit, Celeste Michelle, and John Louis Lucaites. *Crafting Equality: America's Anglo-African Word.* Chicago: University of Chicago Press, 1993.

Conrad, Ryan, ed. *Against Equality: Queer Revolution Not Mere Inclusion.* Oakland, CA: AK Press, 2014.

Corea, Gena. *The Invisible Epidemic: The Story of Women and AIDS.* New York: HarperCollins, 1992.

Councilor, KC. "Feeding the Body Politic: Metaphors of Digestion in Progessive Era US Immigration Discourse." *Communication and Critical/Cultural Studies* 14, no. 2 (2017): 139–57.

Crimp, Douglas. "How to Have Promiscuity in an Epidemic." *October* 43 (1987): 237–71.

———. *Melancholia and Moralism: Essays on AIDS and Queer Politics.* Cambridge, MA: MIT Press, 2002.

———. "Portraits of People with AIDS." In *Cultural Studies,* edited by Lawrence Grossberg, Cary Nelson, and Paula Treichler, 117–31. New York: Routledge, 1991.

Cunningham-Parmeter, Keith. "Alien Language: Immigration Metaphors and the Jurisprudence of Otherness." *Fordham Law Review* 79 (2011): 613–66.

Cvetkovich, Ann. "Video, AIDS, and Activism." In *Art, Activism, and Oppositionality: Essays from* Afterimage, edited by Grant H. Kester, 182–98. Durham, NC: Duke University Press, 1991.

Dannemeyer, William. *Shadow in the Land: Homosexuality in America*. San Francisco: Ignatius Press, 1989.

Del Castillo, Adelaida R. "Illegal Status and Social Citizenship: Thoughts on Mexican Immigrants in a Postnational World." *Aztlan* 27, no. 2 (2002): 9–32.

DiAna, DiAna. "Talking That Talk." In *Women, AIDS, and Activism*, edited by ACT UP/NY and Women and AIDS Book Group, 219–222. Boston: South End Press, 1990.

Drew, Emily M. "'Coming to Terms with Our Own Racism': Journalists Grapple with the Racialization of Their News." *Critical Studies in Media Communication* 28, no. 4 (2011): 353–73.

Duberman, Martin. *Hold Tight Gently: Michael Callen, Essex Hemphill, and the Battlefield of AIDS*. New York: New Press, 2014.

Eckhardt, Nancy J. "The Impact of AIDS on Immigration Law: Unresolved Issues." *Brooklyn Journal of International Law* 14 (1988): 223–48.

Eisenberg, Avigail, and Patti Tamara Lenard. "The Theory and Politics of the Second-Class Citizenship." *Politics, Groups, and Identities* 8, no. 2 (2020): 213–15.

Elwood, Julia Rivera. *Known Simply to the Rest of the World as Carville—100 Years: 1894–1994*. Carville, LA: United States Public Health Service, Gillis W. Long Hansen's Disease Center, 1994.

Epstein, Steven. *Impure Science: AIDS, Activism, and the Politics of Knowledge*. Berkeley: University of California Press, 1996.

Esparza, René. "Black Bodies on Lockdown: AIDS Moral Panic and the Criminalization of HIV in Times of White Injury." *Journal of African American History* 104, no. 2 (2019): 250–80.

Espinosa, Mariola. "The Threat from Havana: Southern Public Health, Yellow Fever, and the US Intervention in the Cuban Struggle for Independence, 1878–1898." *Journal of Southern History* 72, no. 3 (2006): 541–68.

Fairchild, Amy L. *Science at the Borders: Immigrant Medical Inspection and the Shaping of the Modern Industrial Labor Force*. Baltimore: Johns Hopkins University Press, 2003.

Farmer, Paul. *AIDS and Accusation: Haiti and the Geography of Blame*. 2nd ed. Berkeley: University of California Press, 2006.

———. *Pathologies of Power: Health, Human Rights, and the New War on the Poor*. Berkeley: University of California Press, 2003.

———. *The Uses of Haiti*. 2nd ed. Monroe, ME: Common Courage Press, 2003.

Feagin, Joe, and Zinobia Bennefield. "Systemic Racism and U.S. Health Care." *Social Science and Medicine* 103 (2014): 7–14.

Fernandez, Bettina M. "HIV Exclusion of Immigrants under the Immigration Reform & Control Act of 1986." *La Raza Law Journal* 5 (1992): 65–107.

Finger, Simon. *Contagious City: The Politics of Public Health in Early Philadelphia.* Ithaca, NY: Cornell University Press, 2012.

Flores, Lisa A. *Deportable and Disposable: Public Rhetoric and the Making of the "Illegal" Immigrant.* State College: Pennsylvania State University Press, 2020.

Foster, Kenneth R., Mary F. Jenkins, and Anna Coxe Toogood. "The Philadelphia Yellow Fever Epidemic of 1793." *Scientific American* 279, no. 2 (1998): 88–93.

Friedman, Monroe. *Consumer Boycotts: Effecting Change through the Marketplace and the Media.* New York: Routledge, 1999.

Garland Thomson, Rosemarie. "Introduction: From Wonder to Error—a Genealogy of Freak Discourse in Modernity." In *Freakery: Cultural Spectacles of the Extraordinary Body,* edited by Rosemarie Garland Thomson, 1–22. New York: New York University Press, 1996.

Gaudet, Marcia G. *Carville: Remembering Leprosy in America.* Jackson: University Press of Mississippi, 2004.

Geary, Adam M. *Antiblack Racism and the AIDS Epidemic: State Intimacies.* New York: Palgrave Macmillan, 2014.

Goldstein, Brandt. *Storming the Court: How a Band of Yale Law Students Sued the President—and Won.* New York: Scribner, 2005.

Golumbic, Court E. "Closing the Open Door: The Impact of the Human Immunodeficiency Virus Exclusion on the Legalization Program of the Immigration Reform and Control Act of 1986." *Yale Journal of International Law* 5, no. 1 (1990): 162–89.

Goodnight, G. Thomas. "The Personal, Technical, and Public Spheres of Argument: A Speculative Inquiry into the Art of Public Deliberation." *Journal of the American Forensic Association* 18, no. 4 (1982): 214–27.

Gould, Deborah B. *Moving Politics: Emotion and ACT UP's Fight against AIDS.* Chicago: University of Chicago Press, 2009.

Gramsci, Antonio. *Selections from the Prison Notebooks.* New York: International Publishers, 1971.

Gregg, Richard B. "The Ego-Function of the Rhetoric of Protest." *Philosophy and Rhetoric* 4 (1971): 71–91.

Haiman, Franklyn S. "Nonverbal Communication and the First Amendment: The Rhetoric of the Streets Revisited." *Quarterly Journal of Speech* 68, no. 4 (1982): 371–83.

Halkitis, Perry N. *The AIDS Generation: Stories of Survival and Resistance.* Oxford: Oxford University Press, 2014.

Hallas, Roger. *Reframing Bodies: AIDS, Bearing Witness, and the Queer Moving Image.* Durham, NC: Duke University Press, 2009.

———. "The Witness in the Archive." *Scholar and Feminist Online* 2, no. 1 (2003). www.barnard.edu/sfonline.

Hammonds, Evelynn. "Race, Sex, and AIDS: The Construction of 'Other.'" *Radical America* 20, no. 6 (1987): 28–36.

Hampton, Brock C. "Development of the National Maritime Quarantine System of the United States." *Public Health Reports* 55, no. 28 (1940): 1241–93.

Hannabach, Cathy. *Blood Cultures: Medicine, Media, and Militarisms*. New York: Palgrave MacMillan, 2015.

Harden, Victoria A. *AIDS at 30: A History*. Washington, DC: Potomac Books, 2012.

Harrison, Mark. *Contagion: How Commerce Has Spread Disease*. New Haven, CT: Yale University Press, 2012.

Hartman, Saidiya. *Scenes of Subjection: Terror, Slavery, and Self-Making in Nineteenth-Century America*. New York: Oxford University Press, 1997.

———. *Wayward Lives, Beautiful Experiments: Intimate Histories of Social Upheaval*. New York: W. W. Norton, 2019.

Hartmann, Betsy. *Reproductive Rights and Wrongs: The Global Politics of Population Control*. Boston: South End Press, 1995.

Hildebrand, Lucas. "Retroactivism." *GLQ* 12, no. 2 (2006): 303–17.

Hill, Annie. "Breast Cancer's Rhetoricity: Bodily Border Crisis and Bridge to Corporeal Solidarity." *Review of Communication* 16, no. 4 (2016): 281–98.

———. "SlutWalk as Perifeminist Response to Rape Logic: The Politics of Reclaiming a Name." *Communication and Critical/Cultural Studies* 13, no. 1 (2016): 23–39.

Hoberman, John M. *Black and Blue: The Origins and Consequences of Medical Racism*. Berkeley: University of California Press, 2012.

Hoerl, Kristen. "Cinematic Jujitsu: Resisting White Hegemony through the American Dream in Spike Lee's *Malcolm X*." *Communication Studies* 59, no. 4 (2008): 355–70.

Hong, Grace Kyungwon. "Existentially Surplus: Women of Color Feminism and the New Crises of Capitalism." *GLQ* 18, no. 1 (2012): 87–106.

Honig, Bonnie. *Democracy and the Foreigner*. Princeton, NJ: Princeton University Press, 2001.

Hoppe, Trevor. *Punishing Disease: HIV and the Criminalization of Sickness*. Berkeley: University of California Press, 2017.

Ivie, Robert L. "Speaking 'Common Sense' about the Soviet Threat: Reagan's Rhetorical Stance." *Western Journal of Speech Communication* 48 (1984): 39–50.

James, C. L. R. *The Black Jacobins: Toussaint L'ouverture and the San Domingo Revolution*. 2nd ed., revised ed. New York: Vintage Books, 1989.

Jegede, Ayodele Samuel. "What Led to the Nigerian Boycott of the Polio Vaccination Campaign?" *PLoS Medicine* 4, no. 3 (2007): 417–22.

Johnson, David K. *The Lavender Scare: The Cold War Persecution of Gays and Lesbians in the Federal Government*. Chicago: University of Chicago Press, 2006.

Jones, James H. *Bad Blood: The Tuskegee Syphilis Experiment*. New York: Free Press, 1981.

Jones, Joseph. *Outline of the History, Theory and Practice of Quarantine: Relation of Quarantine to Constitutional and International Law and to Commerce*. New Orleans, LA: E.A. Brandao, 1883.

Juhasz, Alexandra. *AIDS TV*. Durham, NC: Duke University Press, 1995.

———. "Video Remains: Nostalgia, Technology, and Queer Archive Activism." *GLQ* 12, no. 2 (2006): 319–28.

———. "WAVE in the Media Environment: Camcorder Activism and the Making of *HIV TV.*" *Camera Obscura: Feminism, Culture, and Media Studies* 10, no. 1 28 (1992): 134–51.

Kahn, Jeffrey S. *Islands of Sovereignty: Haitian Migration and the Borders of Empire.* Chicago: University of Chicago Press, 2019.

Kennedy, Ronald E. "Political Boycotts, the Sherman Act, and the First Amendment: An Accommodation of Competing Interests." *Southern California Law Review* 55 (1981–1982): 983–1030.

Kerr, Ted. "A History of Erasing Black Artists and Bodies from the AIDS Conversation." *Hyperallergic*, December 31, 2015. https://hyperallergic.com/264934/a -history-of-erasing-black-artists-and-bodies-from-the-aids-conversation/.

Kidder, Rebecca. "Administrative Discretion Gone Awry: The Reintroduction of the Public Charge Exclusion for HIV-Positive Refugees and Asylees." *Yale Law Journal* 106, no. 2 (1996): 389–422. www.jstor.org/stable/797213.

King, Tiffany Lethabo. *The Black Shoals: Offshore Formations of Black and Native Studies.* Durham, NC: Duke University Press, 2019.

Koh, Harold Hongju. "The Enduring Legacies of the Haitian Refugee Litigation." *New York Law School Law Review* 61 (2016–2017): 31–66.

———. "The 'Haiti Paradigm' in United States Human Rights Policy." *Yale Law Journal* 103, no. 8 (1994): 2391–435. www.jstor.org/stable/797051.

Koh, Harold Hongju, and Michael J. Wishnie. "The Story of *Sale v. Haitian Centers Council*: Guantánamo and *Refoulement.*" In *Human Rights Advocacy Stories*, edited by Deena R. Hurwitz and Margaret L. Satterthwaite, 385–432. New York: Thomson Reuters/Foundation Press, 2009.

Koop, C. Everett. *Surgeon General's Report on Acquired Immune Deficiency Syndrome.* Washington, DC: US Department of Health and Human Services, 1986.

Kraut, Alan M. *Silent Travelers: Germs, Genes, and the "Immigrant Menace."* Baltimore: Johns Hopkins University Press, 1994.

Lange, W. R., and E. M. Dax. "HIV Infection and International Travel." *American Family Physician* 36, no. 3 (1987): 197–204.

Lawless, Joseph F. "The Deceptive Fermata of HIV-Criminalization Law: Rereading the Case of 'Tiger Mandingo' through the Juridico-Affective." *Columbia Journal of Gender and Law* 35, no. 1 (2017): 117–59.

Lawless, Robert. *Haiti's Bad Press.* Rochester, VT: Schenkman Books, 1992.

Lee, Erika. *America for Americans: A History of Xenophobia in the United States.* New York: Basic Books, 2019.

———. *At America's Gates: Chinese Immigration during the Exclusion Era, 1882– 1943.* Chapel Hill: University of North Carolina Press, 2004.

Lee, Therese J. "Democratizing the Economic Sphere: A Case for the Political Boycott." *Lecturer and Other Affiliate Scholarship Series* 3 (2012): 1–44. http:// digitalcommons.law.yale.edu/ylas/3.

Leonard, Zoe, and Polly Thistlethwaite. "Prostitution and HIV Infection." In *Women, AIDS, and Activism*, edited by ACT UP/NY and Women and AIDS Book Group, 177–85. Boston: South End Press, 1990.

Leonidas, Jean-Robert, and Nicole Hyppolite. "Haiti and the Acquired Immunodeficiency Syndrome." *Annals of Internal Medicine* 98, no. 6 (1983): 1020–21.

Levina, Marina. *Pandemics and the Media*. New York: Peter Lang, 2012.

Levine, Philippa. *Prostitution, Race and Politics: Policing Venereal Disease in the British Empire*. New York: Routledge, 2003.

Lewis, William F. "Telling America's Story: Narrative Form and the Reagan Presidency." *Quarterly Journal of Speech* 73 (1987): 280–302.

Lindskoog, Carl. *Detain and Punish: Haitian Refugees and the Rise of the World's Largest Immigration Detention System*. Gainesville: University of Florida Press, 2018.

Lowe, Lisa. *Immigrant Acts: On Asian American Cultural Politics*. Durham, NC: Duke University Press, 1996.

Loyd, Jenna M., Matt Mitchelson, and Andrew Burridge, eds. *Beyond Walls and Cages: Prisons, Borders, and Global Crisis*. Athens: University of Georgia Press, 2012.

Loyd, Jenna M., and Alison Mountz. *Boats, Borders, and Bases: Race, the Cold War, and the Rise of Migration Detention in the United States*. Oakland: University of California Press, 2018.

Luibhéid, Eithne. *Entry Denied: Controlling Sexuality at the Border*. Minneapolis: University of Minnesota Press, 2002.

——. "Introduction: Queer Migration and Citizenship." In *Queer Migrations: Sexuality, U.S. Citizenship, and Border Crossings*, edited by Eithne Luibhéid and Lionel Cantú Jr., ix–xlvi. Minneapolis: University of Minnesota Press, 2005.

——. "The 1965 Immigration and Nationality Act: An 'End' to Exclusion?" *positions* 5, no. 2 (1997): 501–22.

——. "Sexuality, Migration, and the Shifting Line between Legal and Illegal Status." *GLQ* 14, no. 2–3 (2008): 289–316.

Lyne, John. "Science Controversy, Common Sense, and the Third Culture." *Argumentation and Advocacy* 42 (2005): 38–42.

Macías-Rojas, Patrisia. *From Deportation to Prison: The Politics of Immigration Enforcement in Post-Civil Rights America*. New York: New York University Press, 2016.

Marciniak, Katarzyna. *Alienhood: Citizenship, Exile, and the Logic of Difference*. Minneapolis: University of Minnesota Press, 2006.

Markel, Howard. *Quarantine! East European Jewish Immigrants and the New York City Epidemics of 1892*. Baltimore: Johns Hopkins University Press, 1997.

——. *When Germs Travel: Six Major Epidemics That Have Invaded America and the Fears They Have Unleashed*. New York: Pantheon Books, 2004.

Markel, Howard, and Alexandra Minna Stern. "The Foreignness of Germs: The Persistent Association of Immigrants and Disease in American Society." *Milbank Quarterly* 80, no. 4 (2002): 757–88.

Marshall, Stephen H. "The Political Life of Fungibility." *Theory & Event* 15, no. 3 (2012). www.muse.jhu.edu/article/484457.

McCormick, Elizabeth Mary. "HIV-Infected Haitian Refugees: An Argument against Exclusion." *Georgetown Immigration Law Journal* 7 (1993): 149–72.

McKay, Richard A. *Patient Zero and the Making of the AIDS Epidemic*. Chicago: University of Chicago Press, 2017.

Mckiernan-González, John. *Fevered Measures: Public Health and Race at the Texas-Mexico Border, 1848–1942*. Durham, NC: Duke University Press, 2012.

McKittrick, Katherine. *Demonic Grounds: Black Women and the Cartographies of Struggle*. Minneapolis: University of Minnesota Press, 2006.

Michael, Jerrold M. "The National Board of Health: 1879–1883." *Public Health Reports* 126, no. 1 (2011): 123–29.

Miles, Suzannah Smith. *Writings of the Islands: Sullivan's Island and Isle of Palms*. Columbia, SC: History Press, 2004.

Mills, Claudia. "Should We Boycott Boycotts?" *Journal of Social Philosophy* 27, no. 3 (1996): 136–48.

Mogul, Joey, Andrea Ritchie, and Kay Whitlock. *Queer (in)Justice: The Criminalization of LGBT People in the United States*. Boston: Beacon Press, 2011.

Molina, Natalia. "Borders, Laborers, and Racialized Medicalization: Mexican Immigration and US Public Health Practices in the 20th Century." *American Journal of Public Health* 101, no. 6 (2011): 1024–31.

———. *Fit to Be Citizens? Public Health and Race in Los Angeles, 1879–1939*. Berkeley: University of California Press, 2006.

Moran, Michelle T. *Colonizing Leprosy: Imperialism and the Politics of Public Health in the United States*. Chapel Hill: University of North Carolina Press, 2007.

Morris, Charles E., III. "Archival Queer." *Rhetoric and Public Affairs* 9, no. 1 (2006): 145–51.

Morrow, Rona. "AIDS and Immigration: The United States Attempts to Deport a Disease." *University of Miami Inter-American Law Review* 20, no. 1 (1988–1989): 131–73.

Moses, Peter, and John Moses. "Haiti and the Acquired Immunodeficiency Syndrome." *Annals of Internal Medicine* 99, no. 4 (1983): 565.

Muñoz, José Esteban. "Ephemera as Evidence: Introductory Notes to Queer Acts." *Women and Performance: A Journal of Feminist Theory* 8, no. 2 (1996): 5–16.

Myers, Peter C. "'A Good Work for Our Race To-Day': Interests, Virtues, and the Achievement of Justice in Frederick Douglass's Freedmen's Monument Speech." *American Political Science Review* 104, no. 2 (2010): 209–25.

Namaste, Viviane. "Five AIDS Histories Otherwise: The Case of Haitians in Montreal." In *AIDS and the Distribution of Crises*, edited by Jih-Fei Cheng, Alexandra Juhasz, and Nishant Shahani, 131–47. Durham, NC: Duke University Press, 2020.

———. *Savoirs créoles: Leçons du sida pour l'histoire de Montréal*. Montréal: Mémoire d'encrier, 2019.

Nelson, Alondra. *Body and Soul: The Black Panther Party and the Fight against Medical Discrimination*. Minneapolis: University of Minnesota Press, 2011.

Nevins, Joseph. *Operation Gatekeeper: The Rise of the "Illegal Alien" and the Making of the U.S.-Mexico Boundary*. New York: Routledge, 2002.

Ngai, Mae M. *Impossible Subjects: Illegal Aliens and the Making of Modern America*. Princeton, NJ: Princeton University Press, 2004.

Oakes, James. *The Radical and the Republican: Frederick Douglass, Abraham Lincoln, and the Triumph of Antislavery Politics*. New York: W. W. Norton, 2008.

O'Daniel, Alyson. *Holding On: African American Women Surviving AIDS*. Lincoln: University of Nebraska Press, 2016.

O'Neill, William G. "The Roots of Human Rights Violations in Haiti." *Georgetown Immigration Law Journal* 7, no. 1 (1993): 87–117.

Ong, Aihwa. *Buddha Is Hiding: Refugees, Citizenship, the New America*. Berkeley: University of California Press, 2003.

———. "Cultural Citizenship as Subject-Making: Immigrants Negotiate Racial and Cultural Boundaries in the United States." *Current Anthropology* 37, no. 5 (December 1996): 737–62.

Opitz, Götz-Dietrich. "Transnational Organizing and the Haitian Crisis, 1991–1994." *Journal of Haitian Studies* 8, no. 2 (2002): 114–25.

Ordover, N. "Defying *Realpolitik*: Human Rights and the HIV Entry Bar." *Scholar and Feminist Online* 10, no. 1–2 (2011/2012). http://sfonline.barnard.edu/a-new-queer-agenda/defying-realpolitik-human-rights-and-the-hiv-entry-bar.

Ordover, Nancy. *American Eugenics: Race, Queer Anatomy, and the Science of Nationalism*. Minneapolis: University of Minnesota Press, 2003.

Orloff, Gordon M. "The Political Boycott: An Unprivileged Form of Expression." *Duke Law Journal* (1983): 1076–93.

Paik, A. Naomi. *Rightlessness: Testimony and Redress in US Prison Camps since World War II*. Chapel Hill: University of North Carolina Press, 2016.

Parascandola, John. *Sex, Sin, and Science: A History of Syphilis in America*. Westport, CT: Praeger, 2008.

Parker, Kunal M. *Making Foreigners: Immigration and Citizenship Law in America, 1600–2000*. New York: Cambridge University Press, 2015.

Parmet, Wendy E. "AIDS and Quarantine: The Revival of an Archaic Doctrine." *Hofstra Law Review* 14, no. 1 (1985): 53–90.

Patton, Cindy. "From Nation to Family: Containing African AIDS." In *The Lesbian and Gay Studies Reader*, edited by Henry Abelove, Michele Aina Barale, and David M. Halperin, 127–38. New York: Routledge, 1993.

———. *Globalizing AIDS*. Minneapolis: University of Minnesota Press, 2002.

———. *Inventing AIDS*. New York: Routledge, 1990.

Perrow, Charles, and Mauro F. Guillén. *The AIDS Disaster: The Failure of Organizations in New York and the Nation*. New Haven, CT: Yale University Press, 1990.

Persson, Asha, and Christy Newman. "Making Monsters: Heterosexuality, Crime and Race in Recent Western Media Coverage of HIV." *Sociology of Health & Illness* 30, no. 4 (2008): 632–46.

Pezzullo, Phaedra C. "Contextualizing Boycotts and Buycotts: The Impure Politics of Consumer-Based Advocacy in an Age of Global Ecological Crises." *Communication and Critical/Cultural Studies* 8, no. 2 (2011): 124–45.

Phelan, Craig. *Grand Master Workman: Terence Powderly and the Knights of Labor.* Westport, CT: Greenwood Press, 2000.

Pivar, David J. *Purity and Hygiene: Women, Prostitution, and the "American Plan," 1900–1930.* Westport, CT: Greenwood Press, 2002.

Puar, Jasbir K. *Terrorist Assemblages: Homonationalism in Queer Times.* Durham, NC: Duke University Press, 2007.

Rand, Erica. *The Ellis Island Snow Globe.* Durham, NC: Duke University Press, 2005.

Ratner, Michael. "How We Closed the Guantanamo HIV Camp: The Intersection of Politics and Litigation." *Harvard Human Rights Journal* 11 (1998): 187–220.

Riemer, Nick. "A Question of Academic Freedom." *Jacobin*, July 31, 2017. www .jacobinmag.com/2017/07/bds-boycott-divest-sanctions-palestine-israel -academic-universities.

Roane, J. T. "Black Harm Reduction Politics in the Early Philadelphia Epidemic." *Souls* 21, no. 2–3 (2019): 144–52.

Roberts, Samuel Kelton, Jr. *Infectious Fear: Politics, Disease, and the Health Effects of Segregation.* Chapel Hill: University of North Carolina Press, 2009.

Robinson, Cedric J. *Black Marxism: The Making of the Black Radical Tradition.* 2nd ed. Chapel Hill: University of North Carolina Press, 2000.

Román, David. *Acts of Intervention: Performance, Gay Culture, and AIDS.* Bloomington: Indiana University Press, 1998.

Rosaldo, Renato. "Cultural Citizenship and Educational Democracy." *Cultural Anthropology* 9, no. 3 (1994): 402–11.

Rosen, George. *A History of Public Health.* Expanded ed. Baltimore: Johns Hopkins University Press, 1993.

Rubenstein, William B. "Law and Empowerment: The Idea of Order in the Time of AIDS." *Yale Law Journal* 98 (1989): 975–97.

Saint, Assotto. *Spells of a Voodoo Doll: The Poems, Fiction, Essays and Plays of Assotto Saint.* New York: Richard Kasak Books, 1996.

Salaita, Steven. "Speaking of Palestine and Academic Freedom." *Mondoweiss*, April 24, 2017. http://mondoweiss.net/2017/04/speaking-palestine-academic.

Sassen, Saskia. *Guests and Aliens.* New York: New Press, 1999.

Schulman, Sarah. *Ties That Bind: Familial Homophobia and Its Consequences.* New York: New Press, 2009.

Scott, James C. *Domination and the Arts of Resistance: Hidden Transcripts.* New Haven, CT: Yale University Press, 1992.

Sexton, Jared. "People-of-Color-Blindness: Notes on the Afterlife of Slavery." *Social Text* 28, no. 2 (2010): 31–56.

Shachar, Ayelet, Rainer Bauböck, Irene Bloemraad, and Maarten Vink, eds. *The Oxford Handbook of Citizenship.* Oxford: Oxford University Press, 2017.

Shah, Nayan. *Contagious Divides: Epidemics and Race in San Francisco's China-town.* Berkeley: University of California Press, 2001.

Shilts, Randy. *And the Band Played On: Politics, People, and the AIDS Epidemic.* New York: St. Martin's Press, 1987.

Skloot, Rebecca. *The Immortal Life of Henrietta Lacks.* New York: Crown, 2010.

Smillie, W. G. "The National Board of Health, 1879–1883." *American Journal of Public Health* 33, no. 8 (1943): 925–30.

Smith, Jesús Gregorio. "The Crime of Black Male Sexuality: Tiger Mandingo and Black Male Vulnerability." In *Home and Community for Queer Men of Color: The Intersection of Race and Sexuality*, edited by Jesús Gregorio Smith and C. Winter Han, 149–71. Lanham, MD: Lexington Books, 2020.

Smith, Susan L. *Sick and Tired of Being Sick and Tired: Black Women's Health Activism in America, 1890–1950*. Philadelphia: University of Pennsylvania Press, 1995.

Snorton, C. Riley. *Black on Both Sides: A Racial History of Trans Identity*. Minneapolis: University of Minnesota Press, 2017.

Solomon, Martha M., ed. *A Voice of Their Own: The Woman Suffrage Press, 1840–1910*. Tuscaloosa: University of Alabama Press, 1991.

Sontag, Susan. *Illness as Metaphor*. New York: Farrar, Straus and Giroux, 1978.

———. *Illness as Metaphor and AIDS and Its Metaphors*. New York: Doubleday, 1990.

Stanley, Eric A., and Nat Smith, eds. *Captive Genders: Trans Embodiment and the Prison Industrial Complex*. Oakland, CA: AK Press, 2011.

Starr, Lynn Acker. "The Ineffectiveness and Impact of the Human Immunodeficiency Virus (HIV) Exclusion in U.S. Immigration Law." *Georgetown Immigration Law Journal* 3 (1989): 87–111.

Stauffer, John. *Giants: The Parallel Lives of Frederick Douglass and Abraham Lincoln*. New York: Twelve, 2008.

Steele, Thomas. "CDC Director Says Announcement of AIDS Cause Is Forthcoming." *New York Native*, April 9–22, 1984, 7.

Stephens, Gregory. "Arguing with a Monument: Frederick Douglass' Resolution of the 'White Man Problem' in His 'Oration in Memory of Lincoln.'" *Comparative American Studies: An International Journal* 13, no. 3 (2015): 129–45.

———. *On Racial Frontiers: The New Culture of Frederick Douglass, Ralph Ellison, and Bob Marley*. Cambridge: Cambridge University Press, 1999.

Stern, Alexandra Minna. "Buildings, Boundaries, and Blood: Medicalization and Nation-Building on the U.S.-Mexico Border, 1910–1930." *Hispanic American Historical Review* 79, no. 1 (1999): 41–81.

———. *Eugenic Nation: Faults and Frontiers of Better Breeding in Modern America*. Berkeley: University of California Press, 2016.

Stern, Scott W. "Rethinking Complicity in the Surveillance of Sex Workers: Policing and Prostitution in America's Model City." *Yale Journal of Law and Feminism* 31, no. 2 (2020): 411–96.

———. *The Trials of Nina McCall: Sex, Surveillance, and the Decades-Long Government Plan to Imprison "Promiscuous" Women*. Boston: Beacon Press, 2018.

———. "The Venereal Doctrine: Compulsory Examinations, Sexually Transmitted Infections, and the Rape/Prostitution Divide." *Berkeley Journal of Gender, Law and Justice* 34 (2019): 149–214.

Stockdill, Brett C. *Activism against AIDS: At the Intersection of Sexuality, Race, Gender, and Class.* Boulder, CO: Lynne Rienner, 2003.

Streitmatter, Rodger. *Unspeakable: The Rise of the Gay and Lesbian Press in America.* Boston: Faber and Faber, 1995.

Thrasher, Stephen W. "'Tiger Mandingo,' a Tardily Regretful Prosecutor, and the 'Viral Underclass,'" *Souls* 21, no. 2–3 (2019): 248–52.

Treichler, Paula A. *How to Have Theory in an Epidemic: Cultural Chronicles of AIDS.* Durham, NC: Duke University Press, 1999.

Tripp, Bernell. *Origins of the Black Press: New York, 1827–1847.* Northport, AL: Vision, 1992.

Vaid, Urvashi. *Virtual Equality: The Mainstreaming of Lesbian and Gay Liberation.* New York: Anchor Books/Doubleday, 1995.

Vogel, Kenneth. "Discrimination on the Basis of HIV Infection: An Economic Analysis." *Ohio State Law Journal* 49 (1989): 965–98.

Vogel, Todd, ed. *The Black Press: New Literary and Historical Essays.* New Brunswick, NJ: Rutgers University Press, 2001.

Wachter, Robert M. *The Fragile Coalition: Scientists, Activists, and AIDS.* New York: Palgrave Macmillan, 1991.

Wah, Tatiana, and François Pierre-Louis. "Evolution of Haitian Immigrant Organizations and Community Development in New York City." *Journal of Haitian Studies* 10, no. 1 (2004): 146–64.

Wald, Priscilla. *Contagious: Cultures, Carriers, and the Outbreak Narrative.* Durham, NC: Duke University Press, 2008.

Washington, Harriet A. *Medical Apartheid: The Dark History of Medical Experimentation on Black Americans from Colonial Times to the Present.* New York: Harlem Moon, 2006.

Watkins-Hayes, Celeste. *Remaking a Life: How Women Living with HIV/AIDS Confront Inequality.* Berkeley: University of California Press, 2019.

Watney, Simon. "Missionary Positions: AIDS, 'Africa,' and Race." *Critical Quarterly* 31, no. 3 (1989): 45–62.

Welsh, Joshua. "Common Sense and the Rhetoric of Technology." *POROI: An Interdisciplinary Journal of Rhetorical Analysis and Invention* 10, no. 1 (2014): Article 3.

Weston, Kath. *Families We Choose: Lesbians, Gays, Kinship.* New York: Columbia University Press, 1991.

Wilson, Kirt H. "Interpreting the Discursive Field of the Montgomery Bus Boycott: Martin Luther King Jr.'s Holt Street Address." *Rhetoric and Public Affairs* 8, no. 2 (2005): 299–326.

Wood, Peter H. *Black Majority: Negroes in Colonial South Carolina from 1670 through the Stono Rebellion.* New York: Knopf, 1975.

Worobey, Michael, Thomas D. Watts, Richard A. McKay, Marc A. Suchard, Timothy Granade, Dirk E. Teuwen, Beryl A. Koblin, Walid Heneine, Philippe Lemey, and Harold W. Jaffe. "1970s and 'Patient 0' HIV-1 Genomes Illuminate Early HIV/AIDS History in North America." *Nature: International Journal of Science* 539 (2016): 98–101.

Young, Anna M., Adria Battaglia, and Dana L. Cloud. "(Un)Disciplining the Scholar Activist: Policing the Boundaries of Political Engagement." *Quarterly Journal of Speech* 96, no. 4 (2010): 427–35.

Young, Elliott. *Alien Nation: Chinese Migration in the Americas from the Coolie Era through World War II*. Chapel Hill: University of North Carolina Press, 2014.

Zarefsky, David. "Four Senses of Rhetorical History." In *Doing Rhetorical History: Concepts and Cases*, edited by Kathleen Turner, 19–32. Tuscaloosa: University of Alabama Press, 2003.

———. "Philosophy and Rhetoric in Lincoln's First Inaugural Address." *Philosophy and Rhetoric* 45, no. 3 (2012): 165–88.

INDEX

A

activism. *See* civil disobedience; letter-writing campaigns; protests
activist journalism, 136, 139, 210n20
ACT NOW, 105, 115–16, 202n8
ACT UP, 11, 15, 48, 52–53, 130–36, 154–56, 206n82, 214n64, 216n99, 216n105; New York, 3, 92–93, 110–11, 145–49, 213n62, 215n78; San Francisco and Golden Gate, 64–66, 85, 90, 103–5, 115–19, 123–27, 205n62, 213n62
ACT UP Immigration Working Group (IWG), 125–28
ACT UP Oral History Project, 145, 148, 154–55
Advocate, 58, 133, 190n97
African swine fever virus (ASFV), 43, 135–42, 211n36
Ahmed, Sara, 7–8, 165
Ahuja, Neel, 144, 154, 174n23, 215n72
AIDS Action Council, 90
AIDS ACTION NOW!, 110
"AIDS: A National Inquiry" on *Frontline*, 55–57
AIDS Community TV, 134, 145–51, 154–55, 212n51
AIDS Control Act of 1993, 93, 201n125
AIDS Federal Policy Act, 85
AIDS National Interfaith Network, 124
AIDS Project, 50, 103–4
AIDS Quilt, 116
AIDS research, 71–72, 81, 86, 93–94, 111, 117, 138, 184n16, 206n83; and boycotts, 106, 119–20; exclusion of women from, 47–48, 109; lack of funding for in Haiti, 141
Alexander, Archer, 167

"alien" (term), 5–7, 38, 159–60
Alton, IL, 52, 187n59
Amendment 37, 94–97. *See also* Nickles, Don
American Association of University Professors (AAUP), 106–7
American Civil Liberties Union (ACLU), 52, 60, 187n57, 214n70
American Congress for Sanitary Reform, 25
American Foundation for AIDS Research (amfAR), 81, 127
American Medical Association (AMA), 74, 87–88, 195n33
American Plan, 20, 39, 48
American Public Health Association, 25, 87, 179n38
Americans for Immigrant Justice, 213n63
analogies, 45, 72–74, 126, 161. *See also* metaphors
And the Band Played On, 43
anti-Black racism, 43–44, 48–49, 96–99, 150–51, 166–68, 174n25, 188n68
anti-Chinese racism, 10, 27–29, 32–34
anti-Mexican racism, 9, 27, 33, 36–37, 115
anti-migrant sentiment, 28–34. *See also* nativism
anti-Semitism, 29–32, 126
archives, 5, 13–15, 49, 124, 145–49, 213n62, 215n73, 215n80; recentering people in, 156, 160, 166
Aristide, Jean-Bertrand, 3, 91, 133, 142, 145, 151, 154
Arnoux, Emmanuel, 138, 211n32
Asian migrants, 27–28, 35. *See also* anti–Chinese racism

Association des Réfugiés Politiques Haïtiens, 144
Atlanta, GA, 107–9, 117
Austin, Duane "Duke," 70, 103, 144, 152–53
Awe, Robert, 56
AZT, 71, 103, 135

B

Baker, James, 104
Baldwin, Peter, 40
Bauer, Gary, 71–72
Bauman, Zygmunt, 7, 164
Bay Area Physicians for Human Rights, 119
Beam, Joseph, 188n68
Beauval, Fernand, 126
Benedic, Jean, 147
Bennett, William, 46–47, 71–72
Berger, Michele Tracy, 11
Berlant, Lauren, 153–54
Bernstein, Robert, 54, 57–58
Black AIDS Mobilization (BAM!), 91, 122, 150
Blackness, 13–14, 49, 60, 158–60, 165–68. See also anti–Black racism
Blacks Educating Blacks About Sexual Health Issues (BEBASHI), 188n68
Black sex workers, 4, 14, 41–42, 47–60, 189n78. See also sex workers
blood donations, 41–45, 59, 86, 141, 146, 193n7, 199n102
blood tests, 61, 212n49
Bosniak, Linda, 8
Bost, Darius, 13, 49
Boston, MA, 15, 90, 121–25, 167, 207n104
Bowen, Otis R., 69
Boxer, Barbara, 98
boycotts, 15, 86–87, 90, 104, 129–31; of 1990 IAC, 112–21, 204n48; of 1992 IAC, 122–27; of New York Native, 136, 210n19; as strategy, 105–8, 202n13
Bracero program, 37
Bridges, Fabian K., 54–58, 189n78
Brier, Jennifer, 46, 73, 75, 86, 176n36, 192n2, 195n19
Briggs Initiative, 62
Brimelow, Peter, 157–66
Broberg, Bro, 148

Browning, Edmond, 124
Brutus, Bob, 143
bubonic plague, 33–34, 38
Buetell, Alfred, 32
Bush, George H. W.: and boycotts, 113, 116–18, 122–27, 129; and Haitian prison camp, 132, 142–43, 146, 150–51; and migrant ban, 64–65, 81, 85–87, 90–91, 94, 207n104

C

California Medical Association, 61
Cameron, Paul, 54, 61, 64
Camp Bulkeley, 143
Canadian AIDS Society, 113–14
care, militarization of, 152–53, 159
Carillo Rowe, Aimee, 158
Carville, 32–33, 45
Center for Constitutional Rights (CCR), 144, 214n70, 215n78
Centers for Disease Control and Prevention (CDC), 116, 124–25, 195n33; and activist media, 134–39, 144, 146, 154–55; and migrant ban, 69, 72–74, 78, 86–87, 90, 182n100; and rhetoric of quarantine, 40–44, 47, 59, 185n27
Chamberlain-Kahn Act, 38
Charleston, SC, 19, 23. See also Sullivan's Island
Cheng, Jih-Fei, 12, 16
Chicago Outlines, 197n71
China, 32–33
Chinese Exclusion Act, 27, 29
Chinese migrants, 10, 27–29, 32–34, 181n89. See also anti–Chinese racism
cholera, 25, 28–32, 40, 180n70
Christian Action Network, 89
Christian American Family Association, 45
CIRRS, 70, 85, 90, 105, 115, 125, 127
citizenship, theorization of, 7–12, 28–30, 44, 75, 84, 94, 159–60
civil disobedience, 149, 155. See also protests
Clinton, Bill, 92–93, 130, 143, 146–47, 159
Coalition Against AIDS Propaganda (KAPAIDS), 214n67

coalition politics as method, 158
Coalition to Lift the Bar, 130–31
Cohen, Cathy J., 155
Column, Terry Hughes, 52
Committee on Labor and Human
    Resources, 78, 85
commonsense rhetoric, 72–73, 78–79,
    88–89, 92–95, 98–99, 159, 166. *See also*
    national common sense
Compas, Jean-Claude, 139–41, 214n67
concentration camps, 3, 61, 132, 144, 153
confidentiality, 70, 75, 82–84, 112–13,
    194n11
Corea, Gena, 48
Cortiñas, Jorge, 66, 92, 122–24
costs of HIV testing and care, 62, 78–79,
    88–90, 94–97, 122–23, 153, 196n38
COVID-19, 16, 168
Cranston, Alan, 104
criminalization of HIV, 4, 39, 58–60,
    63–64, 149–50, 185n30
Crimp, Douglas, 48–49, 135
Crowing Rooster Arts, 213n62
Cuba, 12, 25–27, 91, 132, 150. *See also*
    Guantánamo Bay, Cuba
Cunningham, Tom, 119
Curran, James, 59, 136

D
d'Adesky, Anne-christine, 138, 140–42,
    155, 216n105
Dallard, Jean-Louis, 212n49
Damned Interfering Video Activists
    (DIVA) TV, 132–34, 147–49, 208n4,
    213n62, 215n83
Danforth, John, 78–79, 83, 196n52
"dangerous contagious disease," 29,
    37, 65–69, 72, 81–87, 93, 109,
    201n125
Dannemeyer, William, 42, 61–64, 72,
    87–89, 122–23, 159, 199n102, 206n91
debates, 93–99, 104, 211n36; in 1987
    Senate, 67–68, 70–85, 194n11, 196n40,
    196n52; about 1990 Immigration
    Act, 87, 90, 198n90; and history of
    quarantine, 24–26, 37
DeMayo, Anthony, 50–51
Department of Health and Human
    Services, 65, 68, 89, 108–9

Department of Health and Rehabilitative
    Services (HRS), 63
Department of Justice (DOJ), 89–90, 143
deportation, 4, 9, 11–12, 29, 84, 115,
    125–28, 164, 194n11
Derosier, Wesner, 154
detention camps, 22, 31, 38–39, 84, 103,
    125; at Guantánamo Bay, 12–15,
    91–93, 96–99, 132–34, 142–55, 212n49,
    212n51, 213n62–n63, 214n69
DiAna, DiAna, 52
Dixon, Melvin, 133
Doe, Jane, 52–53, 187n54
Doe v. Sercy, 52
Dolce, Joe, 139
Dole, Bob, 83, 98
"don't ask, don't tell," 103
Douglass, Frederick, 167
drug use, intravenous, 12, 44, 50–52, 64,
    88, 98–99, 116–17, 140, 153, 187n57,
    188n68
Dugas, Gaëtan, 43, 184n7
Duvalier, Jean-Claude, 140–41, 211n47

E
1893 National Quarantine Act, 32
Ellis Island, 19, 29, 35–37, 176n2
Elwood, Julia Rivera, 33
Emancipation Memorial, 167–68
Emancipation Proclamation, 167
Emergency Coalition for Haitian
    Refugees (ECHR), 148
Epstein, Steven, 135
Esparza, René, 48, 185n30
Essex, Max, 43, 123–24, 207n104
eugenics, 34–37, 182n97

F
Fábregas, Tomás, 126–29, 213n62
Face the Nation, 65
Falwell, Jerry, 42, 45, 89, 184n16, 199n102
"family values," 45, 94, 157
Farmer, Paul, 135
Fauci, Anthony, 109–10, 120, 135
Feinstein, Dianne, 98–99
felony charges, 39, 52–58
Fernandez, Bettina, 69–70
First Amendment rights, 106–8
Fish, Hamilton, 198n90

Florence, Italy, 121–24, 206n90–n91,
    207n104
Florida, 61–63, 92, 97, 165, 213n63
Foster, Charles, 31
Foster, James, 112
"4-H club," 47, 73, 134–35. *See also*
    high–risk groups
Frank, Barney, 199n102
freak discourse, 161–62
freedom of speech, 106–8
Friedman, Monroe, 105
Fugitive Slave Act, 167
fugitivity, 4, 48–50, 53, 59, 163, 187n62

G
Gallo, Robert, 109
Garland Thomson, Rosemarie, 161
Gaudet, Marcia, 32–33
Gay and Lesbian Freedom Day, 90
Gay Asian Pacific Alliance, 125
Gay Men's Health Crisis, 56, 136, 139–40,
    188n68
Geary Act, 29
Gillis W. Long Hansen's Disease
    Center, 32
GLBT Historical Society, 15
global coalitions, 104–5, 114–16, 123–25,
    129–30
Goddard, H. H., 36
Goldstein, Brandt, 144
Goodnight, Thomas, 22
Gould, Deborah B., 111, 118, 130, 206n82
Gramsci, Antonio, 84
Griscom, John H., 178n22, 179n37
Guantánamo Bay, Cuba, 12–15, 91–93,
    212n49; resistance at, 96–99, 132–34,
    142–55, 212n51, 213n62–n63, 214n64,
    214n69, 215n72
Guantánamo Memory Project, 214n64
Guerin, Jean-Michel, 141–42

H
Haitian Centers Council, 139, 144,
    214n64
Haitian Coalition on AIDS, 139–40,
    214n67
Haitian Refugee Center, 91
Haitian refugees, 91, 97–99, 132–33,
    142–45, 148–51, 212n49, 215n72

Haiti Solidarity Week, 93
Hallas, Roger, 133
Hammonds, Evelynn, 49
Hansen's disease, 32, 45. *See also* leprosy
Harrison, Benjamin, 28–32
Harrison, Mark, 21
Hart, Gary, 62
Hartman, Saidiya, 50, 183n119
Harvard Human Rights Journal, 146
Harvard University AIDS Institute, 121,
    124–25
Haskin, Frederic J., 36
Hatch, Orrin, 95
Haughton, James, 54–55
Hawaiian Islands, 33, 180n70
health care, militarization of, 152–53, 159
health disparities, 9–10
health insurance, 33, 66, 90, 95–96
health metaphors, 22, 34–37, 45, 57,
    181n94
Health Omnibus Programs Extension
    (HOPE) Act of 1988, 85
Heckler, Margaret, 193n7
Helms, Jesse, 61, 64–65, 68, 71–86,
    93–100, 116, 122, 194n11, 195n24,
    196n52
hemophiliacs, 44–47, 85, 134
hepatitis B, 137
high-risk groups, 11, 43–44, 47, 73, 75,
    80, 139–41
High Tech Gays, 116
Hill, Ray, 56, 189n78
HIV 2, 98
HIV testing, 85–89, 115, 127–28, 184n16,
    188n69, 196n38, 196n52; premarital,
    70–75, 78–82, 195n33
Holocaust analogies, 126
homophobia, 9–11, 20, 73, 91–92, 117, 123;
    and Haitian detention, 139–42, 146,
    150; and rhetoric of quarantine, 54–64
Hong, Grace Kyungwon, 94
Hoppe, Trevor, 60
Horton, Felicia Ann, 52–53, 59, 187n59,
    187n62
Houston, TX, 54–56
HTLV, 135–36
Hubbard, Jim, 148
hunger strike, 93, 99, 144, 146–47
Hunt, Charles, 41

I

Illegal Immigrant Responsibility and Reform Act of 1996, 159
Immigration Acts, 27, 29, 36, 85–87, 117, 160–61, 180n56
Immigration and Nationality Act, 69–71, 83, 201n125
Immigration and Naturalization Service (INS), 13, 69–70, 103–4, 123–25, 144–46, 149–53; protests of, 85–87, 90, 115–16, 121–22, 132–34, 139, 205n62
Immigration Reform and Control Act (IRCA), 66, 69–73, 84, 88, 115, 194n11
Immigration Working Group (ACT UP IWG), 125–28
International AIDS Conference (IAC), 81, 106–10, 113–23, 206n90–n91, 207n102; in San Francisco, 85–87, 90–91, 103–5, 111–12, 115–19, 124–25, 130, 206n83
International AIDS Memorial Quilt, 116
International AIDS Society (IAS), 15, 109, 112–13, 119, 121
Ivie, Robert, 72

J

Jackson, Jesse, 92–93, 147
Jackson, MS, 58–59, 190n102
Jean, Yolande, 93
Jean-Bernard, Herard, 154
Jefferson, Thomas, 23–24, 168
Jeudy, Marie Jo, 92
Jewell, Wilson, 25
Jewish migrants, 29–30, 32, 126
Johnson, Michael, 60
Joseph, Stephen, 110
Juhasz, Alexandra, 12–13, 16, 149, 156

K

Kallings, Lars Olaf, 119–21
Kansas House Bill 2183, 41
Kaplan, Esther, 148
Kaposi's sarcoma, 137
Kassebaum, Nancy, 95
Kaunda, Kenneth, 110
Kearney, Denis, 32–34
Kennedy, Edward, 78, 85, 94–100
Kerr, Ted, 13
King, Tiffany Lethabo, 13, 49, 158
Koh, Harold Hongju, 146, 215n73

Kohl, Herb, 95–96
Koop, C. Everett, 47, 72, 195n22
koupab, 132, 208n2
Kramer, Larry, 119, 206n83
Kraut, Alan M., 22
Krim, Mathilde, 81
KS/AIDS Foundation, 56

L

Lambda Legal Defense Fund, 60
The Lancet, 138
LaRouche, Lyndon, 42, 61–64, 159, 193n7
LAV (lymphadenopathy-associated virus), 135–36
Lawless, Robert, 136
League of Red Cross and Red Crescent Societies, 112, 114
Lee, Therese J., 107
legal scholars, 41, 46, 69, 106, 144, 212n59
leper colony analogy, 42, 45. *See also* analogies; metaphors
leprosy, 32–33, 38, 182n100. *See also* Hansen's disease
Lesbian and Gay Freedom Day Parade, 90, 116
letter-writing campaigns, 89, 115, 123–27, 130, 144, 147–49, 199n98
Levi, Jeff, 81
Levine, Philippa, 38
Lewis, William F., 75–76
Lincoln, Abraham, 157, 162–68
Little, Cheryl, 91
Locklear, Carlotta, 50–51, 53, 58–59, 185n30
Lopez, Diego, 56
Los Angeles Times, 46, 212n49
Lott, Trent, 98–99
Louisiana State Home for Lepers, 32
Lowenstein Human Rights Clinic at Yale, 146, 214n70
Lucas, Sue, 112
lucha contra, 132, 208n2
Lyne, John, 76

M

Mack, Connie, 97
Mann, Jonathan, 74, 126
Marciniak, Katarzyna, 8
Marine Hospital Service (MHS), 27, 29

Markel, Howard, 10, 37, 174n22
Marshall, Stephen H., 50
Martinez, Bob, 63
Martin, Trayvon, 165
Maryland, 23–24, 120
Mason, James O., 65, 69, 78, 87, 135,
    144, 193n7
Mass, Lawrence, 136–37, 210n16, 210n21
Matthews, W. P., 34
Mawyer, Martin, 89
Mayfield, Tommy, 58–59, 190n102
McCance, Charles, 125
McCarran, Pat, 37
McIntyre, James Henry, 58–59, 190n97,
    190n102
McKay, Richard A., 20
McKittrick, Katherine, 13–14
medications, 12, 71, 78–79, 103, 155,
    176n38, 196n38
metaphors: of health, 22, 34–37, 45, 57,
    181n94; of war, 29, 76–79
method of book, 11–13, 158; rhetorical
    criticism as, 5, 104–5, 108, 130, 160;
    rhetorical history as, 20–23, 38, 177n5
Mexican migrants, 9, 27, 33, 36–37, 115
Mexico-U.S. border, 27, 35–36, 97
Milenette, Rigaud, 132, 148
Mills, Claudia, 106–7
Minnesota AIDS Project, 50, 104
Mitterrand, François, 125
Molet, Juan Maria Bandrés, 125
Molina, Natalia, 36, 174n22
Mom . . . Guess What?, 44
Montreal, 104, 109–10, 126, 209n10
Montrose Voice, 55, 189n78
Moral Majority, 42, 45, 89
Morris, Charles E. (III), 160
Morrison, Toni, 19
Mulroney, Brian, 110
Muñoz, José Esteban, 160

N

NAACP v. Clairborne Hardware Co., 106
Namaste, Viviane, 209n10
NAMES Project, 116
National Association of People With
    AIDS, 113
national body, U.S., 8–10, 22, 34–35, 38,
    76–80, 157–66

National Commission on AIDS, 85, 112
national common sense, 35, 42, 96–100;
    theorization of, 67–68, 75–85. See also
    commonsense rhetoric
National Gay and Lesbian Task
    Force (NGLTF), 81, 86, 89, 116,
    194n16
National Institute of Allergy and
    Infectious Diseases, 109, 135
National Institutes of Health
    reauthorization bill, 93
National Institutes of Health
    Revitalization Act, 68, 93
National Leadership Coalition on
    AIDS, 86
National Lesbian and Gay Health
    Conference, 103
national phone zaps, 115, 122, 125, 130
National Quarantine and Sanitary
    Convention, 25, 178n22
nativism, 22, 30–32, 67, 157. See also
    anti–migrant sentiment
Nelson, Bob, 124
news, racialization of, 133–35
New York City Health Department,
    32, 137
New York Native, 133–42, 154–55, 209n7,
    210n16, 210n19, 211n36
New York Times, 46, 57–58, 119; early
    reporting about HIV/AIDS, 69–70,
    72, 89–90, 135–38, 193n7, 210n16;
    and history of quarantine, 25, 30–31,
    180n70
Ngai, Mae, 9, 159, 173n20
Nickles, Don, 80, 94–99
1952 McCarran-Walter Act, 37
1987 Pride march, 3
1987 Senate debates, 67–68, 70–85,
    194n11, 196n40, 196n52
1993 National Institutes of Health
    Revitalization Act, 68, 93
"no-questions-asked" waiver, 86–87

O

O'Daniel, Alyson, 51
Ong, Aihwa, 8
Opitz, Götz-Dietrich, 145–46
Ordover, Nancy, 84, 131, 182n97
orientalism, 128–29

origin myths, of HIV/AIDS, 11, 43–44, 68, 84, 134–39, 184n7
Orloff, Gordon M., 106
Ortleb, Charles, 135–38
Osborn, June E., 112
OUT! (Oppression Under Target!), 87
outlaws, 44, 48, 60–61

P

Page Act, 27
Paik, A. Naomi, 144
Palestine/Israel conflict, 107–8
Pan American Health Organization, 138
Parmet, Wendy, 39
passport stamp, 112–13, 126–27
"Patient Zero," 43
People With AIDS Health Group (PWA), 48–49, 113, 116
Pezzullo, Phaedra C., 105
Philadelphia AIDS Task Force (PATF), 188n68
Philadelphia, PA, 23–25, 167, 188n68, 196n56
phone zaps, 115, 122, 125, 130
Pierre-Louis, François, 214n69
plague, 21–23, 33–34, 38, 177n14, 199n102
Porter, Roger, 122
ports, 10, 21–32, 40, 176n2, 177n14, 180n70, 194n8
poverty, 4, 12, 94, 145, 164; and hygiene, 26, 30, 32, 45, 137; and medical costs, 71, 196n38
Powderly, Terence V., 34–35
Prevent AIDS Now In California, 62
Prevent AIDS Now Initiative Committee (PANIC), 62
privacy. See confidentiality
Project Inform, 207n104
Proposition 64, 62
Proposition 69, 62
Proposition 102, 62–64
Proposition 187, 159, 180n53
Proposition 200, 180n53, 217n9
prostitutes. See sex workers
Protect Arizona Now (Proposition 200), 217n9
protests, 3, 48, 57, 81, 168; and boycotts, 103–5, 110, 127; of Haitian detention, 146–53, 213n62–n63; of INS, 85–87, 90,

115–16, 121–22, 132–34, 139, 205n62; of International AIDS Conferences, 15, 118–20, 129–30, 206n91; and solidarity, 116–17, 214n67
public charge exclusion, 27, 90, 94–97
Public Health and Research Act, 38–39

Q

Quarantine and Sanitary Convention, 25, 178n22
quarantine, definitions of, 21–23, 44
quarantine of goods, 21–24, 32
queer archive activism, 156. See also archives
Queer Nation, 123
queer, reclamation of term, 209n7
quotas, 35–36, 160–61

R

racism, 19–20, 56, 91–92, 116–18, 162; anti-Black, 43–44, 48–49, 96–99, 166–68, 174n25, 188n68; anti-Chinese, 10, 27–29, 32–34; anti-Mexican, 9, 27, 33, 36–37, 115; and isolation of Haitians, 133–38, 149–51, 155
Ramsdell, Sheldon, 117–18
Raphael, Kate, 124
Ratner, Michael, 144–47, 215n78
Reaction SIDA, 110
Reagan, Ronald, 3, 45–47, 69–72, 76–78, 81–82, 117, 193n7, 196n56, 211n47
Red Cross, 55, 112–14
Reed, Alfred C., 35–36
refugees, 8, 36, 69–70, 91–92, 97–98, 215n72; and AIDS activism, 132–33, 136–37, 142–45, 148–53, 213n63
Reimer, Nick, 107
Remsen, Henry, 24
Report on Quarantine, 25
Resistance Haiti, 91
Reyes, Jesus, 115
rhetorical criticism as method, 5, 104–5, 108, 130, 160
rhetorical history as method, 20–23, 38, 177n5
Rioux, Julie, 207n102
Roane, J. T., 188n68
Roberti, David, 82
Rothe, Courland, 57
Russia, 29–31, 120

S

Saint, Assotto, 145, 213n63
Saintil, Joel, 146
Salaita, Steven, 107–8
San Francisco AIDS Foundation, 90,
    125, 127
San Francisco, CA, 27, 32–33, 51, 62,
    214n70; conference boycott in, 66,
    86–91, 103–5, 111–12, 115–19, 124–30,
    206n83
San Francisco Chronicle, 51, 119
San Francisco Interreligious Coalition on
    AIDS, 124
sanitation movement, 24–26, 34, 37
Save Our State, 159
Scott, James C., 105
"second-class citizenship," 8–9
Sencer, David J., 137
sex workers, 14–15, 20, 27, 137, 141,
    185n24, 189n78; and boycotts, 116,
    128–29; and history of quarantine,
    38–44, 187n57, 188n69; and media
    spectacle, 47–59; and political
    discourse, 60–64
Shah, Nayan, 10, 34, 181n89
Shahani, Nishant, 12–13, 16
Shilts, Randy, 43
Shut Down Guantánamo Coalition, 148,
    215n72
Simpson, Alan, 93–97, 194n11
slavery, institution of, 162–64, 167–68
slow death, 153–54
smallpox, 25, 27–28, 36
Smith, Samuel, 24
Smith, Susan L., 10, 174n25
Snorton, 49–50
solidarity, 91–93, 115–19, 124, 134, 142,
    147–49, 158
Sontag, Susan, 10, 32
Spivak, Gayatri Chakravorty, 129
Stahl, Leslie, 65
sterilization, 20, 39
Stern, Alexandra Minna, 10, 37
Stern, Scott W., 39, 48, 50, 183n119,
    188n69
St. John, Ronald K., 138
Stockdill, Brett C., 9, 156
Stoddard, Tom, 60
Stonewall News, 154

Stop AIDS Now or Else, 87
strangers, 5–8, 124, 164–65, 172n10
Success, Silieses, 132, 148, 154
Sullivan, Louis, 87–88, 90, 113, 117–19,
    122, 206n91
Sullivan's Island, 19, 23, 176n2
Supplemental Appropriations Act of 1987,
    71, 122
syphilis, 33, 38–40, 65, 73–74, 138,
    182n100. *See also* venereal disease

T

taboo, homosexuality in Haiti, 139–41
Taylor, Elizabeth, 125, 127
Teas, Jane, 138
Texas Board of Health, 57
Texas-Mexico borderlands, 27. *See also*
    US-Mexico border
Texas Social Hygiene Association, 39
Think Progress, 41
Thompson, Ed, 59
Thornburgh, Dick, 90, 104
Thrasher, Steven W., 60
"Tiger Mandingo." *See* Johnson, Michael
Title 42, Federal Code of Regulations, 69,
    81–83
Treichler, Paula, 10–11, 48
Trump, Donald J., 217n1
tuberculosis, 42, 50, 61, 86, 88, 182n100
Tulisano, Richard D., 50–51
typhus, 25, 36

U

UK AIDS Consortium, 112
US-Mexico border, 27, 35–36, 97
US Public Health Service (PHS), 26–27,
    68–69, 80, 90, 144, 182n100, 212n49

V

vaccination, 27, 34, 37, 81, 106, 181n89,
    206n91
Vaid, Urvashi, 86
Van Gorder, Dana, 207n102
venereal disease, 20, 36, 38–39, 44, 48,
    182n100
Verdieu, Elma, 92, 132, 143, 200n116
Verhoef, Hans-Paul, 103–4
Villanueva, Daniel, 45
Villa, Pancho, 36, 38

Vilsaint, Michel, 93, 200n118
Vinikoor, Robert, 103–4
violence, 9, 50, 118, 163–66; and archives, 13–14; Haitians fleeing, 3, 43, 97
Volberding, Paul, 118, 122

W
Wachter, Robert M., 111
Wah, Tatiana, 214n69
Waldegrave, William, 125
Wald, Priscilla, 184n7
war metaphors, 29, 76–79
Washington Post, 62, 92, 103, 212n49
Watkins-Hayes, Celeste, 53, 188n68
Waxman, Henry A., 86
WCCO-TV, 55–57
Weicker, Lowell, 68, 71–72, 75–80, 82–84, 95, 100, 193n3
Weiss, Ted, 84, 198n90
Welsh, David, 214n64
Wentzy, James, 134, 145, 147, 149
White, Laurens, 61
White, Ryan, 85, 98
white supremacy, 155–56, 162–68
Whitman-Walker Clinic (WWC), 188n68

Wilder, Walt, 148, 213n62
William, Dan, 137
Williams, Betty, 148, 155, 215n78, 216n99
Wilson, Woodrow, 39
Windom, Robert, 69
Wise, Ray, 63
Wishnie, Michael, 214n64
Womack, Anissa, 52
women, exclusion from AIDS research, 47–48, 109
Women's AIDS Network, 90
Woodruff, Judy, 56
World Health Organization, 68, 74, 104, 108–9
Wyman, Walter, 31

Y
Yale Law School Lowenstein Human Rights Clinic, 146, 214n70
yellow fever, 10, 23–27

Z
Zarefzsky, David, 162, 177n5
Zimmerman, George, 165

DECOLONIZING FEMINISMS
Piya Chatterjee, Series Editor

Humanizing the Sacred: Sisters in Islam and the Struggle for Gender Justice in Malaysia, by Azza Basarudin

Power Interrupted: Antiracist and Feminist Activism inside the United Nations, by Sylvanna Falcón

Transnational Testimonios: The Politics of Collective Knowledge Production, by Patricia DeRocher

Asian American Feminisms and Women of Color Politics, edited by Lynn Fujiwara and Shireen Roshanravan

Unruly Figures: Queerness, Sex Work, and the Politics of Sexuality in Kerala, by Navaneetha Mokkil

Resisting Disappearance: Military Occupation and Women's Activism in Kashmir, by Ather Zia

Tea and Solidarity: Tamil Women and Work in Postwar Sri Lanka, by Mythri Jegathesan

Axis of Hope: Iranian Women's Rights Activism across Borders, by Catherine Sameh

The Borders of AIDS: Race, Quarantine, and Resistance, by Karma R. Chávez